How to pass the EDAIC

How to pass the **EDAIC**

Edited by

Andrey Varvinskiy
Consultant Anaesthetist, Torbay and South Devon NHS Foundation Trust, Devon, UK

Mario Zerafa
*Consultant Anaesthetist, Deputy Chairperson, Department of Anaesthesia,
Intensive Care and Pain Medicine, Mater Dei Hospital, Malta*

Sue Hill
*Consultant Neuroanaesthetist (retired), Southampton General Hospital,
Southampton, UK*

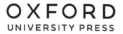

OXFORD
UNIVERSITY PRESS

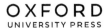

Great Clarendon Street, Oxford, OX2 6DP,
United Kingdom

Oxford University Press is a department of the University of Oxford.
It furthers the University's objective of excellence in research, scholarship,
and education by publishing worldwide. Oxford is a registered trade mark of
Oxford University Press in the UK and in certain other countries

First Edition published in 2023

Published in the United States of America by Oxford University Press
198 Madison Avenue, New York, NY 10016, United States of America

British Library Cataloguing in Publication Data

Data available

Library of Congress Control Number: 2022940780

ISBN 978–0–19–886702–9

DOI: 10.1093/med/9780198867029.001.0001

Printed in the UK by
Ashford Colour Press Ltd, Gosport, Hampshire

DEDICATION

To my wife and my best friend Irina, for all her encouragement and strength.
Andrey Varvinskiy

To my dear wife Josette, for her many sacrifices in the course of my career.
Mario Zerafa

To Hugh, who is always there for me.
Sue Hill

A special thank you to Mr Hugues Scipioni (ESAIC Education & Examinations Manager) for his tireless work in perfecting the smooth running of the EDAIC and his continuous support and friendship.

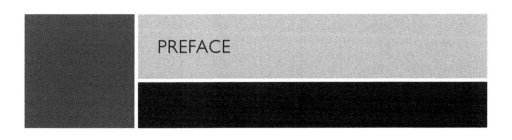

PREFACE

The European Diploma in Anaesthesiology and Intensive Care (EDAIC) is an internationally recognized examination run by the European Society of Anaesthesiology and Intensive Care (ESAIC). The curriculum and specific areas covered by each of the Parts and Papers is available on the ESAIC website alongside the dates and deadlines for application for each of the two Parts of the Examination: https://www.esaic.org/education/edaic.

One of the constant requests received from candidates over past years has been for a book that helps them prepare appropriately. Many of the candidates for the EDAIC work outside of Europe and are not necessarily aware of any differences between their local guidelines and treatment protocols compared with those published by ESAIC. We know that there are many Anaesthesia exam preparation books but all of them address national rather than international examinations and many use different question formats from those encountered in the EDAIC. This book is the first to address the contents of the EDAIC examination and provide examples of typical questions accompanied by answers and explanations. All the questions have been written specifically for this book but are very similar to those encountered in the examination. The contributors all have extensive experience as Examiners for the EDAIC and are best placed to provide an appropriate level of difficulty for each of the practice Papers.

When preparing for the EDAIC, it is important for candidates to use all possible resources: online tutorials, textbooks, local face-to-face or online oral practice sessions as well as exam preparation books. The educational material on the ESAIC website should be used extensively by candidates as it covers European practice. The editors hope that this book will address some of the difficulties experienced by previous EDAIC candidates and suggest ways in which to improve the likelihood of a successful attempt at both Part I and Part II of the EDAIC.

Dr Andrey Varvinskiy MD DA(UK) DEAA FRCA
Past Chairman of the ESAIC Examinations Committee

Dr Mario Zerafa MD DA(UK) DEAA FRCA FERC
Past Chairman of the EDAIC Part II Subcommittee

Dr Sue Hill MA PhD FRCA
Past Chairman of the ESAIC Examinations Committee

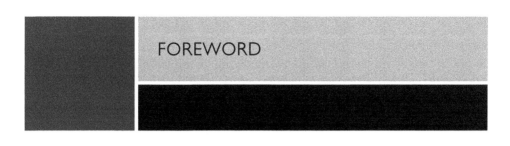

FOREWORD

The history of the European Diploma in Anaesthesiology and Intensive Care (EDAIC) begins in 1984 by the European Academy of Anaesthesiology (EAA), where at the time, this exam was known as the European Diploma in Anaesthesiology (EDA).

Originally created for doctors registered in Europe only, the objective of the exam was to establish a multinational, multilingual European postgraduate diploma examination, which would serve as a means of identifying well-trained anaesthesiologists from any European country. The harmonization of standards and free movement of anaesthesiologists in Europe was of great importance and this exam became the necessary key to create consistency in theoretical and clinical knowledge.

On 1 January 2005, the European Diploma in Anaesthesiology (EDA) moved under the umbrella of ESA as a consequence of the amalgamation of the European Academy of Anaesthesiology, the European Society of Anaesthesiologists, and the Confederation of European National Societies of Anaesthesiology. Diplomates are now known as DESAIC (Diplomates of the European Society of Anaesthesiology and Intensive Care, previously DEAA).

No longer just for doctors registered in Europe, in 2010, the European Diploma opened to candidates from all over the world because of the adoption of the Glasgow Declaration by the ESA. By 2013 the name was officially changed to European Diploma in Anaesthesiology and Intensive Care (EDAIC).

Today, EDAIC is recognized, worldwide, as a high-quality benchmarking tool in anaesthesia and intensive care. As an activity of the ESA, the EDAIC has an educational, non-for-profit purpose. Any profit is either invested in improvements of EDAIC or injected in other educational activities of ESA, which as of 1 October 2020, has become ESAIC (the European Society of Anaesthesiology and Intensive Care), better reflecting our full community and the theoretical skills found within the exam.

EDAIC is organized in most European countries from Iceland and Portugal in the West to Russia and Armenia in the East, but also in other countries in South America, Northern Africa, the Middle East, and Asia. Additionally, it has been officially adopted or recognized in 17 countries in Europe and beyond.

The Society has around 3000 candidates registering for Part I every year, 1200 for Part II and 2000 for the On-Line Assessment (OLA), which was launched as a pilot in 2011 and organized on a yearly basis since 2013. It is an inexpensive but qualitative assessment.

EDAIC Part I (written exam made of 120 multiple-choice questions (MCQs)) and EDAIC Part II (oral exam made of four Structured Oral Examinations, or SOEs) are summative assessments, while the On-Line Assessment (OLA) and In-Training Assessment (ITA) are formative assessments (both made of 120 MCQs). OLA and Part I are organized in 11 languages and Part II is organized in six languages.

One of the most important elements of a successful exam is also to know and to be familiar with the format of the examination procedure. There are different ways to prepare for EDAIC: the

Basic and Clinical Sciences Anaesthetic Course (BCSAC), the OLA, the ITA, the Society's e-learning modules and webinars, and the practice of SOEs and of MCQs that are not in the actual test, but a true reflection of the types of questions to be found on the exam.

This book falls perfectly into the latter category, an area where, based on feedback from previous participants, we found a gap and a need to fill it. It was then decided to provide such a guideline with the highest quality of authors who were previously experienced examiners coming from high positions within the EDAIC structure.

Finally, we are proud to say the Society's Board of Directors fully supports this initiative and are thankful for the excellent work done by the authors. We are confident this book will be advantageous in your preparation for the EDAIC and hope you enjoy it.

Prof. Kai Zacharowski, ESAIC President
[01/01/2020-31/12/2021]
Prof. Stefan De Hert, ESAIC Past President
[01/01/2020-17/03/2021]

CONTENTS

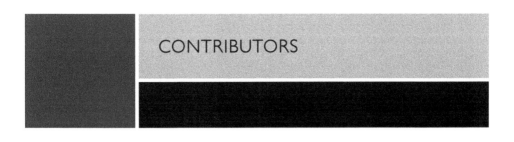

CONTRIBUTORS

Petramay Attard Cortis Anaesthetist, Department of Anaesthesia, Intensive Care and Pain Medicine, Mater Dei Hospital, Msida, MT

Nicolas Brogly Anaesthesiologist, Department of Anaesthesiology, Hospital Universitario La Paz, Hospital Universitario La Zarzuela, Madrid, ES

Mikhail Dziadzko Consultant, Department of Anesthesia, Intensive Care and Pain Management, Hopital de la Croix Rousse, Hospices Civils de Lyon, Université Claude Bernard, Lyon, FR

Vladislav Firago Head of Anesthesia Department, Consultant Anesthesiologist, Department of Anesthesia, Sheikh Khalifa General Hospital, Umm Al Quwain, AE

Svetlana Galitzine Consultant Anaesthetist, Regional and Orthopaedic Anaesthesia Training Lead, Nuffield Department of Anaesthetics, Oxford University Hospitals NHS Foundation Trust, Oxford, UK

Duncan Lee Hamilton Consultant in Anaesthesia & Acute Pain Medicine, James Cook University Hospital, Middlesbrough, UK; Visiting Professor, School of Medicine, University of Sunderland, Sunderland, UK

Sue Hill Retired Consultant Anaesthetist, Anaesthesia and Intensive Care, Southampton General Hospital, Southampton, UK

Krisztina Madach Associate Professor, Department of Anaesthesiology and Intensive Therapy, Semmelweis University, Budapest, HU

Else-Marie Ringvold Head of Department of Anaesthesia, Intensive care, Critical Emergency Medicine and Pain Medicine, Akershus University Hospital, Lörenskog, Norway, Assistant Professor, University of South-East Norway, Norway

Altan Sahin Emeritus Prof., Private Practice, Anesthesiology, Pain Medicine, Hacettepe University, Ankara, TR

Stephen Sciberras Visiting Lecturer, Department of Surgery, University of Malta, Msida, MT

Armen Varosyan Associate Professor, Department of Anaesthesiology and Intensive Care, Yerevan State Medical University, Yerevan, AM

Andrey Varvinskiy Consultant Anaesthetist, Department of Anaesthesia and Intensive Care, Torbay and South Devon NHS Foundation Trust, Torquay, UK

Mario Zerafa Consultant Anaesthetist, Deputy Chairperson, Department of Anaesthesia, Intensive Care and Pain Medicine, Mater Dei Hospital, Msida, MT

ABBREVIATIONS

ABG	Arterial blood gas
AC	Alternating current
ACB	Adductor canal block
ACE	Angiotensin-converting enzyme
ACOG	American College of Obstetricians and Gynecologists
ACS	Acute coronary syndrome
AD	Autonomic dysreflexia
ADH	Anti-diuretic hormone
AED	Automated external defibrillator
AF	Atrial fibrillation
AFE	Amniotic fluid embolism
AKI	Acute kidney injury
ALI	Acute lung injury
AMI	Acute myocardial infarction
ANP	Atrial natriuretic peptide
AP	Anterior-posterior
APACHE	Acute Physiology and Chronic Health Evaluation
APE	Acute pulmonary embolism
APL	Adjustable pressure limiting
ARDS	Acute respiratory distress syndrome
ARF	Acute renal failure
ASA	American Society of Anesthesiologists
AST	Aspartate transaminase
BAEP	Brainstem auditory evoked potentials
BBB	Blood-brain barrier
BCSAC	Basic and Clinical Sciences Anaesthesia Course
BIS	Bispectral Index
BMI	Body mass index
BMR	Basal metabolic rate
BNP	B-type natriuretic peptide
BP	Blood pressure

BSAC   Basic Sciences Anaesthesia Course
CBF   Cerebral blood flow
CC   Closing capacity
CEMACH Confidential enquiry into Maternal and Child Health
CENSA   Confederation of European National Societies of Anaesthesiologists
CF   Cystic fibrosis
CI   Confidence interval
CICO   Can't intubate can't oxygenate
CIED   Cardiovascular implantable electronic devices
CM   Chiari malformations
CMR   Cerebral metabolic rate
CNB   Central neuraxial blockade
CNS   Central nervous system
CO   Cardiac output
COMT   Catechol O-methyl transferase
COPD   Chronic obstructive pulmonary disease
COSHH Control of Substances Hazardous to Health
CPB   Cervical plexus block
CPG   Central pattern generator
CPP   Cerebral perfusion pressure
CRP   C-reactive protein
CRRT   Continuous renal replacement therapy
CSF   Cerebrospinal fluid
CT   Computed tomography
CTEPH   Chronic thromboembolism pulmonary hypertension
CVP   Central venous pressure
DAS   Difficult Airway Society
DBS   Double burst stimulation
DCT   Distal convoluted tubule
DESA   Diplomate of the European Society of Anaesthesiology
DIC   Disseminated intravascular coagulopathy
DK   Don't Know
DLT   Double-lumen tube
EAA   European Academy of Anaesthesiology
EC   European Community
ECG   Electrocardiogram
EDAIC   European Diploma in Anaesthesiology and Intensive Care
EEC   European Economic Community
EJA   European Journal of Anaesthesiology

ER	Emergency room
ERC	European Resuscitation Council
ERS	European Respiratory Society
ESA	European Society of Anaesthesiology
ESAIC	European Society of Anaesthesiology and Intensive Care
ESC	European Society of Cardiology
ESICM	European Society of Intensive Care Medicine
ETC	European Trauma Course
ExC	Examination Committee
FAST	Focused assessment with sonography in trauma
FONA	Front of neck access
FRC	Functional residual capacity
FRCA	Fellowship of the Royal College of Anaesthetists
FVC	Forced vital capacity
GA	General anaesthesia
GABA	Gamma amino butyric acid
GBS	Guillain–Barré syndrome
GCS	Glasgow Coma Scale
GFR	Glomerular filtration rate
GIT	Gastro-intestinal tract
GOLD	Global Initiative for Obstructive Lung Disease
GPCR	G-protein-coupled receptors
HELLP	Haemolysis elevated liver enzymes and low platelets
HFA	Heart Failure Association
HFV	High-frequency ventilation
HME	Heat-moisture exchanger
HPV	Hypoxic pulmonary vasoconstriction
HSCT	Haematopoietic stem cell transplantation
IABP	Intra-aortic balloon pump
ICAROS	International Consensus on Anaesthesia-Related Outcomes after Surgery
ICD	Implantable cardioverter-defibrillator
ICF	Intracellular fluid
ICP	Intracranial pressure
ICU	Intensive care unit
INR	International normalized ratio
ITU	Intensive therapy unit
LA	Local anaesthetic
LAD	Left anterior descending
LBBB	Left bundle branch block

LCCA	Left circumflex coronary artery
LDCT	Low dose computerized tomography
LED	Light emitting diodes
LIA	Local infiltration analgesia
LMA	Laryngeal mask airway
LMWH	Low molecular weight heparin
LV	Left ventricle
LVEF	Left ventricular ejection fraction
MAC	Minimum alveolar concentration
MAP	Mean arterial pressure
MCQ	Multiple-choice question
MEP	Motor evoked potentials
MI	Myocardial infarction
MIDCAB	Minimally invasive direct coronary artery bypass
MILA	Metformin-induced lactic acidosis
MILS	Manual in line stabilization
MRI	Magnetic resonance imaging
MTF	Multiple true-false
NA	Neuraxial anaesthesia
NDMR	Non-depolarizing muscle relaxants
NIV	Non-invasive ventilation
NMDA	N-methyl-D-aspartate
NSAID	Non-steroidal anti-inflammatory drug
NSTEMI	Non-ST-elevation myocardial infarction
NYHA	New York Heart Association
ODC	Oxygen dissociation curve
OHSA	Occupational Health and Safety Act
OLA	On-Line Assessment
OPCAB	Off-pump coronary artery bypass
ORIF	Open reduction and internal fixation
PA	Postero-anterior
PAC	Pulmonary artery catheter
PACU	Post-anaesthesia care unit
PAH	Pulmonary arterial hypertension
PAOP	Pulmonary artery occlusion pressure
PAP	Pulmonary arterial pressure
PASMC	Pulmonary artery smooth muscle cells
PCI	Percutaneous coronary intervention
PDA	Posterior descending coronary artery

PDPH	Post-dural puncture headache
PE	Pulmonary embolism
PEA	Pulseless electrical activity
PEEP	Positive end-expiratory pressure
PESI	Pulmonary Embolism Severity Index
PG	Pressure gradient
PH	Pulmonary hypertension
PPI	Proton pump inhibitor
PRES	Posterior reversible leukoencephalopathy syndrome
PTC	Post-tetanic count
PVR	Pulmonary vascular resistance
RA	Regional anaesthesia
RAAS	Renin-angiotensin-aldosterone system
RASS	Richmond Agitation-Sedation Scale
RBF	Renal blood flow
RCA	Right coronary artery
RCT	Randomized controlled trials
RF	Radio frequency
RHC	Right heart catheterization
ROSC	Return of spontaneous circulation
RSI	Rapid sequence induction
RV	Residual volume (*also* Right ventricular)
RVLM	Rostral ventrolateral medulla
RVOT	Right ventricle outflow tract
SBA	Single best answer
SEM	Standard error of the mean
SIADH	Syndrome of inappropriate antidiuretic hormone
SID	Strong ion difference
SIG	Strong ion gap
SIMV	Synchronized intermittent mandatory ventilation
SIRS	Systemic inflammatory response syndrome
SMFM	Society of Maternal-Fetal Medicine
SOE	Structured oral examination
SOFA	Sequential Organ Failure Assessment
SSRI	Selective serotonin reuptake inhibitors
STEMI	ST-elevation myocardial infarction
SVC	Superior vena cava
SVP	Saturated vapour pressure
SVR	Systemic vascular resistance

TAP	Transversus abdominis plane
TAPSE	Tricuspid annular plane systolic excursion
TARN	Trauma Audit and Research Network
TBG	Thyroxine-binding globulin
TBI	Traumatic brain injury
TIPSS	Transjugular intrahepatic portosystemic shunt
TIVA	Total intravenous anaesthesia
TOF	Train of four
TPR	Total peripheral resistance
TSH	Thyroid-stimulating hormone
VAE	Venous air embolism
VC	Vital capacity
VEGF	Vascular endothelial growth factor
VF	Ventricular fibrillation
VILI	Ventilator induced lung injury
VSD	Ventricular-septal defect
VT	Ventricular tachycardia
WFNS	World Federation of Neurological Surgeons
WPW	Wolff-Parkinson-White

section

1

INTRODUCTION AND ADVICE

INTRODUCTION

This book is the first attempt to put together some training material to help candidates prepare for Part I and Part II of the European Diploma in Anaesthesiology and Intensive Care (EDAIC). We, as authors, also act as trainers and advisers to many candidates in our own institutions and beyond and have known for a long time that no dedicated text existed for this purpose. This is why we decided to offer you this book that will provide a few useful tips and strategies about how to approach written and oral examinations together with examples of Multiple True-False (MTF) questions with explanations and full narratives of the oral examinations with model answers.

The EDAIC has a long history that goes as far back as the days of the European Academy of Anaesthesiology (EAA), an organization that was established on 5 September 1978 and held its first General Assembly in Paris after two years of preparatory work[1]. This preparatory work began in 1976 after a group of anaesthesiologists met during the World Congress in Mexico City to discuss the consequences of Medical Directives of the European Economic Community (EEC) that were adopted by the Council of Ministers in June 1975[2]. Medical Directive 75/362/EEC governed mutual recognition of basic medical qualifications throughout the EEC. This mutual recognition became the basis for the free movement of medical practitioners within the EEC. The minimum requirements for specialist training were described in Article 2 of Medical Directive 75/363/EEC. This Directive also laid down, in Article 4, a minimum length of training for all specialties, which for anaesthesiology was set at three years[3].

The newly formed EAA set itself the following objectives:

1. Raise the standards of practice of anaesthesiology
2. Improve the training of anaesthesiologists
3. Encourage scientific meetings
4. Encourage research in anaesthesiology
5. Promote exchanges between anaesthesiologists in different countries
6. Advise relevant European organizations[4]

The first President of the EAA was Professor J. Lassner (France), who was elected by the initial 42 delegates. The delegates also elected 11 Senators and formed six Committees. In 1984, the EAA started its own journal, *The European Journal of Anaesthesiology*, which over the years has become a very well-respected journal with a recent impact factor of 4.14. Also, in the same year, the EAA introduced the EDAIC consisting of two parts and established the Examinations Committee, led by John Zorab (UK).

The first two EDAIC Part I examinations (written) took place in Oslo and Strasbourg in 1984 followed by the EDAIC Part II examination (oral) in 1985 in the same European cities. The main purpose of the EDAIC was to establish a multinational, multilingual European postgraduate diploma examination that would serve as a means of identifying well-trained anaesthesiologists from any European country. In its original format, this examination could be taken in four languages. At that time, it was known as the European Diploma in Anaesthesiology and Intensive Care but abbreviated simply as EDA. The successful candidates were given the right to use the title of Diplomate of the European Academy of Anaesthesiology (DEAA).

In 2005 the EAA merged with the former European Society of Anaesthesiology (ESA), which was originally established in 1992, and the Confederation of European National Societies of Anaesthesiologists (CENSA), established in 1998, and adopted the common name of the ESA. As a result of this merger, the abbreviated name of the examination was then changed to EDAIC and the title of the successful candidates to Diplomate of the European Society of Anaesthesiology (DESA), and more recently DESAIC.

In 1984 only 101 candidates took Part I followed by 25 candidates who took Part II in 1985. In comparison in 2019 (35 years later) as many as 2720 candidates attempted Part I in 11 languages, in 76 centres across 42 countries and 1175 candidates registered for Part II across 15 exam centres. EDAIC Part II can now be taken in six languages.

Today the objectives of the EDAIC are:

1. To assess knowledge
2. To improve and harmonize training programmes
3. To assist in career progression
4. To help in the evaluation of non-European medical graduates
5. To provide evidence when there is competition for permanent posts
6. Mutual recognition of other diploma examinations

In recent years the EDAIC was opened to the rest of the world and quickly became a truly global phenomenon. In order to sit Part I, a candidate must simply be a medical school graduate and to be eligible for Part II should be either a certified anaesthesiologist in any country or a trainee in the final year of their training in anaesthesiology in one or more of the European member states according to the World Health Organization[5].

The Examination Committee (ExC) of the ESA introduced the On-Line Assessment (OLA) in 2011. This new modality serves as a preparatory knowledge test helping candidates to understand what the EDAIC Part I consists of, using exactly the same layout and format, but a separate bank of MTF questions. Several countries now use OLA to assess the level of knowledge of their trainees year by year. Another initiative of the ExC was the introduction of a Basic and Clinical Sciences Anaesthesia Course (BCSAC) that is run annually during the Euroanaesthesia Annual Congress.

References

1. Spence, A. Editorial, European Academy of Anaesthesiology. *Br J Anaesth*, 1978;50(12):1172.

2. European Economic Community. Council directives. *Official Journal of the European Communities*, 1975;18:No. L167.

3. Zorab, J.S.M., and Vickers, M.D. The European Academy of Anaesthesiology—1992 and beyond. *J R Soc Med*, 1991;84:704–708.

4. Zorab, J.S.M. The European Diploma in Anaesthesiology and Intensive Care. *Acta Anaesthesiol Scand*, 1988;32:597–601.

5. European Diploma in Anaesthesiology and Intensive Care. How to prepare. Available at: https://www.esaic.org/uploads/2022/04/how-to-prepare-for-the-edaic-2022english.pdf

chapter
2

STRUCTURE OF THE EDAIC (PARTS I AND II)

The European Diploma in Anaesthesiology and Intensive Care examination (EDAIC) is a multilingual, two-part examination covering the relevant basic sciences and clinical sciences topics appropriate for a specialist anaesthesiologist.

Part I

The examination is held annually in September simultaneously in several centres and different languages as listed in the annual examination calendar. Part I languages are English, French, German, Italian, Polish, Portuguese, Romanian, Russian, Scandinavian, Spanish, and Turkish.

The Part I examination comprises two multiple-choice question (MCQ) papers. Each paper has 60 questions and is of two hours duration (or 90 minutes if the examination is taken online). The MCQ format adopted is that of a stem with five responses, where each may be either true or false. This format is also known as multiple true-false (MTF).

Paper A concentrates on the basic sciences

1. Physiology and biochemistry (normal and pathological): respiratory, cardiovascular, and neurophysiology. Renal physiology and endocrinology. Physiological measurement: measurement of physiological variables such as blood pressure, cardiac output, lung function, renal function, hepatic function, etc.
2. Pharmacology: basic principles of drug action. Principles of pharmacokinetics and pharmacodynamics, drug–receptor interaction, physicochemical properties of drugs and their formulations, drug actions, and drug toxicity. Pharmacology of drugs used, especially in anaesthesia and in internal medicine.
3. Anatomy: the anatomy of the head, neck, thorax, spine, and spinal canal. The anatomy of peripheral nervous and vascular systems. Surface markings of relevant structures.
4. Physics and principles of measurement: SI system of units. Properties of liquids, gases, and vapours. Physical laws governing gases and liquids as applied to anaesthetic equipment such as pressure gauges, pressure regulators, flowmeters, vaporisers, and breathing systems. Relevant electricity, optics, spectrophotometry, and temperature measurement together with an understanding of the principles of commonly used anaesthetic and monitoring equipment. Electrical, fire, and explosion hazards in the operating room.
5. Statistics: Basic principles of data handling, probability theory, population distributions, and the application of both parametric and non-parametric tests of significance.

Paper B focuses on internal and emergency medicine, general anaesthesia, regional anaesthesia, and special anaesthesia including pain and intensive care medicine

Clinical anaesthesiology (including obstetric anaesthesia and analgesia):

1. Preoperative assessment of the patient, their presenting condition, and any concomitant diseases. Interpretation of relevant X-rays, electrocardiogram (ECG), lung function tests,

cardiac catheterization data, and biochemical results. Use of scoring systems, e.g. American Society of Anesthesiology (ASA).

2. Techniques of both general and regional anaesthesia, including agents, anaesthetic equipment, monitoring and monitoring equipment, and intravenous infusions. Complications of anaesthesia. Obstetric anaesthesia and analgesia including management of complications related to obstetric anaesthesia and analgesia. Neonatal resuscitation. Special requirements of anaesthesia for other surgical subgroups such as paediatrics or the elderly, cardiothoracic, or neurosurgery.

3. Postoperative care of the patient including the management of postoperative analgesia.

Resuscitation and emergency medicine:

1. Cardiopulmonary resuscitation. Techniques of Basic Life Support and Advanced Life Support as per the latest European Resuscitation Council/International Liaison Committee on Resuscitation (ERC/ILCOR) guidelines.

2. Emergency medicine. Prehospital care. Immediate care of patients with a medical or surgical emergency including trauma.

Intensive care:

1. Diagnosis and principles of management of patients admitted to a general intensive care unit with both acute surgical and medical conditions. Use of assessment and prognostic scoring systems.

2. Management of circulatory and respiratory insufficiency including artificial ventilation.

3. Management of infection, sepsis, and use of antimicrobial agents.

4. Management of fluid and electrolyte balance. Administration of crystalloids and colloids including blood and blood products. Parenteral and enteral nutrition.

5. Management of biochemical disturbances such as acid-base imbalance, diabetic ketoacidosis, hyperosmolar syndrome, and acute poisoning.

6. Management of renal failure including dialysis.

7. Management of acute neurosurgical/neurological conditions.

8. Management of patients with multiple injuries, burns, and/or multiorgan failure.

9. Principles of ethical decision-making.

Management of chronic pain:

1. The physiology of pain.

2. The range of therapeutic measures available for the management of pain. The psychological management of pain patients. The concept of multidisciplinary care.

3. The principles of pain and symptom control in terminal care.

The candidate enters his/her responses on answer sheets that are marked by a computer (or into the computer directly if the examination is available online). The marking method is that each correct response earns one positive mark. Each incorrect response carries no mark. Each blank response carries no mark. Please note that negative marking, i.e. when one mark is deducted from the total score for an incorrect answer, was abolished in 2008. The computer assessment produced is then analysed by the Examinations Committee.

In order to provide some 'feedback' information, both successful and unsuccessful candidates are provided with a Candidate Report. From this, candidates can see how well or badly they have performed in each paper of the examination and in various subject areas. This information can be particularly useful to those who have failed the examination and wish to prepare themselves to re-sit. It should be noted that pass/fail marks are evaluated separately for each complete paper and both papers must be passed in order to pass the Part I examination.

Part II

1. Up to 2019, the Part II examinations were held annually between February and November in several centres and different languages as listed in the examination calendar. Part II languages are English, French, German, Portuguese, Scandinavian, and Spanish. Owing to the COVID-19 pandemic, since 2020, the Part II exam has been held online from virtual centres between February and December. Once the pandemic is over, Part II will resume in a face-to-face format, but the online version is likely to continue for those candidates unable to attend in person.
2. The examination of each candidate is held on a single day during which there are four separate 25-minute structured oral examinations (SOE). In each of these SOEs, the candidate is examined by two examiners, thereby meeting eight examiners in all.
3. The SOE embraces the same range of basic science and clinical topics covered in Part I.
4. 'Guided Questions' are used in all four of the SOEs. For the first question of each SOE, the candidates are given ten minutes to make a brief written presentation before meeting the examiners. The subsequent examination will then begin by concentrating on the problems arising from this presentation. Two of the SOEs will concentrate on the basic sciences and two on clinical topics. In the clinical SOEs, X-rays, computed tomography scans, magnetic resonance imaging and ultrasound images, including echocardiography, are also used.

Marking system

Part II examiners use a marking system that is divided into three marks. The marks are 0 for fail, 1 for borderline, and 2 for pass. For each of the 20 topics of the day, each examiner can award one of the three marks. All the marks of the eight examiners (two examiners for each of the four sessions) will be added up to give the final score for each of the candidates. To be successful, the candidate needs to obtain:

1. a score of at least 25 out of 40 in the morning sessions (SOE 1 + SOE 2)
2. a score of at least 25 out of 40 in the afternoon sessions (SOE 3 + SOE 4)
3. an overall score of at least 60 out of 80

It is therefore most important that candidates should try to achieve a consistent and broad range of knowledge rather than become experts in narrow fields. At the end of each day, the examiners meet, and the marks are declared and reviewed. Until this time, no examiner knows how the candidate has performed in other parts of the examination. Following this meeting, the results are handed to the candidates.[1]

Reference

1. European Society of Anaesthesiology and Intensive Care. Education. How to prepare for the exam. EDAIC Preparation Guide. Available at: https://www.esaic.org/uploads/2022/04/how-to-prepare-for-the-edaic-2022english.pdf

HOW TO ANSWER MULTIPLE-CHOICE QUESTIONS (MCQs)

The written papers for the European Diploma in Anaesthesiology and Intensive Care examination (EDAIC) are designed to test knowledge of both Basic Science, in Paper A, and Clinical Practice, in Paper B. Basic Science has three sections: physiology; pharmacology; physics, equipment, methods of measurement and statistics. Clinical Practice will cover general anaesthesia, regional anaesthesia, and specialty areas of anaesthesia including chronic pain, intensive care, internal medicine, and emergency medicine. Each of these papers consists of 60 MCQ questions.

There are many types of multiple-choice question (MCQ), including: one-from-five; extended matching; single best answer (SBA); and multiple true-false (MTF). In the EDAIC written papers, the questions are all of the MTF type. This is no longer a common format in many other examinations and much has been written about the advantages and disadvantages of the different types of question and their ability to discriminate between the competent and incompetent candidate. There is very little written about the impact of using multiple translations for the different types of questions on candidate performance. One-from-five is perhaps the most commonly encountered type of question, which is purported to be easier to write because only one of the five options is correct, however, it limits the amount of material that can be examined in a single paper unless the number of questions is increased well above the current use of 60 questions in each EDAIC paper. From the experience of the Examination Committee, it is extremely difficult to write SBA type questions and achieve the same subtlety among the choices in all 11 languages into which the papers are translated. In our anaesthetic practice, it is important to be in possession of knowledge covering many disciplines in basic science as well as in the practice of medicine. It is therefore considered more appropriate to retain the MTF type of question where each of the five sub-questions is independent of the other four that make up a single question so that more material can be examined in a relatively small total number of questions. In addition, the Examinations Committee is very familiar with this form and has an extensive databank from which to draw questions, along with statistical analysis of the performance of those questions in previous cohorts of candidates.

The first rule of preparation for any examination is to be familiar with the format of the examination and the type of questions that will be used. The MTF question used in the examination consists of a 'stem' and five associated questions. Each of the five questions is independent, so the word or phrase that constitutes the stem should be read with each of the five-question parts in turn. For example, consider the following question:

1. The antihypertensive agent

    A. atenolol is an agonist at beta-1 adrenoceptors
    B. verapamil blocks L-type calcium channels in arterial smooth muscle
    C. hydralazine inhibits nitric oxide synthase
    D. ramipril is a non-competitive inhibitor of acetylcholine esterase
    E. losartan is an angiotensin II receptor antagonist

To answer this question completely, you need to answer each of the following five independent questions:

A. The antihypertensive agent atenolol is an agonist at beta-1 adrenoceptors
B. The antihypertensive agent verapamil blocks L-type calcium channels in arterial smooth muscle
C. The antihypertensive agent hydralazine inhibits nitric oxide synthase
D. The antihypertensive agent ramipril is a non-competitive inhibitor of acetylcholine esterase
E. The antihypertensive agent losartan is an angiotensin II receptor antagonist

Once you have decided on the answers to each of these questions, you will mark the appropriate part of the answer sheet for question 1, for which there will be options of 'True' (T), 'False' (F), 'Don't Know' (DK) for each of the five parts: 1A, 1B, 1C, 1D, 1E. There are 60 questions in each of the MTF papers both in Basic Science and in Clinical Practice, making a total of 300 points maximum per paper. Each part of one question, for example, question 1B, will contribute 0.33% to the overall score on that paper.

It should be clear that there are no indirect clues to the answer to one part of a question from the answers to the other four parts. The answers to any question can all be true (TTTTT) or all false (FFFFF) or any combination in between. In the example above, 1A is false (F) because atenolol is a beta-1 receptor antagonist, not an agonist, and if you answered this correctly one point will be scored. If you answered incorrectly, you score zero. Since there is no penalty for an incorrect answer, it should be obvious that you should answer all the questions, whether you actually know the answer or are guessing. We will come back to 'guessing' later.

There are several types of questions that can be used in MTF papers. The example given above is the simplest type, a single fact is being tested in each of the five associated questions and they all relate to the mechanism of action of the various antihypertensive drugs. You either know the answer or you do not—there is no way of working it out from first principles. These are the easiest questions to write and translate.

The second type of question is one where you need to know two pieces of information in order to get the answer correct: one-step reasoning. For example:

2. Which of the following intravenous fluids have an osmolality greater than plasma osmolality
   A. Ringer lactate (Hartmann's solution)
   B. 0.18% sodium chloride with 4% dextrose
   C. 4.5% human albumin solution
   D. 0.9% sodium chloride
   E. 5% glucose

In order to answer this question correctly, you need to know both the osmolality of plasma in a normal person and the composition of each of the fluids and therefore the osmolality of each solution. This brings us to the question of absolute values and ranges of values. The questions posed are not designed around an absolute value for a physiological variable such as plasma osmolality. We know that it can vary from individual to individual and under different circumstances. In addition, we often calculate osmolarity and use this to approximate osmolality. The one thing we must remember here is that we must consider the normal adult person—not someone dehydrated or seriously ill. There is a range of normal values (280–300 mOsm/kg is commonly quoted) so answer the question with this in mind. In the example above, the most contentious answer will be that to 2D: the osmolality of 0.9% sodium chloride is around 308, so definitely higher than normal plasma osmolality—yet it is often referred to as isotonic. The answer here would be 'True'.

Before moving on, this question raises an important issue—it is important to remember that all questions should be answered for a normal adult person who is NOT anaesthetised unless the question states otherwise. This is particularly important for basic science, where the questions are about a normal adult not an anaesthetised patient, nor a patient on the intensive care unit.

One-step reasoning may also require some kind of simple calculation to reach the answer. In a statistics question, for example:

3. The following readings of diastolic blood pressure (in mmHg) were taken from six consecutive patients attending a medical clinic: 85, 75, 90, 70, 95, 90. In summarizing these observations
   A. the median value is 90
   B. the modal value is 90
   C. the mean value is 90
   D. the variance is less than 100 mmHg
   E. the standard deviation is more than 5 mmHg

In this question, not only do you need to know the definition of the five different statistical terms, but you also need to know how to calculate them correctly from actual data. In fact, exact answers are not required, just an answer to the stated question. Note that the answers to all the first three questions *could* be true, so are not mutually exclusive, but depend on the data presented (but they are not all true in this case!). If calculations are needed, they should be simple and not require a calculator.

There are also more complex reasoning questions that need more than two pieces of information to answer correctly. In general, there are very few of these included in a paper. Consider this question:

4. Blood gases from a patient: pH 7.3, PaO$_2$ 14.5 kPa, PaCO$_2$ 3.2 kPa

A. This patient could be breathing room air

In this question, several pieces of knowledge are required: the alveolar gas equation and how to use the arterial values to approximate the alveolar values; the value of the saturated water vapour partial pressure (6.3 kPa); the normal respiratory quotient (0.8); the FiO$_2$ of air (0.21); and barometric pressure (101 kPa). This is quite difficult to calculate without pencil and paper although the numbers do work well if you have a head for mental arithmetic. This would be a tricky question—and more likely to be a question in the oral examination since the written examination is not testing mental arithmetic ability. It also serves to introduce another important point: the units here are given in kilopascals (kPa). In the real examination, all values would also be given in millimetres of mercury (mmHg).

Having dealt with the type of MCQ question used in the EDAIC, how should you prepare? The answer may be different for different types of people. Some like to use a limited number of small textbooks; others use online resources including lectures from their own or other medical schools and most will use published MCQ books for exams such as the British Fellowship of the Royal College of Anaesthetists (FRCA). All of these are useful resources and have their place. However, broad background knowledge is required to answer a sufficient number of questions correctly. It is very important to look at the syllabus of the examination to know what is expected. If you fail to appreciate that there will be statistics questions in the Basic Science paper for example, then you may not have read enough to give yourself the chance of scoring full marks. There is a suggested reading list on the European Society of Anaesthesiology and Intensive Care (ESAIC) website. This is not meant to be exhaustive but is extensive and some of the recommended texts are for reference only, to read more around a specific topic than to be read from cover to cover. Before the exam, it is important to find out what you know well and what you know little about. One way to do this is to use your everyday clinical practice to test your current level of knowledge. For example, you may choose to revise your knowledge of pharmacology on one day every week, wherever you are working. In this case you should ask yourself about every drug you administer to a patient: how it is prepared; the dose and any contraindications to its use; how it works both in terms of physiological effects and its site and mechanism of action; and the unwanted effects that it could produce. As we use many drugs together in clinical practice you should also check that you know any significant drug interactions and why they occur. In addition, most patients are taking regular medication, and a few are substance abusers, so you should also know how these other drugs work and how they might interact with and alter your choice of anaesthetic agents and their adjuncts. Making a written list of things you don't know will help direct your reading: often we find it easier to recall facts that we have looked-up specifically, rather than from a general re-reading of an entire chapter. You should also ask questions of your teachers—do not expect them to know everything, but they will be able to help you find the information you are looking for. Behaving like a four-year-old child who is always asking 'Why?' will help improve your knowledge—but will exhaust your teacher, so be careful how often you ask. With the ready availability of internet access, it is often possible to find the answer to questions both you and your teacher are unsure about.

Many examination candidates find it useful to study with someone else who is also taking the same examination: a 'study buddy'. This can be done face-to-face or through online video calling. For the MCQ examinations, this may focus on your both having attempted a certain number of questions in a particular preparation book and discussing your answers—especially those you both answered incorrectly.

However you prefer to prepare for the examination, remember that not everything you read in textbooks or online is true. For many of you, particularly if you are unfamiliar with the MTF type of MCQ question, I would suggest taking the On-Line Assessment (OLA) preparatory examination run by the ESAIC Examinations Committee in the year before you take the real examination. This will mimic the conditions you will encounter in the real examination. The composition of the papers and the questions used are very similar to the real examination papers and the online format is the same as that used in the real examination, should you choose to sit the examination electronically. Your overall results for Paper A and Paper B are displayed onscreen immediately after you have completed the examination. A breakdown of performance in different sections will then be sent to you somewhat later. However, you will no doubt know which questions you found easy and which areas you need to work on.

Having understood the type of question used in the EDAIC written papers and prepared accordingly, what strategy should be used on the day of the examination itself? There are two ways of sitting the examination: a paper-based examination or the same questions in an online examination. They are a little different: it will be clear which centres are using the paper-based and which the online format.

The paper-based examination consists of a question booklet, with the questions presented in your chosen language as well as the English master-copy questions opposite, and an answer sheet that will be marked electronically. The questions in the booklet will be presented in a specific order that is the same for every candidate taking the paper-based examination. Read the questions carefully; it is suggested that you initially mark your answers on the question booklet before transferring them to the answer sheet. It takes a minimum of 20–30 minutes to transfer your answers. Make sure you fill the whole bubble for each of the 300 items. If you do not fill the bubble fully or make so many changes that the computer cannot tell what is being marked as correct then the question will be rejected, and no mark awarded.

The online examination uses exactly the same questions as the paper-based examination but there are differences: no paper question booklet; questions presented in random order with the five parts of each question also randomized; a shorter time to complete the examination. The randomization is to prevent covert cheating by observing someone else's screen and the shorter time because no transfer from paper to answer sheet is required.

Finally, what strategy should you use when answering? Is it different for the written compared with the online format? Taking the second question first: the main difference is simply the time element: if you are taking the paper-based examination, then you must leave at least 20 minutes to transfer your answers as no extra time will be allowed if you have not finished this process when time is called. There is a potential small advantage with the paper-based exam in that you have a booklet on which you can scribble notes and make calculations against the questions they refer to.

In my experience, after many years of running MTF-type examinations, I suggest the following strategy:

a. Read through each question carefully, the stem with each associated question, before marking the answer you have chosen.

b. Firstly, go through the entire paper and answer every question you *know* the answer to, and identify those you need to return to. The more preparation you have done, the more questions you will answer on this first run-through. If you are at all unsure, leave the question for later.

c. Secondly, go through the paper again. This time answer questions you have thought about and are now fairly sure of the answer; the more preparation you have done, the more questions you will cover on the second run-through.

d. Thirdly, identify all those questions you have not answered because you do not know the specific answer to the question, but know something about the topic and give the answer that seems most likely: an informed guess.

e. Finally, answer all the questions you have no knowledge about at all: there is no penalty for a wrong answer.

f. Do not alter the answers you have decided upon unless you are very, very sure you were incorrect when you first answered the question. This is particularly important when completing the computer-marked answer sheet since the computer may reject a paper that is incorrectly filled in.

Using this strategy, if you have prepared properly, you are likely to know the answer to around 50–60% of the questions, remember or work out the answers to a further 20–25%, and make an informed guess on around a further 10%. There will always be a few questions you do not know the answer to and have no knowledge of that subject: what strategy should you use here to optimize 'free' points? There are several things to consider. Firstly, it is easier to write a question with the answer 'True' as these are facts written in textbooks that can be referenced and all question writers are asked to reference their answers. This means that in general there are more questions with the answer 'True' than the answer 'False'; the difference is not large but around 51–52% answers are of the 'True' type and 48–49% the 'False' type. One possible strategy, therefore, is to answer all the remaining questions as 'True'—some will be correct, and it is possible that slightly more will be correct than incorrect. This will only be of benefit if the number of questions you know nothing about is small. A second consideration is that it is easier to identify correct answers than incorrect ones since you will have encountered the content of a correct question several times in different contexts if you have been preparing properly. It is possible that in the case of some of the 'informed guesses', where you are really unsure despite having some knowledge of the topic, the statement is incorrect, and the correct answer is 'False'. Thirdly, it is useful to understand how questions are written as sometimes the wording of the question will help in deciding the correct answer. Here are a few useful tips:

1. Questions where the words 'always' or 'never' are used are commonly incorrect, so the answer 'False' is the best choice

2. Use of the word 'may' commonly indicates that the statement is correct, so the answer 'True' is the best choice

3. Any question that seems ambiguous should be interpreted in the most obvious way, the question is not trying to be difficult. If you can read the English version, then this may not be as ambiguous.

It is also important to know if you are good or bad at guessing: the more knowledge you have, the better you tend to be at guessing as well as having fewer questions that you need to guess the answers to. Using examination practice books, such as this, and the online questions on the European Society of Anaesthesiology (ESA) website, could help you find out.

One of the questions we are asked continually is, 'What is the pass score?', which is an important question. The pass score will vary from year to year depending on the difficulty of the questions—it is almost impossible to have entire question papers of equal difficulty every single year. However, the Examinations Committee use a methodology to identify the difficulty of the paper and the ability of the cohort sitting the papers by comparing question performance in previous years with current performance. This is not the place to discuss how the pass score is set: remember that there is no fixed pass score and the percentage of candidates passing is not fixed before the examination is taken. In general, pass scores will be somewhere between 75–80% for each paper. Since there are five parts to each question, this equates to answering four of the five parts correctly in the majority of the questions. This emphasizes that you need broad knowledge across all sections of both papers.

Good luck!

No. I don't believe in luck—just prepare well.

Key points

1. All MCQ questions are of the MTF type, each with a stem and five associated, independent, questions
2. When answering a question, assume it refers to a normal adult person unless stated otherwise
3. MTF questions may be purely factual or require some reasoning to come to the correct answer
4. Values will be given in all commonly used systems of units (e.g., kPa and mmHg for blood gases)
5. Prepare well, using a variety of resources; question your teachers to help clarify understanding
6. There is both a paper-based and online version of the MCQ examination
7. Have a strategy for completing the paper
8. Answer every question: there is no penalty for an incorrect answer

Introduction

Once you have passed the European Diploma in Anaesthesiology and Intensive Care (EDAIC) Part I, you should consider sitting for Part II within as short a time as possible while most of the knowledge you have gained for Part I is still fresh in your mind. However, passing the EDAIC Part II involves much more than reading widely and practising multiple-choice questions (MCQs). Part II is an oral (*viva voce*) examination which means you will have to speak to the examiners clearly, logically, and without too much hesitation. In each of the four oral exams, you have only a short time with each examiner to demonstrate your understanding of the question material. Language itself is not being assessed but you need to avoid long silences and repeated requests to clarify each question, so practice is essential. The oral exam is structured so that every candidate will be asked the same questions in the same order. For any particular question the introductory question will be the same for everyone, but how the discussion develops depends on each individual candidate, although there are specific aspects of that topic that should be covered for success. Unlike Part I, which tests factual knowledge, Part II tests your ability to use that knowledge to convince the examiner you understand the topic under discussion.

Understanding the oral examination

The Part II examination consists of four Structured Oral Examinations (SOE), two in the morning and two in the afternoon. The morning SOEs concentrate on the Basic Sciences and the afternoon ones concentrate on Clinical Anaesthesia and Intensive Care. Each SOE lasts 25 minutes and consists of five questions and there will be two examiners present, each of whom will score your performance independently on **all** the questions asked, not just those **they** ask. Each examiner has 12 ½ minutes to ask questions, so they may change over partway through the third question. Don't let this disturb you—just continue your explanations but address the second examiner.

The Examination Board understands that the oral examination is stressful, particularly if you need to speak in a language that is not your own. To help with this, the first question of each SOE is given to you 10 minutes before the actual examination. Furthermore, it is usually a complicated question that needs some thinking about and preparation. This preparation means you should be able to answer the first question clearly and succinctly, giving yourself sufficient time to cover four more topics. Use these ten minutes wisely. Make sure you extract from the wording of the question as much information as possible: these questions have been discussed beforehand by a panel of examiners, so the wording is very carefully selected. Organize this information so that you can present it to the examiner clearly and promptly at the start of the oral exam.

In the Basic Sciences SOE 1 and 2, your answer may involve a diagram or a graph. Try to anticipate this and prepare the drawings—make them large enough to be seen easily by the examiners, especially if you are taking the exam online—labelling them clearly, particularly the axes of graphs. If you do not anticipate that drawings are needed, and the examiner needs to prompt you for one, then time can be wasted both thinking about what is required and while drawing the appropriate diagram.

For SOEs 3 and 4 the lead-in statement that you are given beforehand is a clinical scenario. Again, use the time wisely to organize the information and prepare a differential diagnosis, a list of further investigations and a management plan. At the start of each clinical viva, the first question is often to summarize the case. Do not simply read back the scenario to the examiner—the examiner already has a copy, and you are wasting precious time—instead, you should identify aspects of the case or abnormal test results that will influence your management of the patient. Since the opening scenarios in SOE 3 and SOE 4 tend to be complex situations with several different challenges for the anaesthesiologist or intensivist, the second question in these afternoon sessions is almost always related to the initial scenario so that these complex cases are discussed for at least ten minutes. Hence your detailed preparation prior to the start of the SOE will also stand you in good stead for the second question.

Subjects covered by each SOE

In the current format of the Part II Exam, SOE 1 deals with physiology (four questions) and anatomy (one question). Cardiovascular and respiratory physiology are considered of paramount importance in anaesthesiology and intensive care and these topics will invariably feature every time in SOE 1. The level of knowledge and understanding expected is high. Do not be misled by the term 'Basic Sciences' as you will need much more than basic knowledge of these topics. There will also be questions about other relevant physiology such as renal, hepatic, and neurophysiology and again the depth expected is significant. In the anatomy question, the topics will relate to anatomical regions of special interest to the anaesthesiologist, especially where invasive procedures are commonly encountered, such as central line placement, regional anaesthetic blocks (both for acute and chronic pain management), transoesophageal echocardiography, and bronchoscopy.

SOE 2 covers pharmacology (four questions) and physics with clinical measurement (one question). General pharmacology principles (pharmacokinetics and pharmacodynamics) always feature prominently here, and you should be well prepared. Since these topics may be quite a challenge to talk fluently about, you should practise explaining these topics out loud. This is especially important if you are taking the examination in a language which is not your mother tongue. The main classes of anaesthetic drugs including intravenous hypnotics, inhalational agents, analgesics, neuromuscular blockers, and local anaesthetics will always feature, so make sure you come to the exam well prepared—any gaps in knowledge are likely to be exposed. Besides anaesthetic drugs, questions will be asked about other medications that patients may be taking or may be prescribed by anaesthesiologists in their practice. Make sure you understand how these drugs work, including antiarrhythmics, diuretics, anticoagulants, antiemetics, steroids, antibiotics, hypoglycaemics, and medication for psychiatric conditions. SOE 2 always has one question on a physics or clinical measurement topic. This is considered a very relevant part of the syllabus, as a practising anaesthesiologist is expected to have a good working knowledge of the equipment they are using every day. Therefore, questions about blood pressure measurement (both invasive and non-invasive), gas concentration, pulse oximetry, echo- and electrocardiography are to be expected. This is not an exhaustive list, and you should take an interest in the workings of whatever equipment you are using in the operating theatre or intensive care unit. If, in your day-to-day clinical work during your preparation for the exam, you have forgotten how a piece of equipment works, remember to look it up.

SOE 3 will cover anaesthetic practice and pain management. Important features and concerns related to the lead-in scenario will be covered in the first question and the second question will often concern your chosen management of the patient in question. It is important that you outline *your* management plan, not what you've read in a textbook. If you have never encountered the particular surgery before, it is fine to say so, but you then need to present a logical plan based on your theoretical knowledge. There will also be a question to test your management of a critical incident, which may or may not be related to the scenario discussed in the first two questions. If it is a different case, then the examiner should make this very clear. It is extremely important that this is dealt with safely and logically. If there are European Guidelines for managing such an incident, then you must be familiar with them. Regional anaesthesia and/or pain management will be covered in a separate question and a final question will cover one of the specialty areas of anaesthesia such as neuroanaesthesia, cardiac, or paediatric anaesthesia. The examiners appreciate that you may not be entirely comfortable with every anaesthesia specialty, but you must understand the principles that make these areas of anaesthesia different from more general cases and be able to discuss common operations and potential pitfalls and complications.

SOE 4 covers Critical Care, Internal, and Emergency Medicine. The lead-in scenario may involve a theatre case or an emergency department patient where the patient requires immediate treatment. Just as for all SOEs, there is a ten-minute preparation time that is crucial to use effectively. The first question is usually about the assessment of the patient's condition with the second question covering management—very similar to SOE 3 in this respect. There will be two questions covering different topics in emergency and internal medicine and one question will require the interpretation of two clinical images. The images presented to you may include an ECG, a chest X-ray, MRI, CT, or ultrasound image. It is important to report your findings in a logical manner rather than a scatter-gun approach. Often it is not important to get the exact diagnosis, but to show how you look at each type of image to identify important features using a logical, structure-based approach.

Preparation for Part II

It is important to read the syllabus for the EDAIC as there are areas that are more likely to be covered in Part II that are not easily examined in Part I.

Make sure you appreciate the structure of the examination. Factual knowledge is not sufficient to be successful: Part II is all about demonstrating your understanding by logically linking facts, whether that is by discussing cardiac function, how the equipment works, or why you make certain clinical decisions. Remember that 'a picture paints a thousand words' and, particularly in SOE 1 and 2, diagrams and graphs are the best way to demonstrate understanding if you construct them logically. For example, if you want to draw a graph always start by drawing the axes, labelling them with appropriate units, followed by putting on specific, important points that can then be joined together.

As mentioned before, some topics are trickier to discuss than others and it is important to practise speaking out loud. It is clear to examiners which candidates have prepared appropriately and those who have not. Start by practising on your own—talk to a favourite teddy bear who can't judge you! Once you feel comfortable with the language you have chosen, see if a colleague is also preparing for the exam and ask each other questions. These days the internet allows for face-to-face discussions even if you are miles and time zones apart. It can be useful to decide a few days in advance what topics you both want to cover, so you feel comfortable with the facts but are concentrating on viva technique. Identify in advance those topics you find difficult to explain out loud and get a colleague to listen and offer advice in their feedback at the end of your viva practice. Please remember that the examiner will not help during the exam (although you might be given one hint). Try to practise answering each question within five minutes, the time allowed per question in the actual oral examination, since this will help you select key information and helps to improve fluency and avoid too much hesitation. It is also important to ask your trainers to ask you questions informally, based on cases you might be doing together. Closer to the examination, if possible, attend an oral preparation course, although not everyone is fortunate enough to have access to such a course. It is also helpful to ask a more senior colleague with experience of the examination to give you formal SOE practice, where you are asked five questions in 25 minutes and then given formal feedback. If an EDAIC examiner is willing to help, then *you* should suggest some possible topics and related questions, so you cannot be accused of gaining an advantage by being asked actual exam questions. Do not embarrass that examiner by asking him or her to use real questions.

There are resources on the European Society of Anaesthesiology and Intensive Care (ESAIC) and the ESAIC Academy websites that can be of great help including: videos of how and how not to answer SOE questions; e-Learning sessions; links to European Guidelines for the management of commonly encountered critical areas of anaesthetic practice, such as management of major haemorrhage. This is a European Exam, so it is essential that if you come from a country outside of Europe you familiarize yourself with European Guidelines, including the European Resuscitation Council Guidelines.

Behaviour during the exam

On the day of the oral examination, you will be nervous, but try and remain calm. Last-minute cramming outside the door rarely pays dividends. Please arrive in good time: travel the day before unless you are being examined very close to home, as late arrival leads to increased stress, anxiety, and failure to perform to your best ability. Remember to leave all phones and Bluetooth earpieces outside the preparation and exam room if you are taking the exam face-to-face and switch all phones off if presenting online. Each exam starts with a ten-minute preparation time after which you will meet your examiners. They will introduce themselves and check your candidate number, but you should not give your name or that of the hospital/country in which you work. Give the examiners a smile and take a deep breath. You have already prepared for the first, and possibly the second, question so be confident in your answers.

Speak clearly, do not rush your words, and allow the examiner to interrupt if necessary—often they will let you speak continuously until there is a need to change direction or get you to explain further. If you are hesitant or continually repeat the same information, the examiner will prompt you to help move the discussion forward but if this happens too often you cannot cover sufficient aspects of that topic and will be marked down. This is why practice is so important; it improves fluency and allows you to show the true level of your knowledge and understanding. When asked about a specific aspect of a larger topic, do not give every single fact you can recall about that topic and expect the examiner to pick out the relevant facts. This scatter-gun approach is not the way to demonstrate understanding and is irritating to the examiner. Instead, think about the question briefly and make a statement that identifies the key information required and then explain each of these points in turn. The examiner will then guide you to those aspects that they wish to cover. Remember that facts alone are not sufficient to ensure success. If you feel you are in unfamiliar territory or on unsure ground, do not fall into the temptation of half-heartedly mentioning a key word (such as the name of a procedure or a medication) about which you only have a very vague idea. Once mentioned by you, it is almost certain that the examiner will ask you to clarify or elaborate. Similarly, with drugs that you do not use often, it is wiser to say you do not know the dose/infusion rate from memory and would check before you administer it rather than offer a dosage that may be considered dangerous. Remember the examiner can only judge you on what you say.

You may be asked about a topic that you have not encountered for some time, which requires you to think before you answer. In such a case it is better to say something such as 'I haven't thought about this for a while' to give your brain time to bring your knowledge to the front of your mind and to avoid an awkward silence. Do not take too long to think, silence uses up valuable time that should be used to cover the question material. Too many silences lead to failure, so if you really can't remember or do not know the answer own up and say so. The examiner is likely to give you a single hint, but if that does not help, they will move on to a different topic. Do not panic if you cannot answer one of the questions: it does not necessarily imply immediate failure, just smile ruefully and let the examination continue. As long as this does not happen in every SOE you can still have a chance of success—just do well in the other questions. The scoring system used by the examiners has been explained in Chapter 2, so make sure you understand how this is used. A very poor performance in either the morning or afternoon session cannot be compensated by a good performance in the other session, so prepare evenly across the Basic Sciences and Clinical Practice.

Please remember that many of the examiners are also asking questions in a language that is not their mother tongue. If you do not understand what the examiner has asked, please ask them to re-phrase the question or define a particular word you are unfamiliar with. However, this does waste a little time so make every effort to listen carefully to the question. Sometimes an examiner will ask you to repeat what you have said. This will only be the case if they really haven't heard you and it does not imply that you were incorrect, just that the examiner didn't quite catch what you said.

Common pitfalls—why you might fail!

There are many reasons for failure in the Part II exam, but please remember that the examiners are doing *their* best to get you to do *your* best. The examiners will ask themselves the following questions to decide upon their mark for each question:

- Does the candidate have a good foundation of knowledge? Can the candidate apply that knowledge and understand its relevance to the practice of anaesthesia and intensive care?
- How does the candidate approach a problem? Is the approach logical and well thought out?
- Have alternative options been explored and understood?
- Is the candidate dangerous?
- Is the candidate able to correct their own errors?

There is no substitute for preparation, both in terms of factual knowledge and practice in speaking clearly, without hesitation in the language you have chosen for the examination. However, despite adequate preparation, some candidates will still fail because they are unable to perform on the day. Examiners are asked not to tell you how well (or badly) you are performing during the oral but to remain neutral in the way they react to your answers and simply thank you at the end of each SOE. This can be difficult if you have not experienced this beforehand and cannot gauge how well you are doing. Examiners will encourage you and prompt you occasionally, but remember that if you frequently need prompting to produce the required facts and explanations this indicates an inadequate performance.

In the clinical SOEs, it is important that your management plan is safe for the patient being discussed. If the examiners judge that you have selected an inappropriate, possibly dangerous approach to the clinical problem, then you are likely to fail that question. In the stress of an examination, it is easy to forget the simple things such as administering oxygen and asking for help if appropriate. The examiners make no assumptions about early steps in patient care, so always start with the basics and work logically through a scenario.

You must cover sufficient material during each oral exam, so avoid long silences, frequent hesitation, and multiple requests for the examiner to repeat the question. All these waste time and time is very limited as you have on average only five minutes to convince the examiner you understand the topic presented. Each question is scored individually by each examiner, so more than one poor question will make it difficult for you to recover on that SOE, which puts pressure on you for the remaining ones. However, do not assume you have failed if you *think* you have done badly partway through the exam. It can sometimes be hard to know how you are performing: if you are asked a very difficult question at the end of a topic it can mean you've done well, and the examiner wants to know how far your knowledge goes! There have been candidates who have left the exam before the afternoon session, yet they would have had every chance to pass if they had done well in the clinical SOEs. It makes sense to try your best in all four SOEs, even if you think that you have underperformed in one of them. If at the end of the day you are not successful, you have at least gained very valuable experience in the depth and breadth of knowledge that is required to pass and can be better prepared when making your next, hopefully successful, attempt.

Finally, the most important word for success: PRACTICE!

PRACTICE FOR PART I: PAPER A

The following five chapters cover the major areas of the basic science written paper. In the actual examination there will be a total of 60 questions: 20 questions on physiology and anatomy; 20 questions on pharmacology and the remaining 20 questions cover physics, clinical measurement, equipment and statistics.

5 Physiology *Armen Varosyan*

6 Pharmacology *Sue Hill*

7 Anatomy *Mikhail Dziadzko*

8 Physics *Andrey Varvinskiy*

9 Statistics *Sue Hill*

PHYSIOLOGY

QUESTIONS

1. **Increased ventilation in response to activation of peripheral chemoreceptors occurs in response to**
   A. reduced arterial PO_2
   B. alkalaemia
   C. hypoperfusion
   D. hypothermia
   E. carbon monoxide

2. **Central chemoreceptors**
   A. are located deep in the dorsolateral part of the medulla
   B. are located outside of the blood-brain barrier
   C. respond mainly to short-term and rapid changes in arterial PCO_2
   D. are stimulated by a decrease in pH
   E. are not sensitive to blood PO_2

3. **Pulmonary vascular resistance (PVR)**
   A. is lower than the resistance in the systemic circulation
   B. is at its lowest at functional residual capacity (FRC)
   C. is decreased by prostaglandins via the activation of G-protein-coupled receptors
   D. is increased by vasoactive intestinal peptide
   E. is decreased by nitric oxide (NO)

4. **Hypoxic pulmonary vasoconstriction (HPV)**
   A. does not occur in the transplanted lung
   B. is controlled by the central nervous system
   C. is an inherent property of pulmonary endothelial cells
   D. can lead to irreversible pulmonary hypertension in long-term hypoxia
   E. is enhanced by endothelin

5. **Regarding central control of respiration**
   A. the dorsal respiratory group is responsible for the timing of the respiratory cycle
   B. both Bötzinger and pre-Bötzinger complexes are located in the ventral respiratory group
   C. the central pattern generator (CPG) is believed to be located in the pre-Bötzinger complex
   D. the ventral respiratory group has both inspiratory and expiratory functions
   E. the pontine respiratory group is important in controlling the timing of the respiratory cycle

6. **General anaesthesia**
   A. reduces functional residual capacity (FRC)
   B. decreases ventilation/perfusion (V/Q) ratio in dependent parts of the lung
   C. increases dead space ventilation in non-dependent parts of the lung
   D. with spontaneous breathing, depresses diaphragm contraction more than that of intercostal muscles
   E. with positive pressure ventilation does not impair carbon dioxide excretion

7. **Regarding dead space**
   A. physiological dead space is the difference between anatomical and alveolar dead space
   B. alveolar dead space can be measured using Fowler's method with a nitrogen or CO_2 washout technique
   C. physiological dead space is measured using the alveolar air equation
   D. anatomical dead space is increased by increasing the length of the expiratory limb of the anaesthesia circle system
   E. physiological dead space is primarily influenced by changes in anatomical dead space

8. **Regarding physiological changes in respiratory function associated with ageing**
   A. alveoli are dilated
   B. residual volume is increased
   C. the work of breathing is increased
   D. respiratory centre sensitivity to hypoxaemia is increased
   E. adequate gas exchange at rest and during exertion is maintained throughout life

9. **Regarding physiological changes at high altitude**
   A. the O_2 dissociation curve is shifted to the right at moderate altitudes
   B. the O_2 dissociation curve is shifted to the left at very high altitudes
   C. the maximum breathing capacity decreases
   D. hypoxic pulmonary vasoconstriction is not beneficial
   E. hyperventilation occurs because of hypercapnia

10. **Oxygen affinity of haemoglobin is increased by**
    A. hyperthermia
    B. hypercapnia
    C. acidaemia
    D. an increase in concentration of 2,3-diphosphoglycerate (DPG)
    E. the presence of carbon monoxide in the blood

11. **The metabolic functions of the lung include**
    A. synthesis of bradykinin
    B. inactivation of serotonin
    C. conversion of angiotensin II to angiotensin I
    D. activation of noradrenaline (norepinephrine)
    E. degradation of adrenaline (epinephrine)

12. Regarding coronary blood supply

A. in 20% of people the posterior descending coronary artery (PDA) arises from the right coronary artery (RCA)
B. occlusion of the left anterior descending artery (LAD) artery may cause right ventricle (RV) ischaemia or infarction
C. acute occlusion of the RCA may cause bradyarrhythmias
D. the proximal portion of the ventricular conduction system is less vulnerable to ischaemia
E. the right ventricular veins drain into the coronary sinus

13. Bradycardia may be caused by

A. the baroreceptor reflex
B. the Bainbridge reflex
C. the Bezold–Jarisch reflex
D. increased intracranial pressure
E. the oculocardiac reflex

14. Regarding hormones affecting cardiac function

A. adrenomedullin has direct positive chronotropic and inotropic effects
B. angiotensin II causes cardiac hypertrophy
C. natriuretic peptide receptors are G-protein-coupled receptors (GPCRs)
D. B-type natriuretic protein (BNP) is released from the atria in response to volume overload
E. aldosterone may cause cardiac fibrosis

15. Regarding neural regulation of cardiac function

A. ventricles have more intense parasympathetic innervation than atria
B. at rest the heart has no parasympathetic tone
C. activation of muscarinic receptors increases pacemaker activity
D. β_2-adrenoreceptors can couple to G protein-independent pathways to modulate cardiac function
E. α_1-adrenoreceptors mediate cardiac hypertrophy

16. Noradrenaline (norepinephrine)

A. is the principal catecholamine synthesized by the adrenal medulla
B. is less potent at α_1-receptors than adrenaline (epinephrine)
C. has prominent β_2 agonist effects
D. concentration in the plasma is increased in older adults
E. is not metabolized by the enzyme catechol-O-methyltransferase (COMT)

17. In left ventricular diastole

A. left ventricular volume is constant during isovolumetric relaxation
B. atrial systole is the first phase of ventricular diastole
C. atrial systole normally generates 15% to 25% of the final stroke volume
D. the early rapid filling phase of diastole is not important in determining stroke volume
E. diastasis is the least important phase contributing to stroke volume

18. Determinants of cardiac output include
A. heart rate
B. myocardial contractility
C. ejection fraction
D. preload
E. afterload

19. In the cardiac cycle
A. ventricular systole begins on the peak of the R wave and ends just before the T wave
B. ventricular ejection begins when the aortic valve opens
C. most ventricular filling occurs during atrial systole
D. during isovolumetric contraction, left ventricular volume and shape are unchanged
E. ventricular diastole is composed of four phases

20. The differences in contraction of the left and right sides of the heart include the following
A. left atrial systole precedes right atrial systole
B. contraction of the right ventricle (RV) typically begins before that of the left ventricle
C. left ventricular ejection precedes right ventricular ejection
D. the RV contracts less homogenously than the left ventricle
E. the RV normally generates a pressure approximately half that of the left ventricle

21. On the central venous pressure waveform
A. two upstroke waves and three descents are described
B. the 'a' wave is absent in atrial fibrillation
C. the 'c' wave results from the direct influence of the carotid pulsation
D. the 'v' wave results from ventricular contraction
E. the 'y' descent occurs during ventricular filling

22. Systemic vascular resistance
A. is the resistance to blood flow offered by the systemic vasculature including the pulmonary circulation
B. under physiological conditions is almost equal to the pulmonary vascular resistance
C. is normally higher than total peripheral resistance
D. is decreased by endothelin
E. is inversely proportional to the diameter of the vessel

23. Cerebral blood flow (CBF)
A. decreases in hypocapnia
B. increases in hypoxia
C. increases in anaemia
D. is not influenced by blood viscosity
E. does not change with age in healthy individuals

24. Regarding the arterial blood supply to the brain

A. the external carotid arteries give rise to the anterior circulation

B. the posterior circulation is formed by two vertebral arteries

C. basilar arteries are formed by the connection of internal carotid and vertebral arteries on each side

D. the circle of Willis is located at the base of the brain

E. blood from the anterior and posterior circulations normally do not mix

25. Cerebrospinal fluid (CSF)

A. is produced primarily by the arachnoid granulations in the dural sinuses

B. reabsorption occurs primarily via the choroid plexus in the lateral ventricles

C. production is an exclusively passive process

D. is mostly produced during normal sleep

E. density varies between individuals depending on gender

26. In the blood supply to the spinal cord

A. there are two posterior spinal arteries but only one anterior spinal artery

B. segmental spinal arteries typically originate directly from the aorta

C. the anterior portion of the spinal cord is most prone to ischaemia

D. the artery of Adamkiewicz is the largest anterior segmental medullary artery

E. anterior arteries supply the anterior two-thirds of the spinal cord

27. The cerebral metabolic rate (CMR)

A. is usually expressed in terms of carbon dioxide production

B. is greatest in the grey matter of the cerebral cortex

C. normally is not related to glucose consumption

D. may dramatically increase in body temperature above 42°C

E. is indirectly proportional to neuronal activity

28. The following is true for neurotransmitters in the central nervous system

A. L-glutamate is an inhibitory neurotransmitter

B. gamma aminobutyric acid (GABA) is the major excitatory neurotransmitter in the brain

C. glycine is a major inhibitory neurotransmitter

D. GABA is the major neurotransmitter in the basal ganglia

E. acetylcholine has only ionotropic receptors

29. The Cushing reflex

A. is caused by elevated intracranial pressure (ICP)

B. increases cerebral perfusion pressure (CPP)

C. may contribute to an increase in ICP

D. is clinically manifest by severe systemic hypotension

E. may be a result of brain herniation

30. Glucocorticoids have multiple actions, including

A. stimulation of protein synthesis
B. decreasing glucose utilization
C. depletion of hepatic glycogen stores
D. decreasing the circulating lymphocyte count
E. promoting osteoporosis

31. Triiodothyronine (T3)

A. is the primary hormone secreted by the thyroid
B. has lower biological activity than thyroxine (T4)
C. is generated mainly in the thyroid gland by de-iodination of T4
D. is not bound to thyroxine-binding globulin (TBG)
E. is catabolized by de-iodination

32. In the normal kidneys

A. blood flow is approximately 40% of the total cardiac output
B. oxygen extraction is less than 2 ml/100 ml arterial blood
C. the cortex receives the major proportion of renal blood flow
D. the medulla has a higher oxygen content than the cortex
E. the tubular system has a high energy requirement

33. A gallstone blocking the sphincter of Oddi will increase the plasma levels of

A. conjugated bile acids
B. cholesterol
C. phosphatidylcholine
D. amylase
E. unconjugated bile acids

34. In the anhepatic phase of liver transplantation, a rise in the blood level of the following substances would be expected

A. glucose
B. fibrinogen
C. 25-hydroxycholecalciferol
D. conjugated bilirubin
E. oestrogens

35. Hyponatraemia

A. is defined as a plasma Na^+ less than 120 mEq/l
B. is always associated with low serum osmolality
C. when euvolaemic, may be associated with an excess of antidiuretic hormone (ADH)
D. cannot be associated with hypovolaemia
E. is a recognized complication in postoperative patients

36. Plasma ionized calcium concentration

A. is increased by hyperventilation
B. is unaffected by calcitonin
C. is increased by 1,25-dihydroxycholecalciferol
D. is decreased by parathyroid hormone
E. drop may cause skeletal muscle weakness

37. Ketone bodies

A. are normal by-products of carbohydrate metabolism
B. are present in the blood, where acetone is the major type
C. are increased in prolonged starvation
D. are formed from acetyl coenzyme A
E. are measured in urine as β-hydroxybutyrate

38. Tonicity

A. is the osmotic pressure gradient between two solutions
B. expresses the osmolal activity of solutes restricted to the extracellular compartment
C. is determined by all solutes in a solution
D. is not affected by urea
E. is affected by ethanol but not by mannitol

39. The Stewart physicochemical theory of physiological acid-base balance includes the following biochemical parameters

A. strong ion difference (SID)
B. total weak acid concentration
C. chloride ion
D. the strong ion gap
E. bicarbonate ion

40. Basal metabolic rate (BMR)

A. is determined during sleep
B. of a 70 kg human subject is about 3000 kcal/day (12,500 kJ/day)
C. is increased during prolonged starvation
D. is higher in children than in elderly people
E. is increased with a rise in body temperature

41. With respect to thermoreceptors

A. cold and heat receptors are innervated by different types of nerve fibres
B. the skin has more cold than heat receptors
C. at normothermia, most afferent input comes from cold receptors
D. central thermoreceptors are mainly located in the brainstem
E. afferent thermal signals from heat receptors are transmitted to the anterior hypothalamus

42. In naturally occurring anticlotting mechanisms

A. activated protein C proteolyses activated factors V and VIII
B. antithrombin inhibits the action of activated factors IX, X, XI, XII
C. antithrombin does not affect the extrinsic coagulation pathway
D. the action of antithrombin is enhanced by heparin
E. conversion of plasminogen to plasmin is an essential part of fibrinolysis

43. A hypercoagulable state induced by pregnancy is characterized by

A. decreased fibrinolysis
B. decreased bleeding time
C. a slight increase in clotting factor XIII level
D. an essential increase in clotting factor VII level
E. the greatest increase in clotting activity occurs at the time of delivery

44. Respiratory changes in pregnancy include

A. a reduction in airway resistance
B. a significant increase in arterial pH due to respiratory alkalosis during the second and third trimesters
C. a shift of the oxyhaemoglobin dissociation curve to the left
D. an increased minute ventilation mainly due to an increase in respiratory frequency
E. a reduced functional residual capacity to closing capacity (FRC/CC) ratio by term

45. Concerning immune cells

A. unlike granulocytes, mast cells are not granulated
B. tissue macrophages are derived from monocytes
C. Kupffer cells of the liver are a type of tissue macrophage
D. T lymphocytes are responsible for forming antibodies
E. B lymphocytes provide humoral immunity

Question 1: Answer

A. True. Glomus (type I) cells within the carotid body are in synaptic contact with neurons of the glossopharyngeal nerve. The discharge rate in the afferent nerves from the carotid body increases exponentially in response to falling arterial PO_2.

B. False. Ventilation is increased in acidaemia. Elevated arterial PCO_2 or hydrogen ion concentration both stimulate ventilation. The change produced by elevated PCO_2 on the peripheral chemoreceptors is only about one-sixth of that caused by the action on the central chemoreceptors. This response occurs very rapidly and develops only when a 'threshold' value of arterial PCO_2 is exceeded.

C. True. Stimulation of peripheral chemoreceptors by hypoperfusion can occur as a result of severe systemic hypotension, possibly by causing a 'stagnant hypoxia' of the chemoreceptor cells.

D. False. Ventilation is increased in hyperthermia. An increase in body temperature increases the rate of firing from peripheral chemoreceptor neurons.

E. True. Carbon monoxide causes increased ventilation blocking the cytochrome system and thus preventing oxidative metabolism.

Lumb, A.B. and Horncastle, E. Pulmonary physiology. In: H.C. Hemmings, Jr., and T.D. Egan (eds.). *Pharmacology and Physiology for Anesthesia: Foundations and Clinical Application*, 2nd edition. Elsevier, 2019: p. 595

Question 2: Answer

A. False. Central chemoreceptors are located 0.2 mm below the ventrolateral surface of the medulla in the retrotrapezoid nucleus inside the blood-brain barrier.

B. False. See explanation above for A.

C. False. The central chemoreceptors are regarded as monitors of steady-state arterial PCO_2 and tissue perfusion in the brain, while the peripheral chemoreceptors respond more to short-term and rapid changes in arterial PCO_2.

D. True. The mechanism by which a change in pH causes stimulation of chemoreceptor neurons remains controversial: the retrotrapezoid nucleus might contain pH-sensitive K^+ channels, and the release of adenosine triphosphate (ATP) has been proposed.

E. True. They are sensitive to the PCO_2 but not PO_2 of blood.

Lumb, A.B. and Horncastle, E. Pulmonary physiology. In: H.C. Hemmings, Jr., and T.D. Egan (eds.). *Pharmacology and Physiology for Anesthesia: Foundations and Clinical Application*, 2nd edition. Elsevier, 2019: p. 594.

Question 3: Answer

A. True. As blood flow through the two circulations is virtually identical, this range of flow can normally be achieved with a minimal increase in pulmonary vascular pressures, owing to the considerably lower PVR, which is only one-tenth that of the systemic circulation.

B. True. As lung volume increases, some pulmonary capillaries become narrowed and stretched, whereas a reduction in lung volume makes some capillaries more tortuous or kinked, both of which increase PVR, therefore the PVR has its lowest value at FRC.

C. False. Prostaglandins dilate pulmonary vessels by acting directly on smooth muscle cells via the cyclic adenosine monophosphate (cAMP) second-messenger system. In contrast, vasoconstrictors activate G-protein-coupled receptors.

D. False. Vasoactive intestinal peptide is a vasodilator and acts by a similar mechanism to prostaglandins (see the previous question explanation).

E. True. NO acts as a final common pathway for relaxation of pulmonary vascular smooth muscle. It diffuses from the site of production to the smooth muscle cell, where it activates guanylyl cyclase to produce cyclic guanosine monophosphate (cGMP), which in turn activates protein kinase G causing relaxation by a combination of effects on cytosolic Ca^{2+} levels and the activity of enzymes controlling myosin activity.

Lumb, A.B. and Horncastle, E. Pulmonary physiology. In: H.C. Hemmings, Jr., and T.D. Egan (eds.). *Pharmacology and Physiology for Anesthesia: Foundations and Clinical Application*, 2nd edition. Elsevier, 2019: pp. 590, 592.

Question 4: Answer

A. False. Neural connections to the lung are not required as HPV occurs in isolated lung preparations and in humans following lung transplantation.

B. False. See explanation above for A.

C. False. Uncertainties remain regarding the exact cellular mechanisms of HPV, but there is now agreement that contraction of pulmonary artery smooth muscle cells (PASMCs) in response to hypoxia is an inherent property of these cells and that pulmonary endothelial cells act only to modulate the PASMC response.

D. True. Long-term HPV, either continuous or intermittent, can lead to remodelling of the pulmonary vasculature and irreversible pulmonary hypertension.

E. True. Endothelin is released by endothelial cells in response to hypoxia. It is a potent vasoconstrictor peptide, and has a prolonged effect on pulmonary vascular tone such that this mechanism is probably involved in the second slow phase of HPV.

Lumb, A.B. and Horncastle, E. Pulmonary physiology. In: H.C. Hemmings, Jr., and T.D. Egan (eds.). *Pharmacology and Physiology for Anesthesia: Foundations and Clinical Application*, 2nd edition. Elsevier, 2019: pp. 592–593.

Question 5: Answer

A. True. The dorsal respiratory group lies close to the nucleus tractus solitarius, which is the area of the brain where visceral afferents from cranial nerves IX and X terminate. This group consists mainly of inspiratory neurons and is responsible for the timing of the respiratory cycle.

B. True. The ventral respiratory group is a column of respiratory neurons divided into four subgroups, two of which are Bötzinger and pre-Bötzinger complexes.

C. True. The pre-Bötzinger complex is believed to be the anatomic location of the central pattern generator, while the Bötzinger complex is within the nucleus retrofacialis and has widespread expiratory functions.

D. True. The caudal subgroup of the ventral respiratory group has both inspiratory and expiratory functions in addition to controlling the force of contraction of the contralateral inspiratory muscles.

E. False. The pontine respiratory group, previously known as the pneumotaxic centre, was believed to be important in controlling the timing of the respiratory cycle. It is no longer considered essential for generation of the respiratory rhythm but exerts fine control over medullary neurons, for example, setting the lung volume at which inspiration is terminated.

Lumb, A.B. and Horncastle, E. Pulmonary physiology. In: H.C. Hemmings, Jr., and T.D. Egan (eds.). *Pharmacology and Physiology for Anesthesia: Foundations and Clinical Application*, 2nd edition. Elsevier, 2019: p. 593.

Question 6: Answer

A. True. Following induction of anaesthesia, changes in the dimensions of the thoracic cavity occur due to muscle relaxation, in particular loss of tonic activity in the diaphragm, leading to a 10% to 20% reduction in FRC.

B. True. As FRC approaches CC, areas of collapse (atelectasis) develop in the dependent regions of the lung, resulting in areas of lung that are perfused but not ventilated, increasing shunt and therefore impairing oxygenation in most patients during general anaesthesia. Even in dependent areas without atelectasis, the V/Q ratio is less than 1.

C. True. Non-dependent areas of lung are well ventilated relative to dependent regions. General anaesthesia commonly leads to low cardiac output and pulmonary hypotension, resulting in reduced perfusion to non-dependent regions. As a result, V/Q ratios in non-dependent regions are normally greater than 1, and there are some areas with ventilation but no perfusion, which constitutes alveolar dead space.

D. False. With spontaneous breathing, intercostal activity is depressed, and diaphragm contraction is preserved. This leads to uncoordinated activity, with diaphragm contraction causing indrawing of the upper ribcage in early inspiration.

E. False. Irrespective of the mode of ventilation, there are increases in areas of both high and low ventilation/perfusion (V/Q) ratio, with the former increasing alveolar dead space and so impairing CO_2 excretion and the latter increasing venous admixture.

Andrew B. Lumb and Elizabeth Horncastle. Pulmonary physiology. In: Hugh C. Hemmings, Jr., and Talmage D. Egan. *Pharmacology and physiology for anesthesia: foundations and clinical application*, 2nd ed. Elsevier, 2019: p. 591.

Question 7: Answer

A. False. Physiological dead space equals the sum of anatomical and alveolar dead spaces.

B. False. Anatomical but not alveolar dead space can be measured using Fowler's method with a nitrogen or CO_2 washout technique.

C. False. The alveolar air equation is used to calculate oxygen concentration in an ideal alveolus. Physiological dead space is measured using the Bohr equation, which is based on the assumption that the volume of expired CO_2 must equal the volume of CO_2 breathed out from ventilation of ideal alveoli (assuming inspired CO_2 is negligible).

D. False. Anatomic dead space is modified by large lengths of ventilator tubing between the tracheal tube and the ventilator Y-piece. Ventilation occurs because gas flows into and out of the alveoli. In contrast, the inspiratory or expiratory limb of the anaesthesia circle system has unidirectional flow, and therefore, is not a component of anatomic dead space ventilation.

E. **False.** In clinical situations, changes in physiological dead space are usually a result of altered alveolar dead space as anatomical dead space is approximately fixed provided any artificial airway is unchanged. Since disease produces little change in anatomical dead space, physiological dead space is primarily influenced by changes in alveolar dead space. Rapid changes in physiological dead space ventilation most often arise from changes in pulmonary blood flow, resulting in decreased perfusion to ventilated alveoli.

Lumb, A. and Kumara, P. Respiratory system. In: J. Thompson, I. Moppett, and M. Wiles (eds.). *Smith and Aitkenhead's Textbook of Anaesthesia*, 7th edition. Elsevier, 2019: pp. 189–190.

Question 8: Answer

A. True. Physiological ageing of the lung is associated with dilation of the alveoli, enlargement of the airspaces, decrease in exchange surface area, and loss of supporting tissue.

B. True. Changes in the ageing lung and chest wall result in decreased lung recoil (elastance) creating an increased residual volume and FRC.

C. True. The compliance of the chest wall diminishes, and respiratory muscle strength decreases with ageing, thereby increasing the work of breathing compared with younger subjects.

D. False. With ageing, respiratory centres in the nervous system demonstrate decreased sensitivity to hypoxaemia and hypercapnia resulting in a blunted ventilatory response when challenged by heart failure, airway obstruction, or pneumonia.

E. True. Despite changes with age, the respiratory system is normally able to maintain adequate gas exchange at rest and during exertion throughout life, with only modest decrements in PaO_2 and no change in $PaCO_2$.

Tamul, P.C. and Ault, M. Respiratory function in anesthesia. In: P.G. Barash et al. (eds.). *Clinical Anesthesia (Barash)*, 8th edition. Wolters Kluwer, 2017: p. 952.

Question 9: Answer

A. True. There is a rightward shift of the O_2 dissociation curve at moderate altitudes that results in better unloading of oxygen in venous blood at a given PO_2. The cause of the shift is an increase in concentration of 2,3-diphosphoglycerate, which develops primarily because of the respiratory alkalosis.

B. True. At higher altitudes, there is a leftward shift in the dissociation curve caused by the respiratory alkalosis, and this assists in the loading of oxygen in the pulmonary capillaries.

C. False. Maximum breathing capacity increases because the air is less dense, and this allows for a very high ventilation rate (up to 200 l/min) during exercise.

D. True. Pulmonary vasoconstriction occurs in response to alveolar hypoxia. This increases the pulmonary arterial pressure and the work done by the right heart. The hypertension is exaggerated by polycythaemia, which raises the viscosity of the blood. Hypertrophy of the right heart may develop. There is no physiological advantage in this response, except that the topographical distribution of blood flow becomes more uniform. Pulmonary hypertension is sometimes associated with pulmonary oedema, although the pulmonary venous pressure is normal. The probable mechanism is that the arteriolar vasoconstriction is uneven, and leakage occurs in unprotected, damaged capillaries. The oedema fluid has a high protein concentration, indicating that the permeability of the capillaries is increased.

E. False. Hyperventilation is the most important feature of acclimatization to high altitude; however, the mechanism of hyperventilation is hypoxic stimulation of the peripheral chemoreceptors.

West, J.B. *Respiratory Physiology: The Essentials*, 9th edition. Wolters Kluwer, 2012: p. 146.

Question 10: Answer

A. False. The oxygen dissociation curve is shifted to the right by an increase in hydrogen ion concentration, carbon dioxide partial pressure (PCO_2) and temperature, which means that the oxygen affinity of haemoglobin is reduced.

B. False. Please see the explanation given in A above. In addition, the effect of PCO_2, which is known as the Bohr effect, can be attributed to its action on hydrogen ion concentration.

C. False. A simple way to remember the shifts of the oxygen dissociation curve, and the unloading of oxygen to tissues, is the following: an exercising muscle is acidic, hypercarbic, and hot, and it benefits from increased unloading of oxygen from its capillaries.

D. False. 2,3-DPG is an end product of red cell metabolism, an increase in its concentration shifts the O_2 dissociation curve to the right facilitating the unloading of oxygen to peripheral tissues and reducing the oxygen affinity of haemoglobin. Its concentration is increased in chronic hypoxia, for example, at high altitude or in the presence of chronic lung disease. By contrast, stored blood in a blood bank may be depleted of 2,3-DPG and unloading of oxygen is impaired.

E. True. A small amount of carbon monoxide added to blood increases its oxygen affinity causing a leftward shift of the O_2 dissociation curve and thus interfering with the unloading of oxygen.

West, J.B. *Respiratory Physiology: The Essentials*, 9th edition. Wolters Kluwer, 2012: pp. 80–82.

Question 11: Answer

A. False. Bradykinin is largely inactivated in the lungs (up to 80%), and the enzyme responsible is angiotensin-converting enzyme (ACE).

B. True. The lung is the major site for inactivation of serotonin (5-hydroxytryptamine), but this is not by enzymatic degradation but by an uptake and storage process. Some of the serotonin may be transferred to platelets in the lung or stored in some other way and released during anaphylaxis.

C. False. The only known example of biological activation by passage through the pulmonary circulation is the conversion of the relatively inactive polypeptide angiotensin I to the potent vasoconstrictor angiotensin II, which is up to 50 times more active than its precursor and is unaffected by passage through the lung. The conversion of angiotensin I is catalysed by ACE located in small pits in the surface of the capillary endothelial cells.

D. False. Up to 30% of noradrenaline (norepinephrine) is taken up by the lung.

E. False. Adrenaline (epinephrine) passes through the lungs without significant gain or loss of activity.

West, J.B. *Respiratory Physiology: The Essentials*, 9th edition. Wolters Kluwer, 2012: pp. 52–54.

Question 12: Answer

A. False. The major epicardial coronary vessel that feeds the PDA determines the 'dominance' of the coronary circulation. A 'right dominant' circulation (RCA supplies blood to the PDA) is observed in approximately 80% of the human population, whereas a 'left dominant' circulation (left circumflex coronary artery (LCCA) perfuses the PDA) occurs in the remaining 20%.

B. True. Distal diagonal and septal branches of the LAD artery perfuse the RV anterior wall. Therefore, LAD artery occlusion may cause RV ischaemia or infarction with resulting contractile dysfunction.

C. True. The RCA usually supplies blood to the atrioventricular (AV) node, but the LCCA may also perfuse the AV node depending on the coronary circulation's right or left dominance, therefore critical stenosis or acute occlusion of either the RCA or LCCA may interrupt normal atrial or AV node conduction and cause bradyarrhythmias.

D. False. The coronary capillary network distribution is quite uniform throughout the atria and ventricles except in the AV node and interventricular septum, where it is substantially reduced, which explains why the proximal portion of the RV and left ventricular (LV) conduction system is more vulnerable to ischaemia.

E. False. Approximately 85% of total coronary blood flow returning from the left ventricle empties into the coronary sinus, the remaining flow drains directly into the atrial and ventricular cavities through the Thebesian veins. The RV veins drain into the anterior cardiac veins that empty individually into the RA.

Pagel, P.S. and Stowe, D.F. Cardiac anatomy and physiology. In: P.G. Barash et al. (eds.). *Clinical Anesthesia (Barash)*, 8th edition. Wolters Kluwer, 2017: p. 747.

Question 13: Answer

A. True. Baroreceptors are stimulated by the stretch of the vessel wall because of increased transluminal pressure. Impulses originating in the baroreceptors inhibit the discharge of sympathetic nerves to the heart and blood vessels and facilitate the discharge of the vagus nerve to the heart. A rise in arterial pressure reduces baroreceptor afferent activity, resulting in further inhibition of the sympathetic and facilitation of parasympathetic output. This produces vasodilation and reductions in stroke volume, heart rate, and cardiac output, which combine to normalize arterial pressure.

B. False. The Bainbridge reflex is elicited by stretch receptors located in the right atrial wall and the cavoatrial junction. An increase in right-sided filling pressure sends vagal afferent signals to the cardiovascular centre in the medulla, which inhibit parasympathetic activity, thereby increasing the heart rate. Acceleration of the heart rate also results from a direct effect on the sinoatrial node by stretching the atrium.

C. True. The Bezold–Jarisch reflex is a response to noxious ventricular stimuli sensed by chemoreceptors and mechanoreceptors within the left ventricular wall by inducing the triad of hypotension, bradycardia, and coronary artery dilatation. The activated receptors communicate along unmyelinated vagal afferent C fibres, which reflexively increase parasympathetic tone invoking bradycardia.

D. True. When ICP is increased, the blood supply to rostral ventrolateral medulla (RVLM) neurons is compromised and the local hypoxia and hypercapnia increase their activity. The resultant rise in systemic arterial pressure (Cushing reflex) tends to restore the blood flow to the medulla. Over a considerable range, the blood pressure rise is proportional to the increase in ICP. The rise in blood pressure causes a reflex decrease in heart rate via the arterial baroreceptors. This is why bradycardia rather than tachycardia is characteristically seen in patients with increased ICP.

E. True. The oculocardiac reflex is provoked by pressure applied to the globe of the eye or traction on the surrounding structures. Stretch receptors located in the extraocular muscles are activated and send afferent signals through the short and long ciliary nerves, which merge with the ophthalmic division of the trigeminal nerve at the ciliary ganglion. The trigeminal nerve carries these impulses to the Gasserian ganglion, thereby resulting in increased parasympathetic tone and subsequent bradycardia.

Barrett, K.E. et al. *Ganong's Medical Physiology Examination & Board Review*. McGraw-Hill Education, Lange, 2018: p. 735.

Sun, L.S. and Davis, N.A. Cardiac physiology. In: M. Gropper et al. (eds.). *Miller's Anesthesia*, 9th edition. Elsevier, 2020: pp. 400–401.

Question 14: Answer

A. True. Adrenomedullin is a recently discovered cardiac hormone that was originally isolated from phaeochromocytoma tissue. It increases the accumulation of cAMP and has direct positive chronotropic and inotropic effects. Adrenomedullin, with interspecies and regional variations, has also been shown to increase nitric oxide production, and it functions as a potent vasodilator.

B. True. Angiotensin II mediates cell growth and proliferation of cardiomyocytes and fibroblasts. Angiotensin II stimulates AT1 subtype receptors, activation of which is directly involved in the development of cardiac hypertrophy and heart failure, as well as adverse remodelling of the myocardium.

C. False. Most hormone receptors expressed in cardiomyocytes are plasma membrane GPCRs. However, natriuretic peptide receptors are guanylyl cyclase-coupled receptors.

D. False. Increased stretch of the myocardium, which may occur in volume overload stimulates the release of atrial natriuretic protein (ANP) from the atria and BNP from the ventricles.

E. True. Aldosterone binds to mineralocorticoid receptors and can increase the expression or activity (or both) of cardiac proteins involved in ionic homeostasis or the regulation of pH. It modifies cardiac structure by inducing cardiac fibrosis in both ventricular chambers and thereby leads to impairment of cardiac contractile function.

Sun, L.S. and Davis, N.A. Cardiac physiology. In: M. Gropper et al. (eds.). *Miller's Anesthesia*, 9th edition. Elsevier, 2020: pp. 397–399.

Question 15: Answer

A. False. Supraventricular tissue receives significantly more intense vagal innervation than the ventricles. The parasympathetic nervous system has a more direct inhibitory effect in the atria and has a negative modulatory effect in the ventricles.

B. False. At rest, the heart has a tonic level of parasympathetic cardiac nerve firing and little, if any, sympathetic activity. Therefore, the major influence on the heart at rest is parasympathetic. During exercise or stress, however, the sympathetic neural influence becomes more prominent.

C. False. The muscarinic receptors in the heart are the principal parasympathetic target neuroeffectors. Their activation reduces pacemaker activity, slows atrioventricular conduction, directly decreases atrial contractile force, and exerts inhibitory modulation of ventricular contractile force.

D. True. Both β_1- and β_2-adrenoreceptors are coupled to the G_s-cAMP pathway. Additionally, β_2-adrenoreceptors can couple to G-protein-independent pathways to modulate cardiac function, and also couple to the inhibitory G-protein (Gi) to activate non-cAMP-dependent signalling pathways. β-adrenoreceptor stimulation increases both contraction and relaxation.

E. True. Cardiac hypertrophy is primarily mediated by α_1-adrenoreceptors. Cardiac hypertrophic responses to α_1-adrenoreceptor agonists involve activation of protein kinase C and mitogen-activated protein kinase through G_q-signalling mechanisms.

Sun, L.S. and Davis, N.A. Cardiac physiology. In: M. Gropper et al. (eds.). *Miller's Anesthesia*, 9th edition. Elsevier, 2020: pp. 395–396.

Question 16: Answer

A. False. The principal catecholamine synthesized by the adrenal medulla is adrenaline (epinephrine).

B. False. Noradrenaline (norepinephrine) has a greater effect at α_1-receptors than adrenaline, thereby creating greater arterial and venous vascular constriction than adrenaline.

C. False. It is a β-receptor agonist, however, β_2 effects are not apparent clinically.

D. True. While the amount of circulating adrenaline and the number of β-adrenergic receptors is not reduced in older adults, the amount of noradrenaline is increased. This leads to a cyclic decline in responsiveness of adrenergic receptors as circulating plasma noradrenaline increases and receptors downregulate, requiring more stimulation.

E. False. Both adrenaline and noradrenaline are metabolized by catechol-O-methyltransferase (COMT) and monoamine oxidase (MAO). COMT is an intracellular enzyme located in postsynaptic neurons.

Ebert, T.J. Autonomic nervous system pharmacology. In: H.C. Hemmings, Jr. and T.D. Egan (eds.). *Pharmacology and Physiology for Anesthesia: Foundations and Clinical Application*, 2nd edition. Elsevier, 2019: p. 287.

Hakeem Yusuff, M. Charlton cardiovascular system. In: J. Thompson, I. Moppett, and M. Wiles (eds.). *Smith and Aitkenhead's Textbook of Anaesthesia*, 7th edition. Elsevier, 2019: pp. 164–165.

Johnson, J.O. Autonomic nervous system: physiology. In: H.C. Hemmings, Jr. and T.D. Egan (eds.). *Pharmacology and Physiology for Anesthesia: Foundations and Clinical Application*, 2nd edition. Elsevier, 2019: p. 278.

Question 17: Answer

A. True. Isovolumetric relaxation is the first phase of left ventricular diastole, left ventricular volume is constant during this phase because both the aortic and mitral valves are closed.

B. False. The first phase of ventricular diastole is isovolumetric relaxation, atrial systole is the final phase of ventricular diastole. Left atrial contraction creates a positive pressure gradient between the left atrium and ventricle and stimulates active blood flow at the end of diastole.

C. True. This percentage increases when delayed left ventricular relaxation or reduced left ventricular compliance is present. It is common for patients with such abnormalities to develop acute hemodynamic instability when left atrial contraction suddenly becomes timed improperly (e.g., atrioventricular conduction block) or disappears entirely (e.g., atrial fibrillation).

D. False. The early filling phase of diastole normally provides 70–80% of the final stroke volume.

E. True. Diastasis is the third phase of diastole, the left atrium acts as a conduit for pulmonary venous blood to flow freely through the open mitral valve into the left ventricle. Less than 5% of total stroke volume enters the left ventricle during diastasis, which may be shortened or eliminated by tachycardia.

Pagel, P.S. and Stowe, D.F. Cardiac anatomy and physiology. In: P.G. Barash et al. (eds.). *Clinical Anesthesia (Barash)*, 8th edition. Wolters Kluwer, 2017: pp. 765–766.

Question 18: Answer

A. True. An increase in heart rate increases cardiac output if ventricular filling is adequate during diastole.

B. True. Contractility is the intrinsic ability of the cardiac myocyte to increase (or decrease) the force of contraction as a result of changes in inotropy independent of loading conditions.

C. False. Ejection fraction is a clinical index of global contractile function of cardiac muscle providing information about systolic pump performance.

D. True. Preload is defined as the initial stretching of the cardiac myocyte to its end-diastolic length. An increase in end-diastolic volume due to enhanced venous return causes an increase in sarcomere length, resulting in a proportional rise in force development and ventricular stroke work.

E. True. Afterload describes the force against which the ventricle must eject and equates to ventricular wall stress. All other things being equal, decreasing afterload will lead to increasing stroke volume and vice versa.

Crystal, G.J., Assaad, S.I., and Heerdt, P.M. Cardiovascular physiology: integrative function. In: H.C. Hemmings, Jr. and T.D. Egan (eds.). *Pharmacology and Physiology for Anesthesia: Foundations and Clinical Application*, 2nd edition. Elsevier, 2019: p. 479.

Hakeem Yusuff, M. Charlton cardiovascular system. In: J. Thompson, I. Moppett, and M. Wiles (eds.). *Smith and Aitkenhead's Textbook of Anaesthesia*, 7th edition. Elsevier, 2019: pp. 157–158.

Question 19: Answer

A. False. Ventricular systole begins near the end of the R wave and ends just after the T wave.

B. True. When ventricular pressure exceeds aorta pressure, the aortic valve opens, and ventricular ejection begins.

C. False. Most ventricular filling occurs prior to atrial systole. Atrial systole normally generates 15–25% of final stroke volume.

D. False. During left ventricular isovolumic contraction, its volume is constant because both the aortic and mitral valves are closed; however, the left ventricular shape becomes more spherical due to a decrease in its longitudinal dimension.

E. True. Isovolumetric relaxation, early ventricular filling, diastasis, and atrial systole are the four phases of ventricular diastole.

Crystal, G.J., Assaad, S.I., and Heerdt, P.M. Cardiovascular physiology: integrative function. In: H.C. Hemmings, Jr. and T.D. Egan (eds.). *Pharmacology and Physiology for Anesthesia: Foundations and Clinical Application*, 2nd edition. Elsevier, 2019: pp. 475–476.

Pagel, P.S. and Stowe, D.F. Cardiac anatomy and physiology. In: P.G. Barash et al. (eds.). *Clinical Anesthesia (Barash)*. 8th edition. Wolters Kluwer, 2017: pp. 763–764.

Question 20: Answer

A. False. Events on the right side of the circulation are similar to those on the left side but are somewhat asynchronous. Right atrial systole precedes left atrial systole.

B. False. Contraction of the RV typically begins after that of the left ventricle.

C. False. Although the contraction of the RV typically begins after that of the left ventricle, because pulmonary arterial pressure is less than aortic pressure, right ventricular ejection precedes that of the left ventricle.

D. True. The pattern of contraction differs for the left and right ventricles. The left ventricle contracts in a relatively homogeneous fashion with both the short and long axes shortening simultaneously. In contrast, the RV contracts in peristaltic fashion sequentially from the inflow tract to the outflow tract.

E. False. The right ventricle normally develops a pressure only 20% of that in the left ventricle.

Pagel, P.S. and Stowe, D.F. Cardiac anatomy and physiology. In: P.G. Barash et al. (eds.). *Clinical Anesthesia (Barash)*, 8th edition. Wolters Kluwer, 2017: p. 764.

Question 21: Answer

A. False. Three upstroke waves named 'a', 'c', and 'v' and two descents 'x' and 'y' are described, reflecting changes in the central venous pressure throughout the cardiac cycle.

B. True. The 'a' wave is generated by atrial contraction and is absent in atrial fibrillation as there is no synchronized atrial contraction.

C. False. The 'c' wave results from the bulging of the tricuspid valve into the right atrium during ventricular contraction.

D. False. The 'v' wave results from atrial filling against a closed tricuspid valve.

E. True. The 'y' descent is caused by passive ventricular filling after opening of the tricuspid valve.

Cross, M.E. and Plunkett, E.V.E. *Physics, Pharmacology and Physiology for Anaesthetists. Key Concepts for the FRCA*, 2nd edition. Cambridge University Press, 2014: p. 276.

Question 22: Answer

A. False. Systemic vascular resistance describes the resistance to blood flow offered by the systemic vasculature to the output of the left side of the heart, thus excluding the pulmonary circulation.

B. False. Under physiological conditions, the pulmonary vascular system is a low-resistance system. Pulmonary arterial pressure therefore remains low despite receiving the same cardiac output as the systemic circulation.

C. False. Systemic vascular resistance is sometimes referred to as total peripheral resistance (TPR).

D. False. Endothelin is a potent vasoconstrictor peptide and increases vascular tone.

E. True. Resistance to flow is inversely proportional to the fourth power of the radius according to the Hagen–Poiseuille equation.

Hakeem Yusuff, M. Charlton cardiovascular system. In: J. Thompson, I. Moppett, and M. Wiles (eds.). *Smith and Aitkenhead's Textbook of Anaesthesia*, 7th edition. Elsevier, 2019: p. 158.

Question 23: Answer

A. True. CBF varies directly with $PaCO_2$. The magnitude of the reduction in CBF caused by hypocapnia is more intense when resting CBF is increased (as might occur during anaesthesia with volatile agents). Conversely, when resting CBF is reduced, the magnitude of the hypocapnia-induced reduction in CBF is decreased slightly.

B. True. Changes in PaO_2 from 60 to more than 300 mmHg have little influence on CBF. A reduction in PaO_2 below 60 mmHg rapidly increases CBF.

C. True. In anaemia, cerebral vascular resistance is reduced and CBF increases. This may result in a compensatory response to reduced oxygen delivery.

D. False. Blood viscosity can influence CBF. Haematocrit is the single most important determinant of blood viscosity. In healthy humans, variation of the haematocrit within the normal range (33–45%) probably results in only modest alterations in CBF. Beyond this range, changes are more substantial.

E. False. Concomitant with the loss of neurons in the normally ageing brain, CBF decreases by 15–20% at the age of 80 years in the healthy aged brain.

Patel, P.M., Drummond, J.C., and Lemkuil, B.P. Cerebral physiology and the effects of anesthetic drugs. In: M. Gropper et al. (eds.). *Miller's Anesthesia*, 9th edition. Elsevier, 2020: pp. 300–307.

Question 24: Answer

A. False. The arterial blood supply to the brain is composed of paired right and left internal carotid arteries, which give rise to the anterior circulation, and paired right and left vertebral arteries, which give rise to the posterior circulation.

B. True. Please see the explanation above.

C. False. There is only one basilar artery, which is formed by the connection of the two vertebral arteries.

D. True. The internal carotid arteries and the basilar artery connect to form a vascular loop called the circle of Willis at the base of the brain that permits collateral circulation between both the right and left and the anterior and posterior perfusing arteries.

E. True. Under normal circumstances, blood from the anterior and posterior circulations does not admix because the pressures in the two systems are equal.

Patel, P.M., Drummond, J.C., and Lemkuil, B.P. Cerebral physiology and the effects of anesthetic drugs. In: M. Gropper et al. (eds.). *Miller's Anesthesia*, 9th edition. Elsevier, 2020: p. 295.

Question 25: Answer

A. False. CSF is produced primarily by the choroid plexus in the lateral, third, and fourth ventricles; there are small contributions from the endothelial cells and from fluid that is produced as a consequence of metabolic activity.

B. False. CSF reabsorption occurs primarily via the arachnoid granulations present in the dural sinuses. A smaller proportion of CSF, which tracks along cranial and peripheral nerves, perivascular routes, and along white matter tracts, gains access to the cerebral venous system by transependymal flow.

C. False. CSF production is the result of hydrostatic efflux from capillaries into the perivascular space, and then active transport into the ventricles.

D. True. CSF production is under the influence of a circadian rhythm, with peak production of CSF occurring during sleep.

E. True. The density of CSF is lower in women compared with men.

Brull, R., Macfarlane, A.J.R., and Chan, V.W.S. Spinal, epidural, and caudal anesthesia. In: M. Gropper et al. (eds.). *Miller's Anesthesia*, 9th edition. Elsevier, 2020: p. 295, 1424.

Question 26: Answer

A. True. Blood is partially supplied to the spinal cord from one anterior spinal artery (originating from the vertebral artery), two posterior spinal arteries (originating from the inferior cerebellar artery).

B. False. The segmental spinal arteries typically originate from the intercostal and lumbar arteries.

C. True. The anterior portion of the spinal cord is most prone to ischaemia (leading to anterior horn motor neuron injury, or anterior spinal syndrome) because there are fewer anterior medullary feeder vessels than posterior feeder vessels.

D. True. The artery of Adamkiewicz is the major medullary branch of the spinal arteries, variably entering between T7 and L4 typically on the left, supplying the lower thoracic and upper lumbar regions.

E. True. The anterior two-thirds of the spinal cord are supplied by the anterior arterial branches and the posterior one-third by the posterior branches.

Brull, R., Macfarlane, A.J.R., and Chan, V.W.S. Spinal, epidural, and caudal anesthesia. In: M. Gropper et al. (eds.). *Miller's Anesthesia*, 9th edition. Elsevier, 2020: p. 1415.

Question 27: Answer

A. False. The CMR is usually expressed in terms of oxygen consumption ($CMRO_2$) and averages 3–3.8 ml/100 g/min (50 ml/min) in adults.

B. True. CMR is greatest in the grey matter of the cerebral cortex and generally parallels cortical electrical activity.

C. False. CMR normally parallels glucose consumption. This relationship is not maintained during starvation, when ketone bodies (acetoacetate and β-hydroxybutyrate) also become major energy substrates.

D. False. Hyperthermia leads to substantial increases in CMR and CBF. However, above 42°C a dramatic reduction in CMR occurs, possibly because of neuronal injury and protein denaturation.

E. False. CMR is directly proportional to neuronal activity. Although the mechanism is not entirely understood, an increase in neuronal activity and CMR is tightly coupled to increased CBF. This physiologic process, wherein blood flow and metabolism are matched, is referred to as flow-metabolism coupling.

Butterworth, J.F., Mackey, D.C., and Wasnick, J.D. *Morgan and Mikhail's Clinical Anesthesiology*, 6th edition. McGraw-Hill Education, Lange, 2018: p. 584.

Lemkuil, B.P., Drummond, J.C., and Patel, P. Central nervous system physiology: cerebrovascular. In: H.C. Hemmings, Jr. and T.D. Egan (eds.). *Pharmacology and Physiology for Anesthesia: Foundations and Clinical Application*, 2nd edition. Elsevier, 2019: p. 176.

Question 28: Answer

A. False. L-glutamate is a major excitatory transmitter in the brain.

B. False. GABA is the major inhibitory neurotransmitter in the brain and activates both ionotropic and metabotropic receptors, $GABA_A$ and $GABA_B$ receptor types respectively.

C. True. Glycine is a major inhibitory neurotransmitter, primarily in the spinal cord. It is released by local inhibitory interneurons and activates ligand-gated Cl⁻ channels.

D. True. The nuclei in basal ganglia are unique in that GABA is the major neurotransmitter used both locally by interneurons as well as by the projection neurons creating a variety of inhibitory and disinhibitory responses (inhibition of inhibition that leads to excitation).

E. False. Acetylcholine has both ionotropic and metabotropic receptors, nicotinic, and muscarinic receptors respectively. Nicotinic receptors are ionotropic and are present in the central nervous system (CNS) in addition to their well-known role at the neuromuscular junction and at ganglia in the autonomic nervous system. There are several types of metabotropic muscarinic G-protein-coupled receptors.

Raz, A. and Perouansky, M. Central nervous system physiology: neurophysiology. In: H.C. Hemmings, Jr. and T.D. Egan. *Pharmacology and Physiology for Anesthesia: Foundations and Clinical Application*, 2nd edition. Elsevier, 2019: pp. 157–159.

Question 29: Answer

A. True. The Cushing reflex is a nervous system physiological response to increased ICP.

B. True. The Cushing reflex increases CPP in response to an increase in ICP by first producing reflex systemic hypertension and tachycardia and then bradycardia.

C. True. Despite its compensatory mechanism the Cushing reflex also contributes to an increase in ICP.

D. False. Please see the explanation for B.

E. True. Very severe intracranial hypertension may lead to brain herniation, and the presence of the Cushing reflex indicates a need for immediate care.

Nathanson, M. Neurosurgical anaesthesia. In: J. Thompson, I. Moppett, and M. Wiles (eds.). *Smith and Aitkenhead's Textbook of Anaesthesia*, 7th edition. Elsevier, 2019: p. 759.

Question 30: Answer

A. False. Glucocorticoids cause protein breakdown and prevent muscle protein synthesis. At high circulating levels, glucocorticoids cause catabolism and breakdown of lean body mass, including bone and muscle.

B. True. This is one of the mechanisms of hyperglycaemia caused by glucocorticoids.

C. False. Glucocorticoids increase hepatic glycogen synthesis.

D. True. Glucocorticoids decrease the circulating lymphocyte count and the size of the lymph nodes and thymus by inhibiting lymphocyte mitotic activity. They reduce the secretion of cytokines. The reduced secretion of the cytokine IL-2 leads to reduced proliferation of lymphocytes, and these cells undergo apoptosis.

E. True. Glucocorticoid excess leads to bone dissolution by decreasing bone formation and increasing bone resorption. This leads to osteoporosis, a loss of bone mass that leads eventually to collapse of vertebral bodies and other fractures.

Barrett, K.E., Barman, S.M., Boitano, S., and Reckelhoff, J.F. *Ganong's Medical Physiology Examination & Board Review*. McGraw-Hill Education, Lange, 2018: pp. 479–480.

Forkin, K.T., Huffmyer, J.L., and Nemergut, E.C. Endocrine physiology. In: H.C. Hemmings, Jr. and T.D. Egan (eds.). *Pharmacology and Physiology for Anesthesia: Foundations and Clinical Application*, 2nd edition. Elsevier, 2019: pp. 700–701.

Question 31: Answer

A. False. The primary hormone secreted by the thyroid is thyroxine (T4), along with a much lower amount of triiodothyronine (T3).

B. False. In spite of its lower plasma level, T3 has much greater biological activity than T4 and is believed to be the primary mediator of the physiological effects of thyroid secretion.

C. False. T3 is generated at its site of action in peripheral tissues by de-iodination of T4.

D. False. More than 40% of T3 is bound to TBG and most of the remainder to albumin, with very little binding to the protein called transthyretin.

E. True. T4 and T3 are de-iodinated in the liver, the kidneys, and many other tissues. These de-iodination reactions catabolize the hormones but also provide a local supply of T3.

Barrett, K.E., Barman, S.M., Boitano, S., and Reckelhoff, J.F. *Ganong's Medical Physiology Examination & Board Review*. McGraw-Hill Education, Lange, 2018: pp. 451–455.

Question 32: Answer

A. False. The kidneys receive about 20% of the cardiac output.

B. True. Despite receiving 20% of the total cardiac output, kidneys extract relatively little oxygen. The renal arteriovenous oxygen difference is only 1.5 ml/dl.

C. True. The kidney cortex receives 85–90% of the renal blood flow (RBF).

D. False. The medulla receives only 6% of the RBF and has an average oxygen tension (PO_2) of just 8 mmHg. Thus, severe hypoxia could develop in the medulla despite a relatively adequate total RBF; the metabolically active medullary thick ascending loop of Henle is particularly vulnerable.

E. True. In normal kidneys, 80% of the energy is required for Na^+/K^+-ATPase that maintains the osmotic gradient needed for the resorption of filtered molecules. Despite this high energy demand, the tubular system is supplied by only 10–15% of the RBF—a key reason for acute tubular necrosis after hypotension.

Pino, R.M. and Sonny, A. Renal anatomy, physiology, pharmacology, and evaluation of function. In: M. Gropper et al. (eds.). *Miller's Anesthesia*, 9th edition. Elsevier, 2020: pp. 445–447.

Question 33: Answer

A. True. When the sphincter of Oddi is blocked, substances that are normally eliminated in the bile including conjugated bile acids, cholesterol, and phosphatidylcholine will reflux into the systemic circulation where they accumulate; thus, the plasma levels of these substances will increase.

B. True. See the explanation above.

C. True. See the explanation above.

D. True. The location of the gallstone will also prevent the release of pancreatic secretions and the level of amylase and other pancreatic products will rise in the circulation.

E. False. Since bile cannot reach the small intestine, conjugated bile acids cannot be deconjugated by intestinal bacteria and the level of unconjugated bile acids in the circulation should fall.

Barrett, K.E., Barman, S.M., Boitano, S., and Reckelhoff, J.F. *Ganong's Medical Physiology Examination & Board Review.* McGraw-Hill Education, Lange, 2018: p. 646.

Question 34: Answer

A. False. With the loss of the glucose buffer function, as well as the capacity to synthesize plasma proteins, hypoglycaemia and a fall in fibrinogen would be expected with an acute reduction in liver function.

B. False. See the explanation above.

C. False. 25-hydroxycholecalciferol is produced in the liver from cholecalciferol produced in the skin.

D. False. As bilirubin is conjugated in hepatocytes this reaction will not occur in the anhepatic phase and the level of conjugated bilirubin will not increase.

E. True. As the liver is responsible for metabolizing steroid hormones, oestrogen levels will rise.

Barrett, K.E., Barman, S.M., Boitano, S., and Reckelhoff, J.F. *Ganong's Medical Physiology Examination & Board Review.* McGraw-Hill Education, Lange, 2018: p. 644.

Question 35: Answer

A. False. Hyponatraemia is defined as a level of Na^+ less than 135 mEq/l; plasma Na^+ less than 120 mEq/l is considered severe hyponatraemia.

B. False. Hyponatraemia may occur with a normal or high serum osmolality, this may result from the presence of a non-sodium solute, such as glucose or mannitol, which holds water within the extracellular space and results in dilutional hyponatraemia.

C. True. Euvolaemic hyponatraemia is usually associated with exogenous ADH administration, pharmacologic potentiation of ADH action, drugs that mimic the action of ADH in the renal tubules, or excessive ectopic ADH secretion.

D. False. The underlying mechanism of hypovolaemic hyponatraemia is secretion of ADH in response to volume contraction with ongoing oral or intravenous intake of hypotonic fluid. Angiotensin II also decreases renal free water clearance. Thiazide diuretics, unlike loop diuretics, promote hypovolaemic hyponatraemia by interfering with urinary dilution in the distal tubule of the nephron.

E. True. Although patients retain sodium perioperatively, they retain proportionately more electrolyte-free water. Careful postoperative attention to fluid and electrolyte balance can minimize the occurrence of symptomatic hyponatraemia.

Svensen, C. Electrolytes and diuretics. In: H.C. Hemmings and Jr., T.D. Egan (eds.). *Pharmacology and Physiology for Anesthesia: Foundations and Clinical Application,* 2nd edition. Elsevier, 2019: pp. 814–818.

Question 36: Answer

A. False. In hyperventilation there is a fall in plasma ionized calcium but a slight increase in total plasma calcium. Hyperventilation increases pH, plasma proteins are more ionized when pH is high, thus providing more protein anions to bind with Ca^{2+}.

B. False. Calcitonin is a hormone secreted primarily by the thyroid gland that lowers the calcium level in plasma.

C. True. 1,25-dihydroxycholecalciferol is a steroid hormone formed from vitamin D in the liver and kidneys. Its primary action is to increase calcium absorption from the intestine increasing plasma ionized calcium level.

D. False. The main action of parathyroid hormone is to mobilize calcium from bone. After parathyroidectomy, there is a steady decline in plasma calcium levels.

E. False. A decrease in extracellular Ca^{2+} exerts a net excitatory effect on nerve and muscle cells. The result is hypocalcaemic tetany characterized by extensive spasms of skeletal muscle, involving especially muscles of the extremities and the larynx.

Barrett, K.E., Barman, S.M., Boitano, S., and Reckelhoff, J.F. *Ganong's Medical Physiology Examination & Board Review*. McGraw-Hill Education, Lange, 2018: pp. 491–492.

Question 37: Answer

A. False. Ketone bodies are normal by-products of fat metabolism. They are produced when fatty acids are metabolized by the liver when glucose is unavailable as an energy source.

B. False. There are three ketone bodies: acetoacetate, β-hydroxybutyrate, and acetone, however, acetone is not the main form. The quantitative distribution of ketone body formation is the following: acetone (<2%), acetoacetate (20%), and β-hydroxybutyrate (βOHB) (78%).

C. True. In situations where fat becomes the primary source of energy, for example in starvation or low-carbohydrate diets, an increase in circulating ketone bodies occurs that can be measured in blood and in urine.

D. True. In many tissues acetyl coenzyme A units condense to form acetoacetyl coenzyme A. Free acetoacetate is formed in the liver through the action of deacylase. This β-keto acid is converted to β-hydroxybutyrate and acetone.

E. False. Urinary ketone sticks measure only acetoacetate. The absence of ketones in the urine does not eliminate the diagnosis of ketoacidosis particularly if it is not associated with diabetes.

Barrett, K.E., Barman, S.M., Boitano, S., and Reckelhoff, J.F. *Ganong's Medical Physiology Examination & Board Review*. McGraw-Hill Education, Lange, 2018: pp. 42, 44.

Neligan, P.J. Perioperative acid-base balance. In: M. Gropper et al. (eds.). *Miller's Anesthesia*, 9th edition. Elsevier, 2020: pp. 1540–1541.

Question 38: Answer

A. True. Tonicity is used to describe the effective osmotic pressure of a solution relative to that of plasma; it is the osmotic pressure gradient between two solutions. This is the effective osmolality of a solution with respect to a particular semipermeable membrane and takes into account solutes that do not exert an *in vivo* osmotic effect.

B. True. Tonicity expresses the osmolal activity of solutes restricted to the extracellular compartment; that is, those which exert an osmotic force affecting the distribution of water between intracellular fluid (ICF) and extracellular fluid (ECF).

C. False. The critical difference between osmolality and tonicity is that all solutes contribute to osmolality, but only solutes that do not cross the cell membrane contribute to tonicity.

D. True. As urea diffuses freely across cell membranes, it does not alter the distribution of water between these two body fluid compartments and does not contribute to tonicity.

E. False. Ethanol and methanol, both of which distribute rapidly throughout the total body water contribute to plasma osmolality but not tonicity. In contrast, mannitol and sorbitol are restricted to the ECF and contribute to both osmolality and tonicity.

Edwards, M.R. and Grocott, M.P.W. Perioperative fluid and electrolyte therapy. In: M. Gropper et al. (eds.). *Miller's Anesthesia*, 9th edition. Elsevier, 2020: p. 1482.

Williams, G. Fluid, electrolyte and acid-base balance. In: J. Thompson, I. Moppett, and M. Wiles (eds.). *Smith and Aitkenhead's Textbook of Anaesthesia*, 7th edition. Elsevier, 2019: p. 217.

Question 39: Answer

A. True. The SID is one of the biochemical parameters that contribute to the Stewart theory of physiological acid-base balance. It is quantitatively the total concentration of fully dissociated cations minus the total concentration of fully dissociated anions: SID = ($[Na^+]$ + $[K^+]$ + $[Mg^{2+}]$ + $[Ca^{2+}]$)— ($[Cl^-]$ + [lactate]).

B. True. Total weak acid concentration (A_{TOT}) = 2.43 × [total protein], this includes associated and dissociated ions (predominantly albumin). Within this theory, it is not just the function of the lungs (CO_2) and the kidneys (SID) being modelled but also the organs determining A_{TOT}, namely the gastrointestinal tract and liver.

C. True. The Stewart equation emphasizes the importance of the chloride ion $[Cl^-]$ as a key determinant of SID and therefore pH. An increasing $[Cl^-]$ in relation to $[Na^+]$ will decrease SID (with a normal strong ion gap (SIG)) and thereby decrease pH.

D. True. The SID equates to about 40 mmol/l (i.e., a net positive charge). This is the apparent SID (SID_a). However, the plasma cannot be charged, and SID_a is offset by the effective SID (SID_e), which is generated by poorly dissociated weak acids (albumin, phosphate, and sulphate). The difference between SID_a and SID_e is the SIG, which is analogous but superior to the anion gap as it also takes into account total weak acid, in particular albumin.

E. False. Stewart's theory rejects HCO_3^- as an independent variable and therefore a determinant of pH, as in the classical model, being altered by both changes in $PaCO_2$ and SID.

Williams, G. Fluid, electrolyte and acid-base balance. In: J. Thompson, I. Moppett, and M. Wiles (eds.). *Smith and Aitkenhead's Textbook of Anaesthesia*, 7th edition. Elsevier, 2019: p. 233–234.

Question 40: Answer

A. False. BMR is determined at complete mental and physical rest in a room at a comfortable temperature in the thermoneutral zone 12–14 h after the last meal. It falls about 10% during sleep.

B. False. The BMR of an adult human subject of average size is about 2000 kcal/day (8368 kJ).

C. False. The BMR falls up to 40% during prolonged starvation.

D. True. A child younger than 5 years of age may have twice the BMR of a man or woman over 70 years old.

E. True. The BMR rises about 14% for each degree Celsius elevation of body temperature.

Andrzejowski, J. and Riley, C. Metabolism, the stress response to surgery and perioperative thermoregulation. In: J. Thompson, I. Moppett, and M. Wiles (eds.). *Smith and Aitkenhead's Textbook of Anaesthesia*. 7th edition. Elsevier, 2019: p. 234, 239.

Barrett, K.E., Barman, S.M., Boitano, S., and Reckelhoff, J.F. *Ganong's Medical Physiology Examination & Board Review*. McGraw-Hill Education, Lange, 2018: p. 608.

Question 41: Answer

A. True. Cold-specific receptors are innervated by Aδ fibres, heat receptors are innervated by C fibres.

B. True. Cold receptors in the skin outnumber heat receptors tenfold and are the major mechanism by which the body protects itself against cold temperatures.

C. True. Blockade of this afferent input by regional anaesthesia explains why the lower limbs are often perceived by the patient as feeling warm when the regional block is established.

D. False. Central thermoreceptors are mainly located in the hypothalamus.

E. True. The reflex responses activated by warmth are controlled primarily from the anterior hypothalamus; stimulation causes cutaneous vasodilation and sweating. Lesions in this region cause hyperthermia.

Andrzejowski, J. and Riley, C. Metabolism, the stress response to surgery and perioperative thermoregulation. In: J. Thompson, I. Moppett, and M. Wiles (eds.). *Smith and Aitkenhead's Textbook of Anaesthesia*. 7th edition. Elsevier, 2019: p. 245.

Barrett, K.E., Barman, S.M., Boitano, S., and Reckelhoff, J.F. *Ganong's Medical Physiology Examination & Board Review*. McGraw-Hill Education, Lange, 2018: p. 424.

Question 42: Answer

A. True. The thrombin-thrombomodulin complex activates protein C, which proteolyses activated factors V and VIII. Activated factor V increases the rate of conversion of prothrombin to thrombin, and activated factor VIII is a cofactor in the generation of activated factor X.

B. True. Antithrombin is a circulating serine protease inhibitor found in high concentrations in plasma. It inhibits the action of activated factors IX, X, XI, XII, and thrombin.

C. False. Antithrombin also inhibits activated factor VII from the extrinsic (tissue factor) pathway.

D. True. Heparin binds to antithrombin to increase the inactivation of thrombin by a factor of more than 2000.

E. True. Naturally occurring fibrinolysis involves the conversion of plasminogen to plasmin, which in turn degrades fibrin. Plasminogen can be activated by a naturally occurring tissue plasminogen activator and urokinase.

Wake, P. Blood, coagulation and transfusion. In: J. Thompson, I. Moppett, and M. Wiles (eds.). *Smith and Aitkenhead's Textbook of Anaesthesia*. 7th edition. Elsevier, 2019: pp. 251–252.

Question 43: Answer

A. True. Fibrinolysis decreases as a result of decreased activity of tissue plasminogen activator because of inhibitors produced by the placenta.

B. False. Bleeding time remains within normal limits during pregnancy.

C. False. The level of clotting factor XIII is decreased by 40–50% in late pregnancy.

D. True. There is a 10-fold increase in factor VII level.

E. True. The increase in clotting activity is greatest at the time of delivery with placental expulsion releasing thromboplastic substances, which stimulate clot formation to stop maternal blood loss.

Pillai, A. Obstetric anaesthesia and analgesia. In: J. Thompson, I. Moppett, and M. Wiles (eds.). *Smith and Aitkenhead's Textbook of Anaesthesia*. 7th edition. Elsevier, 2019: p. 805.

Question 44: Answer

A. True. The airway resistance decreases because of the dilation of larger airways.

B. False. The respiratory alkalosis is accompanied by a decrease in plasma bicarbonate concentration resulting from renal excretion and arterial pH does not change significantly.

C. False. The oxyhaemoglobin dissociation curve is shifted to the right because the increase in red cell 2,3-diphosphoglycerate concentration outweighs the effects of a low PCO_2, which would normally shift the curve to the left.

D. False. The larger minute ventilation is attained primarily as a result of a larger tidal volume and a slight increase in respiratory frequency.

E. True. The expanding uterus forces the diaphragm cephalad and creates a 20% decrease in FRC by term. However, closing capacity (CC) remains unchanged and creates a reduced FRC/CC ratio resulting in more rapid small airway closure with reduced lung volumes, and in the supine position FRC can be less than CC for many small airways giving rise to atelectasis.

Pillai, A. Obstetric anaesthesia and analgesia. In: J. Thompson, I. Moppett, and M. Wiles (eds.). *Smith and Aitkenhead's Textbook of Anaesthesia*. 7th edition. Elsevier, 2019: pp. 802–803.

Sharpe, E.E. and Arendt, K.W. Anesthesia for obstetrics. In: M. Gropper et al. (eds.). *Miller's Anesthesia*, 9th edition. Elsevier, 2020: p. 2009.

Question 45: Answer

A. False. Mast cells are heavily granulated connective tissue cells that are abundant beneath epithelial surfaces. Their granules contain proteoglycans, histamine, and many proteases.

B. True. Monocytes enter the blood from the bone marrow and circulate for about 72 h. They then enter the tissues and become tissue macrophages, which persist in tissues for about 3 months.

C. True. Tissue macrophages include Kupffer cells of the liver, which line the liver sinusoids forming an effective particulate filtration system so that almost none of the bacteria from the gastrointestinal tract pass from the portal blood into the general systemic circulation.

D. False. T lymphocytes are responsible for forming the activated lymphocytes that provide cell-mediated immunity. B lymphocytes are responsible for forming antibodies that provide humoral immunity.

E. True. See the explanation above.

Barrett, K.E., Barman, S.M., Boitano, S., and Reckelhoff, J.F. *Ganong's Medical Physiology Examination & Board Review*. McGraw-Hill Education, Lange, 2018: p. 107.

Hall, J.E. and Hall, M.E. *Guyton and Hall Textbook of Medical Physiology*, 14th edition. Elsevier, 2021: p. 460.

1. **Responses to an infusion of glyceryl trinitrate (GTN) include**
   A. an increase in the P-R interval
   B. a decrease in the height of the QRS complex
   C. tachycardia
   D. headache
   E. increased splanchnic blood flow

2. **Tachycardia is associated with**
   A. venlafaxine
   B. phenylephrine
   C. salmeterol
   D. levothyroxine
   E. amiodarone

3. **Pharmacological treatment of acute, life-threatening supraventricular tachycardia includes**
   A. atropine
   B. lidocaine
   C. adenosine
   D. sotalol
   E. an infusion of magnesium sulfate

4. **Contractility of the left ventricle**
   A. is reduced during sevoflurane anaesthesia
   B. is increased by atropine
   C. is unaffected by ketamine
   D. is reduced by sildenafil
   E. is increased by beta-1 adrenergic blockade

5. **Blood flow to cardiac muscle**
   A. is increased by vecuronium
   B. is increased by milrinone
   C. is increased by prostacyclin
   D. is unaffected by heparin infusion
   E. is increased by cocaine

6. **Nicorandil**
    A. is a myocardial potassium channel inhibitor
    B. has a low bioavailability of less than 15%
    C. causes venodilatation to reduce preload
    D. prolongs the QTc (corrected QT) interval
    E. has no effect on atrioventricular conduction

7. **Calcium channel blockade by**
    A. diltiazem affects both myocardial and vascular channels
    B. nifedipine has a greater effect on blood pressure than on contractility
    C. verapamil increases atrioventricular conduction time
    D. nifedipine makes it more effective anti-anginal therapy than verapamil
    E. nimodipine is more effective than nifedipine in the central nervous system due to higher lipid solubility

8. **The beta-adrenergic antagonist**
    A. atenolol is cardioselective
    B. esmolol is metabolized by plasma cholinesterase
    C. propranolol prevents the peripheral conversion of thyroxine T4 to T3
    D. metoprolol has no intrinsic sympathomimetic activity
    E. sotalol has Vaughan-Williams class III anti-arrhythmic activity

9. **Dobutamine**
    A. is an indirect-acting beta-1 adrenergic agonist
    B. increases cardiac contractility
    C. reduces systemic vascular resistance
    D. increases myocardial oxygen demand
    E. is excreted unchanged in the urine

10. **Propofol**
    A. reduces the cerebral metabolic rate for oxygen ($CMRO_2$)
    B. reduces the rate of cerebrospinal fluid production
    C. has no effect on cerebral autoregulation
    D. is a $GABA_A$ receptor antagonist
    E. decreases intraocular pressure

11. **Sevoflurane**
    A. increases the duration of the QRS complex in the electrocardiogram (ECG)
    B. increases the dead space to tidal volume ratio (V_D/V_T)
    C. reduces the rate of gastric emptying
    D. increases splanchnic blood flow
    E. reduces jugular venous oxygen partial pressure ($SjvO_2$)

12. Ketamine

A. has analgesic activity
B. has an active metabolite
C. increases blood pressure by direct action on alpha adrenoceptors
D. is an antiemetic
E. acts at histamine H_1 receptors

13. Isoflurane

A. is more water-soluble than sevoflurane
B. is more lipid-soluble than sevoflurane
C. undergoes 2% metabolism by CYP450 enzymes
D. sensitizes the myocardium to catecholamines
E. increases cerebral blood flow above one MAC (minimum alveolar concentration)

14. Propofol

A. is more lipid-soluble than fentanyl
B. has a pKa of 7.4
C. is more water-soluble than remifentanil
D. is more plasma protein-bound than rocuronium
E. has a lower molecular weight than morphine

15. The benzodiazepine

A. midazolam is an anticonvulsant
B. temazepam is an inhibitor of the $GABA_A$ receptor
C. diazepam induces hepatic CYP450 enzymes
D. lorazepam has active metabolites
E. flumazenil has inverse agonist properties

16. Gabapentin

A. inhibits presynaptic voltage-gated calcium channels in the central nervous system
B. undergoes more than 60% hepatic metabolism
C. is a first-line drug for the treatment of generalized seizures
D. is used to treat neuropathic pain in doses more than three times higher than used for seizure control
E. is associated with ataxia at high dose

17. Remifentanil

A. has a steady-state volume of distribution that is smaller than the extracellular fluid volume
B. is metabolized by muscle and plasma esterases
C. has a context-sensitive half-time that doubles if the duration of infusion increases from two to four hours
D. clearance is reduced in renal failure
E. is an inducer of CYP2D6 in the liver

18. Morphine

A. is a more potent analgesic than fentanyl

B. is an agonist at histamine type 1 receptors

C. increases colonic motility

D. increases myocardial contractility

E. tolerance limits its use in chronic pain

19. Sufentanil

A. has a shorter duration of analgesic action than fentanyl

B. is conjugated by hepatic enzymes prior to elimination

C. is more potent than fentanyl

D. is contraindicated in patients with porphyria

E. has two isomers, only one of which has analgesic activity

20. Rocuronium

A. is a benzylisoquinolinium

B. is excreted unchanged in bile

C. has a volume of distribution similar to cis-atracurium

D. crosses the placenta

E. is more potent than vecuronium

21. Neostigmine

A. is a direct-acting antagonist at neuromuscular nicotinic acetylcholine receptors

B. induces bradycardia

C. prolongs the QT interval

D. inhibits plasma cholinesterase

E. reduces intraocular pressure

22. Vecuronium

A. increases intracellular calcium in cardiac myocytes

B. blocks the afferent limb of the monosynaptic knee-jerk reflex

C. is a muscarinic cholinergic receptor antagonist

D. has a direct antagonist action at the ryanodine receptor

E. acts synergistically with magnesium to reduce striated muscle tone

23. Sugammadex

A. selectively binds aminosteroid neuromuscular blocking agents

B. has a volume of distribution greater than total body water

C. is effective in reversing neuromuscular blockade only when both the first and second twitch can be recorded using a train-of-four monitor

D. is excreted unchanged in the urine

E. reduces the effectiveness of progesterone-containing oral contraceptive medication

24. **Non-steroidal anti-inflammatory drugs**
    A. increase leukotriene production in the lung
    B. produce analgesia by a central action on receptors in the peri-aqueductal grey matter
    C. reduce glomerular filtration rate
    D. reduce daily morphine requirements postoperatively
    E. increase gastric acid production

25. **The following are correctly paired drug and receptor type**
    A. glycopyrrolate and muscarinic cholinergic receptors
    B. morphine and Gs type G-protein-coupled receptors (GPCRs)
    C. insulin and a tyrosine kinase-linked receptor
    D. dobutamine and Gi type GPCRs
    E. cis-atracurium and nicotinic cholinergic receptors

26. **In a three-compartment model**
    A. the steady-state volume of distribution (Vss) is greater than the central compartment volume
    B. at steady state the rate of elimination is equal to the infusion rate multiplied by the administered drug concentration
    C. the volume of the central compartment is equal to plasma volume
    D. the rate constant of elimination is equal to the rate constant for transfer from compartment 3 to the central compartment
    E. the effect compartment volume is assumed to be zero

27. **The drug interaction between**
    A. remifentanil and propofol is synergistic
    B. morphine and methadone is antagonistic
    C. rocuronium and vecuronium is additive
    D. heparin and warfarin is synergistic
    E. ondansetron and omeprazole is additive

28. **Regarding local anaesthetics**
    A. potency is inversely correlated with lipid solubility
    B. duration of action is dependent on pKa
    C. depth of block increases with increased nerve action potential frequency
    D. they act from the inside of the membrane to block voltage-gated sodium channels
    E. the rate of onset of action is positively correlated with pKa

29. **Ropivacaine**
    A. is an ester-type local anaesthetic
    B. is presented as a single enantiomer
    C. is less lipid soluble than bupivacaine
    D. is more potent than lidocaine
    E. produces a greater motor block than bupivacaine

30. Ondansetron

A. acts at the same gastric receptors as omeprazole
B. does not cross the blood-brain barrier
C. reduces gastric hydrogen ion concentration
D. is associated with bradycardia on rapid intravenous administration
E. is less potent than granisetron

31. The anticoagulant

A. heparin is associated with thrombocytopenia
B. warfarin enhances the activity of vitamin K
C. apixaban is a direct-acting inhibitor of factor Xa
D. dabigatran is a direct-acting antithrombin III inhibitor
E. enoxaparin is a direct-acting thrombin inhibitor

32. The antiplatelet agent

A. aspirin irreversibly inhibits adenylyl cyclase
B. clopidogrel is less effective in the presence of omeprazole
C. abciximab has a high affinity for the glycoprotein IIb/IIIa receptor
D. ticagrelor is an agonist at the $P2Y_{12}$ receptor
E. prasugrel inhibits an adenosine diphosphate (ADP) receptor

33. The intravenous fluid

A. Hartmann's solution (Ringer lactate) has a sodium concentration of 131 mmol/l
B. 0.18% sodium chloride/4% glucose has a chloride concentration of 55 mmol/l
C. 5% glucose has a calorie content of 200 kcal/l (837 kJ)
D. Hartmann's solution (Ringer lactate) has a calcium concentration of 1.8 mmol/l
E. 0.9% sodium chloride has a pH of 7.4

34. The antimicrobial drug

A. gentamicin inhibits bacterial cell wall synthesis
B. teicoplanin inhibits viral protein synthesis
C. ciprofloxacin inhibits bacterial DNA synthesis
D. clindamycin inhibits bacterial protein synthesis
E. acyclovir inhibits viral thymidine kinase

35. Penicillin

A. is a beta-lactam
B. is mainly excreted unchanged by the kidneys
C. has a plasma half-life of more than eight hours
D. is bacteriostatic
E. is effective against Gram-negative bacteria

36. **Tricyclic antidepressant toxicity is associated with**
    A. seizures
    B. sinus bradycardia
    C. prolonged QT interval
    D. mydriasis
    E. hypothermia

37. **Furosemide**
    A. increases free water clearance
    B. increases sodium clearance
    C. decreases potassium clearance
    D. increases chloride clearance
    E. increases phosphate clearance

38. **Thiazide diuretics**
    A. are less potent than furosemide
    B. inhibit sodium-hydrogen exchange in the distal convoluted tubule
    C. increase potassium clearance in the kidney
    D. are uricosuric
    E. may cause hyperglycaemia

39. **In patients with diabetes mellitus**
    A. metformin increases peripheral sensitivity to insulin
    B. gliclazide increases glucagon secretion
    C. glibenclamide is ineffective in insulin-dependent patients
    D. repaglinide increases insulin receptor sensitivity
    E. insulin exerts its effects by activation of Gs type GPCRs

40. **Nitric oxide**
    A. increases vascular tone in the pulmonary arteries
    B. when inhaled, has no effect on the systemic circulation
    C. has a lower affinity for haemoglobin than carbon monoxide
    D. reduces V/Q mismatch when used therapeutically in acute respiratory distress syndrome
    E. is a bronchodilator

41. **Anatomical respiratory dead space**
    A. is increased by atropine
    B. is reduced by salbutamol
    C. is unaffected by histamine
    D. is increased by atenolol
    E. is reduced by prostacyclin

42. In the treatment of asthma

A. prolonged use of salbutamol causes tachyphylaxis
B. montelukast is effective in acute asthma attacks
C. ipratropium bromide is primarily a rescue medication
D. salmeterol inhibits mast cell degranulation
E. inhaled beclometasone is a first-line controller medication

43. Bronchoconstriction occurs with

A. sevoflurane
B. isoflurane
C. nicorandil
D. ephedrine
E. phentolamine

44. Unwanted effects of long-acting beta-2 sympathomimetics include

A. anxiety
B. headache
C. hypokalaemia
D. tremors
E. bradycardia

45. Prednisolone

A. increases lipogenesis
B. reduces inflammation
C. inhibits protein catabolism
D. increases insulin sensitivity in adipocytes
E. in high dose, is associated with osteoporosis

Question 1: Answer

A. False. The P-R interval reflects the time for electrical activity to propagate from the atrium to the ventricle. This is dependent on several factors including heart rate. GTN reduces both pre-load and after-load, which can cause a slight fall in blood pressure and a small reflex increase in heart rate. If anything, this would decrease the P-R interval although there is no significant change in a normal individual.

B. False. The height of the QRS complex depends on the anatomical axis of the heart, which is unchanged by GTN.

C. True. As explained in A, there is a small increase in heart rate even in the normal individual.

D. True. GTN causes vasodilatation and this is frequently associated with headache.

E. True. Nitric oxide is an important regulator of splanchnic blood flow; GTN acts through the nitric oxide system to produce vasodilatation and an increase in splanchnic blood flow.

Peck, T.E. and Hill, S.A. *Pharmacology for Anaesthesia and Intensive Care*, 4th edition. Cambridge University Press, 2014: Chapter 16, Vasodilators: p. 238.

Question 2: Answer

A. True. Venlafaxine is a serotonin re-uptake inhibitor (SSRI) antidepressant. All such drugs commonly cause tachycardia as a side effect.

B. False. Phenylephrine is an alpha-adrenergic agonist and causes reflex bradycardia.

C. True. Salmeterol is a beta-2 adrenergic agonist used in the treatment of asthma. This group of drugs commonly cause tachycardia.

D. True. Thyroxine is commonly associated with tachycardia, especially in overdose.

E. False. The anti-arrhythmic drug amiodarone is used to treat tachyarrhythmias and acts to slow heart rate by several mechanisms.

Peck, T.E. and Hill, S.A. *Pharmacology for Anaesthesia and Intensive Care*, 4th edition. Cambridge University Press, 2014: Chapter 18, Central nervous system: p. 262; Chapter 13, Sympathomimetics: p. 197, 200; Chapter 26, Corticosteroids and other hormone preparations: p. 339; Chapter 15, Anti-arrhythmics: p. 229.

Question 3: Answer

A. False. Atropine is used to treat bradycardia.

B. False. Lidocaine has been used to treat wide-complex tachycardia.

C. True. Adenosine is the first-line pharmacological treatment for paroxysmal supraventricular tachycardia (SVT).

D. True. Beta-blockers, in particular sotalol, are recommended to control heart rate in rapid atrial fibrillation (irregular SVT).

E. True. Magnesium is used in the treatment of tachyarrhythmias associated with hypomagnesaemia.

European Resuscitation Council 2015 guidelines, adult advanced life support. 2015. Available at: https://cprguidelines.eu

European Society of Cardiology 2019 guidelines on the management of SVT. 2019. Available at: https://www.escardio.org/Guidelines/Clinical-Practice-Guidelines/Supraventricular-Tachycardia

Question 4: Answer

A. True. All halogenated volatile anaesthetic agents reduce myocardial contractility, but to varying effects. The effect of sevoflurane is small, but present.

B. False. Atropine significantly increases the heart rate, reduces ventricular filling, and therefore reduces ventricular tension and contractility (Starling mechanism).

C. False. Ketamine increases adrenergic action on the ventricle and increases contractility.

D. False. Sildenafil is used to treat pulmonary hypertension, it has no direct effect on myocardial contractility but may induce a small, reflex, sympathetic-mediated increase in contractility.

E. False. Beta-1 adrenergic blockers have a negative inotropic effect.

Peck, T.E. and Hill, S.A. *Pharmacology for Anaesthesia and Intensive Care*, 4th edition. Cambridge University Press, 2014: Chapter 9, General anaesthetic agents: p. 118, Table 9.8; p. 104; Chapter 14, Adrenoceptor antagonists: p. 211.

Question 5: Answer

A. False. Non-steroidal muscle relaxants have no effect on the cardiovascular system.

B. True. Milrinone causes coronary vasodilatation and increases cardiac blood flow.

C. True. Prostacyclin is a coronary vasodilator as well as causing pulmonary vasodilatation.

D. True. Heparin is an anticoagulant that prevents intravascular clot formation. In the normal individual, with a slow infusion, it has no direct effect on myocardial blood flow.

E. False. Cocaine inhibits noradrenaline re-uptake and causes coronary artery constriction, so reducing myocardial blood flow.

Peck, T.E. and Hill, S.A. *Pharmacology for Anaesthesia and Intensive Care*, 4th edition. Cambridge University Press, 2014: Chapter 12, Muscle relaxants and reversal agents: p. 177; Chapter 13, Sympathomimetics: p. 205; Chapter 24, Drugs affecting coagulation: p. 321, 323; Chapter 11, Local anaesthetics: p. 164.

Question 6: Answer

A. False. Nicorandil is an ATP-sensitive potassium channel activator.

B. False. Nicorandil is used orally, and bioavailability is high, around 75%.

C. True. Vasodilatation with nicorandil reduces both pre-load and after-load.

D. False. Nicorandil has no effect on heart rate, the QT or QTc interval.

E. True. Nicorandil has little effect on the ECG in a normal person or one with angina, the PR interval is unchanged.

Peck, T.E. and Hill, S.A. *Pharmacology for Anaesthesia and Intensive Care*, 4th edition. Cambridge University Press, 2014: Chapter 16, Vasodilators: pp. 239–240.

Question 7: Answer

A. True. Verapamil affects myocardial more than vascular channels, dihydropyridines affect vascular more than myocardial channels and diltiazem is intermediate between these two groups.

B. True. Dihydropyridines are better arteriodilators than myocardial depressants and are used primarily to treat hypertension.

C. True. A-V conduction time is increased with verapamil, making it useful in the treatment of supraventricular tachycardia (SVT).

D. True. Dihydropyridines are potent arterial vasodilators, more than verapamil or diltiazem.

E. True. Nimodipine is more lipid-soluble than nifedipine and is used in the management of cerebral vasospasm following an aneurysmal bleed.

Peck, T.E. and Hill, S.A. *Pharmacology for Anaesthesia and Intensive Care*, 4th edition. Cambridge University Press, 2014: Chapter 16, Vasodilators: pp. 240–243.

Question 8: Answer

A. True. Atenolol, metoprolol, and esmolol all show moderate cardioselectivity.

B. False. Esmolol is metabolized by red cell esterases.

C. True. Peripheral T4 to T3 conversion is inhibited by propranolol but not other beta-adrenergic antagonists.

D. True. Intrinsic activity indicates inverse agonist activity, seen with pindolol but not metoprolol.

E. True. Sotalol prolongs the duration of the action potential by blockade of potassium channels.

Peck, T.E. and Hill, S.A. *Pharmacology for Anaesthesia and Intensive Care*, 4th edition. Cambridge University Press, 2014: Chapter 14, Adrenoceptor antagonists: Table 14.2, p. 211; pp. 214–216.

Question 9: Answer

A. False. Dobutamine is a direct-acting sympathomimetic that is selective for beta-1 adrenergic receptors.

B. True. The increased contractility seen with dobutamine improves systolic blood pressure.

C. True. Dobutamine does have some beta-2 adrenergic activity, which can cause a reduction in systemic vascular resistance.

D. True. The increase in contractility due to dobutamine increases myocardial demand for oxygen.

E. False. Structurally dobutamine is a catecholamine that is metabolized rapidly by catechol O-methyl transferase (COMT) before being excreted renally.

Peck, T.E. and Hill, S.A. *Pharmacology for Anaesthesia and Intensive Care*, 4th edition. Cambridge University Press, 2014: Chapter 13, Sympathomimetics: p. 198.

Question 10: Answer

A. True. Propofol reduces cerebral blood flow (CBF) along with $CMRO_2$.

B. True. The fall in CBF seen with propofol is associated with reduced cerebrospinal fluid (CSF) production.

C. True. Cerebral autoregulation is preserved under propofol administration.

D. False. Propofol enhances gamma-aminobutyric acid (GABA)-induced chloride current by its allosteric activation at the $GABA_A$ receptor.

E. True. Propofol reduces intraocular pressure.

Miller, R.D. et al. *Anesthesia E-Book: Expert Consult*, 7th edition. Churchill Livingstone, 2009: Chapter 13, Cerebral physiology and the effects of anesthetic drugs: Key point 8.

Peck, T.E. and Hill, S.A. *Pharmacology for Anaesthesia and Intensive Care*, 4th edition. Cambridge University Press, 2014: Chapter 9, General anaesthetic agents: p. 95.

Question 11: Answer

Assume this is anaesthesia with sevoflurane alone in a normal person who is breathing spontaneously; otherwise, the question would have specified that the person was intubated and ventilated.

A. False. Sevoflurane has no effect on electrical conduction in the heart.

B. True. Sevoflurane decreases the tidal volume, and causes bronchodilatation thus increasing dead space, so the dead space to tidal volume ratio increases.

C. True. Smooth muscle activity is reduced under volatile anaesthesia and the rate of gastric emptying decreases.

D. False. Sevoflurane causes a reduction in systemic mean arterial blood pressure, but aortic pulse pressure increases, and splanchnic blood flow is preserved.

E. False. Up to one MAC of sevoflurane, CBF is maintained and coupled to $CMRO_2$, so $SjvO_2$ is unchanged or may increase as cerebral activity falls.

Miller, R.D. et al. *Anesthesia E-Book: Expert Consult*, 7th edition. Churchill Livingstone, 2009: Chapter 13, Cerebral physiology and the effects of anesthetic drugs: Key point 7.

Peck, T.E. and Hill, S.A. *Pharmacology for Anaesthesia and Intensive Care*, 4th edition. Cambridge University Press, 2014: Chapter 9, General anaesthetic agents: pp. 117–119.

Question 12: Answer

A. True. Ketamine has good analgesic properties.

B. True. Ketamine is demethylated in the liver to norketamine, which has around 30% activity of the parent compound.

C. False. The effect of ketamine on sympathetic activity is indirect, inhibiting noradrenaline re-uptake.

D. False. Ketamine does not have anti-emetic properties and can cause nausea and vomiting.

E. False. Ketamine acts as an inhibitor at N-methyl-D-aspartate (NMDA) receptors.

Peck, T.E. and Hill, S.A. *Pharmacology for Anaesthesia and Intensive Care*, 4th edition. Cambridge University Press, 2014: Chapter 9, General anaesthetic agents: p. 95; pp. 103–105.

Question 13: Answer

A. False. Isoflurane has a slower onset than sevoflurane, with a blood/gas partition coefficient of 1.4 compared with 0.65 for sevoflurane.

B. True. Isoflurane is more potent than sevoflurane, with an oil/gas partition coefficient of 98 compared with 80 for sevoflurane.

C. False. Only 0.2% of isoflurane is metabolized in the liver by CYP2E1.

D. False. Halothane and, to a lesser extent, enflurane—but not isoflurane—sensitize the myocardium to catecholamines.

E. True. Below one MAC there is little effect on CBF, but above this CBF increases as cerebral vasodilatation increases and autoregulation is lost.

Miller, R.D. et al. *Anesthesia E-Book: Expert Consult*, 7th edition. Churchill Livingstone, 2009: Chapter 13, Cerebral physiology and the effects of anesthetic drugs: Key point 7.

Peck, T.E. and Hill, S.A. *Pharmacology for Anaesthesia and Intensive Care*, 4th edition. Cambridge University Press, 2014: Chapter 9, General anaesthetic agents: p. 115, Table 9.6; p. 110, Table 9.5; p. 118, Table 9.8.

Question 14: Answer

A. True. Propofol is more lipid-soluble than fentanyl.

B. False. Propofol has a pKa of 11.

C. False. Remifentanil is more water-soluble than propofol.

D. True. Less than 50% of rocuronium is plasma protein-bound whereas propofol is more than 95% plasma protein-bound.

E. True. Propofol has a much simpler structure than morphine with a lower molecular weight.

Peck, T.E. and Hill, S.A. *Pharmacology for Anaesthesia and Intensive Care*, 4th edition. Cambridge University Press, 2014: Chapter 9, General anaesthetic agents: pp. 101–102.

Question 15: Answer

A. True. Midazolam is a useful anticonvulsant in acute epilepsy.

B. False. Benzodiazepines are positive allosteric modulators at the $GABA_A$ receptor and increase the affinity of the receptor for GABA so increasing hyperpolarization by increasing the inward chloride current.

C. False. The benzodiazepines are not CYP450 enzyme inducers.

D. False. Unlike some benzodiazepines, lorazepam has no active metabolites.

E. True. Flumazenil is an antagonist at the benzodiazepine receptor site but also has inverse agonist activity.

Peck, T.E. and Hill, S.A. *Pharmacology for Anaesthesia and Intensive Care*, 4th edition. Cambridge University Press, 2014: Chapter 18, Central nervous system: pp. 257–269.

Question 16: Answer

A. True. Gabapentin binds to presynaptic voltage-gated calcium channels to block neurotransmitter release.

B. False. Gabapentin is water-soluble and is excreted unchanged by renal excretion.

C. False. Gabapentin is used as an adjunct for the treatment of partial seizures.

D. False. The dose range required for treatment of neuropathic pain or seizure control is similar.

E. True. Ataxia is frequently seen with high dose gabapentin.

Peck, T.E. and Hill, S.A. *Pharmacology for Anaesthesia and Intensive Care*, 4th edition. Cambridge University Press, 2014: Chapter 18, Central nervous system: p. 268.

Question 17: Answer

A. True. The steady-state volume of distribution (Vss) of remifentanil is 350 ml/kg—around 25 L for a 70 kg person. The extracellular fluid volume is around 42 L.

B. True. Several types of esterase can metabolize remifentanil.

C. False. The context-sensitive half-time of remifentanil increases only a little with an increased duration of infusion; it is effectively context-insensitive.

D. False. Remifentanil clearance does not rely on renal excretion.

E. False. Codeine is metabolized by CYP2D6, but remifentanil is not a hepatic inducer of CYP450 enzymes.

Peck, T.E. and Hill, S.A. *Pharmacology for Anaesthesia and Intensive Care*, 4th edition. Cambridge University Press, 2014: Chapter 7, Applied pharmacokinetic models: pp. 72–73; Chapter 10, Analgesics: pp. 136–137; Chapter 2, Absorption, distribution, metabolism and excretion: p. 19, Table 2.1; p. 21, Table 2.2.

Product information for Ultiva™ (n.d.). Available at: https://www.medicines.org.uk/emc/product/800/smpc

Question 18: Answer

A. False. Fentanyl is approximately 100 times more potent than morphine.

B. False. Morphine can cause histamine release but is not a histamine-receptor agonist.

C. False. Morphine reduces intestinal motility by its inhibitory action on the myenteric plexus.

D. False. Morphine does not have a direct negative inotropic action in the normal person. Morphine may cause a small decrease in pre-load that could cause a slight indirect reduction in contractility by the Starling mechanism.

E. True. In chronic pain, the perception of noxious stimuli is different compared with acute pain, morphine is of limited value in its treatment and tolerance occurs with prolonged use.

Peck, T.E. and Hill, S.A. *Pharmacology for Anaesthesia and Intensive Care*, 4th edition. Cambridge University Press, 2014: Chapter 10, Analgesics: pp. 128–131.

Question 19: Answer

A. True. Sufentanil has a high hepatic clearance and a shorter duration of action than fentanyl.

B. False. Sufentanil is metabolized by oxidative N- and O-dealkylation, not conjugated.

C. True. Sufentanil is more potent than fentanyl.

D. False. Sufentanil has no effect in porphyria.

E. False. There are multiple isomers of most opioid drugs, but there is little evidence of any relationship between different isomers of sufentanil and potency.

Barash, P.G. et al. *Clinical Anesthesia (E-Book)*, 6th edition. Lippincott Williams & Wilkins, 2011: Chapter 19, Opioids, Table 19-3.

The Drug Database for Acute Porphyria (n.d.). Available at: http://www.drugs-porphyria.org

Question 20: Answer

A. False. Rocuronium is an aminosteroid neuromuscular blocking agent.

B. True. Rocuronium is eliminated unchanged mainly through the liver.

C. True. All non-depolarizing muscle relaxants (NDMR) are permanently charged molecules and their volumes of distribution are similar and small, around 150–200 ml/kg, due to minimal lipid solubility.

D. False. Rocuronium is a permanently ionized drug that does not cross the placental membrane.

E. False. Vecuronium is more potent than rocuronium: the more potent the neuromuscular blocking agent, the slower the onset, so rocuronium has a faster onset than vecuronium.

Peck, T.E. and Hill, S.A. *Pharmacology for Anaesthesia and Intensive Care*, 4th edition. Cambridge University Press, 2014: Chapter 12, Muscle relaxants and reversal agents: p. 175 and pp. 178–179.

Question 21: Answer

A. False. Neostigmine reverses neuromuscular blockade by increasing acetylcholine concentration in the synaptic cleft by inhibiting acetylcholinesterase.

B. True. Acetylcholinesterase is inhibited by neostigmine throughout the body, at myocardial muscarinic receptors the increased concentration of acetylcholine causes bradycardia.

C. False. The QT interval reflects repolarization of the myocardium and is not affected directly by neostigmine, although the R-R' interval is increased.

D. True. Neostigmine inhibits both acetylcholinesterase and plasma cholinesterase so can prolong the neuromuscular block produced by succinylcholine.

E. False. In the eye, increased acetylcholine activity following neostigmine administration leads to pupillary constriction and a reduction in intraocular pressure.

Peck, T.E. and Hill, S.A. *Pharmacology for Anaesthesia and Intensive Care*, 4th edition. Cambridge University Press, 2014: Chapter 12, Muscle relaxants and reversal agents: pp. 183–184.

Question 22: Answer

A. False. Vecuronium has no effect on cardiac muscle cells.

B. False. The afferent limb is sensory, so unaffected by vecuronium.

C. False. Vecuronium is a nicotinic neuromuscular cholinergic receptor antagonist with no action on muscarinic receptors.

D. False. Ryanodine receptor antagonists such as dantrolene are muscle relaxants but vecuronium does not enter myocytes so cannot affect the intracellular ryanodine receptor.

E. True. Magnesium is a physiological antagonist of calcium and has an intracellular depressant effect on muscle contractility, so acts synergistically with neuromuscular blocking agents such as vecuronium and prolongs neuromuscular blockade.

Peck, T.E. and Hill, S.A. *Pharmacology for Anaesthesia and Intensive Care*, 4th edition. Cambridge University Press, 2014: Chapter 12, Muscle relaxants and reversal agents: pp. 175–177.

Question 23: Answer

A. True. Although specifically used to reverse the action of rocuronium, sugammadex also binds vecuronium. The benzylisoquinolinium neuromuscular blocking agents are not bound by sugammadex.

B. False. Sugammadex is a large molecule, does not cross cell membranes and remains largely in the vascular compartment with a volume of distribution around 10 L.

C. False. Sugammadex can reverse deep neuromuscular blockade following rocuronium administration.

D. True. Sugammadex is not metabolized and undergoes renal excretion.

E. True. Progesterone and rocuronium are both steroids and sugammadex can also bind progesterone.

Peck, T.E. and Hill, S.A. *Pharmacology for Anaesthesia and Intensive Care*, 4th edition. Cambridge University Press, 2014: Chapter 12, Muscle relaxants and reversal agents: pp. 185–186.

Question 24: Answer

A. True. Prostaglandins share the same precursors as leukotrienes. Inhibition of cyclo-oxygenase by non-steroidal anti-inflammatory drugs (NSAIDs) increases substrate availability for the leukotriene pathway and can increase production in the lung: the basis of aspirin-induced bronchospasm.

B. False. Opioids, not NSAIDs, act on receptors in the peri-aqueductal grey matter.

C. True. The action of NSAIDs in the kidney is to inhibit prostaglandin-induced vasodilatation, which reduces renal blood flow and hence glomerular filtration rate.

D. True. In the normal person, there is a significant morphine-sparing effect of NSAIDs postoperatively.

E. False. The gastric effects of NSAIDs are to reduce the cytoprotective effect of prostaglandins in gastric mucosa without a direct effect on hydrogen ion secretion.

Peck, T.E. and Hill, S.A. *Pharmacology for Anaesthesia and Intensive Care*, 4th edition. Cambridge University Press, 2014: Chapter 10, Analgesics: pp. 141–144.

Question 25: Answer

A. True. Glycopyrrolate is an antagonist at muscarinic receptors.

B. False. Opioids act as agonists at Gi type (inhibitory) GPCRs.

C. True. The insulin receptor is linked to tyrosine kinase.

D. False. Dobutamine acts at beta-1 receptors that are Gs (stimulatory) GPCRs.

E. True. Cis-atracurium is a non-depolarizing muscle relaxant so is a competitive inhibitor of acetylcholine at neuromuscular nicotinic receptors.

Peck, T.E. and Hill, S.A. *Pharmacology for Anaesthesia and Intensive Care*, 4th edition. Cambridge University Press, 2014: Chapter 19, Antiemetics and related drugs: pp. 275–276; p. 30; p. 223; p. 30; p. 175.

Question 26: Answer

A. True. The steady-state volume of distribution is the sum of all three compartment volumes: central and compartments 2 and 3.

B. True. At steady-state input equals output, the rate of input is the infusion rate multiplied by the concentration of drug in the infused solution.

C. False. The central compartment reflects the behaviour of the plasma concentration of a drug but the volume of the central compartment depends on both drug and patient factors.

D. False. The rate constant of elimination is the rate constant associated with elimination from the central compartment out of the system.

E. True. It may seem strange, but this is the assumption of a model including the effect site.

Peck, T.E. and Hill, S.A. *Pharmacology for Anaesthesia and Intensive Care*, 4th edition. Cambridge University Press, 2014: Chapter 6, Pharmacokinetic modelling: pp. 55–63.

Question 27: Answer

Principle: synergy occurs with drugs having similar activity but different mechanisms of action; additivity if two drugs share the same mechanism of action and effect; antagonism if the drugs have the same activity by a different mechanism and in combination counteract each other's effect.

A. True. Propofol and remifentanil is a well-known example of synergism: the isobologram is concave.

B. False. Morphine and methadone act in the same way and show additivity, not antagonism.

C. True. Rocuronium and vecuronium are both aminosteroid neuromuscular blocking agents acting in the same way so demonstrate additivity.

D. True. Heparin and warfarin act through different mechanisms synergistically.

E. False. Ondansetron and omeprazole have completely different effects and so cannot have additive activity.

Peck, T.E. and Hill, S.A. *Pharmacology for Anaesthesia and Intensive Care*, 4th edition. Cambridge University Press, 2014: Chapter 4, Drug interaction: pp. 42–44.

Question 28: Answer

To answer this question, compare lidocaine with bupivacaine: lidocaine has a lower pKa, lower lipid solubility, lower protein binding, faster onset, and shorter duration of action than bupivacaine.

A. False. Local anaesthetic drugs need to cross the nerve membrane to be active, so lipid solubility is directly correlated with potency.

B. False. Duration of action depends on the degree of protein binding rather than pKa.

C. True. This is use-dependency; access is more rapid the more frequently the channels open.

D. True. The ionized form of a local anaesthetic is active from within the cell.

E. False. The higher the pKa the slower the rate of onset as a higher proportion of the drug is in the ionized form, so there is a negative correlation between speed of onset and pKa.

Peck, T.E. and Hill, S.A. *Pharmacology for Anaesthesia and Intensive Care*, 4th edition. Cambridge University Press, 2014: Chapter 11, Local anaesthetics: pp. 154–157.

Question 29: Answer

A. False. Ropivacaine is an amide local anaesthetic.

B. True. Ropivacaine is presented as the S-enantiomer.

C. True. Ropivacaine is less toxic compared with bupivacaine for this reason.

D. True. Ropivacaine is around four times more potent than lidocaine.

E. False. The motor block is said to be less dense with ropivacaine, but after infusion is likely to be similar to that of bupivacaine.

Peck, T.E. and Hill, S.A. *Pharmacology for Anaesthesia and Intensive Care*, 4th edition. Cambridge University Press, 2014: Chapter 11, Local anaesthetics: pp. 163–164; p. 161.

Question 30: Answer

A. False: Ondansetron is a 5-HT$_3$ receptor antagonist, and omeprazole is a proton pump inhibitor.

B. False: Ondansetron is lipid-soluble and works both peripherally and centrally, so can cross the blood-brain barrier.

C. False. Ondansetron blocks vagal afferent activity as one of its anti-emetic actions but does not alter hydrogen ion formation.

D. True. Bradycardia is a recognized unwanted effect if ondansetron is given by rapid intravenous injection.

E. True. Granisetron is more potent than ondansetron.

Peck, T.E. and Hill, S.A. *Pharmacology for Anaesthesia and Intensive Care*, 4th edition. Cambridge University Press, 2014: Chapter 19, Antiemetics and related drugs: pp. 277–278; Chapter 20, Drugs acting on the gut: p. 282.

Question 31: Answer

A. True. Heparin-induced thrombocytopenia is a recognized complication of therapy.

B. False: Warfarin is an inhibitor of vitamin K-dependent clotting factor production in the liver.

C. True. Apixaban is a reversible direct inhibitor of factor Xa.

D. False. Dabigatran is a direct thrombin inhibitor.

E. False. Enoxaparin is a low-molecular-weight heparin that binds to and potentiates the activity of antithrombin III and indirectly inhibits thrombin.

Peck, T.E. and Hill, S.A. *Pharmacology for Anaesthesia and Intensive Care*, 4th edition. Cambridge University Press, 2014: Chapter 24, Drugs affecting coagulation: pp. 322–328.

Question 32: Answer

A. False. Aspirin irreversibly inhibits cyclo-oxygenase.

B. True. Omeprazole is a commonly encountered inhibitor of CYP2C19 that reduces the conversion of clopidogrel to its active form.

C. True. The monoclonal antibody abciximab is an antagonist with a high affinity for the glycoprotein IIb/IIIa receptor.

D. False. Ticagrelor is an antagonist at the $P2Y_{12}$ receptor.

E. True. Prasugrel, like clopidogrel, inhibits the $P2Y_{12}$ receptor, an ADP receptor.

Peck, T.E. and Hill, S.A. *Pharmacology for Anaesthesia and Intensive Care*, 4th edition. Cambridge University Press, 2014: Chapter 24, Drugs affecting coagulation: pp. 318–321.

Question 33: Answer

A. True. Hartmann's has a sodium concentration of 131 mmol/l.

B. False. 0.18% sodium chloride is one-fifth normal so sodium and therefore chloride concentration is one-fifth of 154 mol/l or 31 mmol/l.

C. True. 5% glucose contains 50 g glucose per litre; 1 g of glucose provides around 4 kilocalories. So, 5 g is equivalent to 200 kcal/l; this is an approximation but close enough for the answer to be true, if it was meant to be false it would be given as a value different by a factor of ten or more. 200 kcal is approximately 837 kJ.

D. True. The calcium content of Hartmann's is 1.8 mol/l.

E. False. All commercial solutions of sodium chloride for medical use are acidic with 0.9% NaCl (normal saline) having a pH of around 5.5. This is largely due to the presence of dissolved carbon dioxide in the atmosphere.

Peck, T.E. and Hill, S.A. *Pharmacology for Anaesthesia and Intensive Care*, 4th edition. Cambridge University Press, 2014: Chapter 21, Intravenous fluids and minerals: p. 288, Table 21.1.

Question 34: Answer

A. False. Gentamicin inhibits ribosomal activity and protein synthesis.

B. False. Teicoplanin inhibits bacterial cell wall synthesis by preventing cross-linkage of peptidoglycans.

C. True. Ciprofloxacin inhibits bacterial DNA gyrase and prevents the separation of DNA strands for replication so inhibiting cell division.

D. True. Clindamycin acts on the 50S ribosome subunit to prevent protein synthesis.

E. False. Viral thymidine kinase is responsible for the formation of acyclovir monophosphate that can subsequently become acyclovir triphosphate, a high-affinity substrate for viral DNA polymerase, which is incorporated into viral DNA but causes chain termination.

Peck, T.E. and Hill, S.A. *Pharmacology for Anaesthesia and Intensive Care*, 4th edition. Cambridge University Press, 2014: Chapter 23, Antimicrobials: pp. 298–313.

Question 35: Answer

A. True. A beta-lactam ring is a structural feature of all penicillins.

B. True. This is the reason probenecid, which reduces penicillin excretion, is added to some penicillin antibiotics.

C. False. Renal excretion is very rapid for penicillin, which explains the need for frequent dosing.

D. False. By causing structural failure of cell wall peptidoglycan cross-linkage, penicillins are bactericidal.

E. False. Gram-negative bacteria have a lipopolysaccharide outer layer that prevents penicillin action.

Peck, T.E. and Hill, S.A. *Pharmacology for Anaesthesia and Intensive Care*, 4th edition. Cambridge University Press, 2014: Chapter 23, Antimicrobials: pp. 300–304.

Question 36: Answer

A. True. Drowsiness and confusion are common with tricyclic antidepressants (TCAs), but seizure activity may also occur.

B. False. TCAs induce sinus tachycardia.

C. True. TCA toxicity causes intraventricular conduction delay, the QRS complex may also be broadened. ·

D. True. Dilated pupils are commonly seen in TCA toxicity.

E. False. TCA overdose is typically associated with hyperthermia.

Peck, T.E. and Hill, S.A. *Pharmacology for Anaesthesia and Intensive Care*, 4th edition. Cambridge University Press, 2014: Chapter 18, Central nervous system: p. 262.

Question 37: Answer

A. True. Free water clearance is defined as that volume of plasma from which solute-free water is excreted per unit time, so if the urine becomes less concentrated than normal, then free water clearance is increased. Loop diuretics disturb the medullary countercurrent mechanism that allows the production of concentrated urine and increases free water clearance.

B. False. Most of the sodium reabsorption is in the proximal tubule; furosemide inhibits the $Na^+/K^+/2Cl^-$ symporter in the thick ascending limb of the renal tubule so more potassium, sodium, and chloride reach the distal convoluted tubule where the sodium is exchanged for potassium and hydrogen ions, but potassium and chloride remain in the renal tubule so a hypokalaemic, hypochloraemic alkalosis can develop.

C. False. Furosemide increases potassium loss as explained above.

D. True. Furosemide blocks chloride uptake as explained above.

E. False. Phosphate is re-absorbed in the proximal and distal tubules, so furosemide has little effect on phosphate clearance: volume depletion also reduces phosphate clearance so there is no effect from fluid depletion caused by furosemide.

Peck, T.E. and Hill, S.A. *Pharmacology for Anaesthesia and Intensive Care*, 4th edition. Cambridge University Press, 2014: Chapter 22, Diuretics: pp. 294–295.

Question 38: Answer

A. True. Furosemide is a more potent diuretic than the thiazides.

B. False. Thiazides inhibit sodium and chloride reabsorption in the early distal convoluted tubule (DCT), which allows enhanced hydrogen and potassium exchange for sodium in the more distal DCT.

C. True. Increased potassium clearance is due to enhanced exchange for sodium in the DCT.

D. False. The reverse is true; thiazides and urate compete for excretion into the renal tubule, so plasma uric acid levels rise, and gout is a complication of thiazide therapy.

E. True. Thiazides reduce insulin secretion and hyperglycaemia is a recognized complication of thiazide therapy.

Peck, T.E. and Hill, S.A. *Pharmacology for Anaesthesia and Intensive Care*, 4th edition. Cambridge University Press, 2014: Chapter 22, Diuretics: pp. 292–294.

Question 39: Answer

A. True. Increasing insulin sensitivity is the main action of metformin.

B. False. Gliclazide is a sulfonylurea, displacing insulin from beta cells in the pancreas.

C. True. Glibenclamide is also a sulfonylurea: in the absence of pancreatic insulin, sulfonylureas are ineffectual.

D. False. Repaglinide is a meglitinide, which increase insulin secretion; it does not alter receptor sensitivity.

E. False. Insulin receptors are coupled to tyrosine kinase, not GPCRs.

Peck, T.E. and Hill, S.A. *Pharmacology for Anaesthesia and Intensive Care*, 4th edition. Cambridge University Press, 2014: Chapter 25, Drugs used in diabetes: pp. 331–335.

Question 40: Answer

A. False. Nitric oxide (NO) is a pulmonary vasodilator.

B. True. NO is very rapidly bound to haemoglobin and does not reach the systemic circulation when inhaled.

C. False. Although carbon monoxide has a high affinity for haemoglobin, NO has an even higher affinity—by a factor of around 1500.

D. True. NO can improve oxygenation by reducing V/Q mismatch but has no effect on mortality when used in ARDS.

E. True. NO is both a vasodilator and a bronchodilator.

Peck, T.E. and Hill, S.A. *Pharmacology for Anaesthesia and Intensive Care*, 4th edition. Cambridge University Press, 2014: Chapter 9, General anaesthetic agents: pp. 122–124.

Question 41: Answer

Principle: bronchodilators cause an increase, whereas bronchoconstrictors are associated with a decrease in anatomical dead space.

A. True. Atropine blocks muscarinic cholinergic receptors reducing resting cholinergic tone with an increase in anatomical dead space.

B. False. Salbutamol is a bronchodilator; it does not reduce anatomical dead space.

C. False. Histamine is a bronchoconstrictor, it decreases dead space.

D. False. Atenolol is a beta-1-selective adrenergic antagonist and has minimal effects on airways although potentially at high doses it could cause bronchoconstriction.

E. False. Prostacyclin is a vasodilator, not a bronchodilator.

Peck, T.E. and Hill, S.A. *Pharmacology for Anaesthesia and Intensive Care*, 4th edition. Cambridge University Press, 2014: Chapter 19, Antiemetics and related drugs: p. 276; Chapter 13, Sympathomimetics: p. 199; Chapter 14, Adrenoceptor antagonists: p. 212; Chapter 24, Drugs affecting coagulation: p. 321.

Question 42: Answer

A. True. Salbutamol should be used for rescue therapy as tachyphylaxis occurs due to down-regulation of beta-2 adrenoceptors with long-term use.

B. False. Montelukast is a leukotriene inhibitor used in prevention of asthma, so is a controller medication.

C. True. Ipratropium bromide is an anticholinergic used in combination therapy for long-term use but is more commonly used as an adjunct in acute therapy.

D. True. Inhibition of mast cell degranulation is an anti-inflammatory effect of beta-2 agonists such as salmeterol.

E. True. Inhaled steroids, such as beclametasone, are the first-line, regular, long-term therapy for asthma in adults.

Asthma medication (2022). Product information. Available at: https://emedicine.medscape.com/article/296301-medication

Peck, T.E. and Hill, S.A. *Pharmacology for Anaesthesia and Intensive Care*, 4th edition. Cambridge University Press, 2014: Chapter 13, Sympathomimetics: pp. 199–200.

Question 43:   Answer

A. False. Sevoflurane causes bronchodilation by a direct effect on smooth muscle.

B. False. Isoflurane is an upper airway irritant and can cause laryngospasm but is a bronchodilator.

C. False. Nicorandil is a potassium channel activator and a vasodilator, with no effect on bronchial muscle.

D. False. Ephedrine is an indirect, non-specific sympathomimetic causing bronchodilation.

E. False. Phentolamine is an alpha-adrenergic antagonist with no effect on the bronchioles; it has been reported that sulphites in the ampoule can cause bronchoconstriction in susceptible people, but this is not a property of phentolamine.

Peck, T.E. and Hill, S.A. *Pharmacology for Anaesthesia and Intensive Care*, 4th edition. Cambridge University Press, 2014: Chapter 9, General anaesthetic agents: p. 118, 114; Chapter 16, Vasodilators: p. 239; Chapter 13, Sympathomimetics: p. 201; Chapter 14, Adrenoceptor antagonists: pp. 207–208.

Question 44:   Answer

A. True. Anxiety is a common side effect of long-acting beta-2 sympathomimetics.

B. True: Headache is a common side effect of long-acting beta-2 sympathomimetics.

C. True. Beta-2 agonists increase potassium uptake into cells, therefore may cause hypokalaemia.

D. True. This is the most commonly encountered unwanted effect of beta-2 sympathomimetics.

E. False. Tachycardia and rarely arrhythmias are occasionally encountered with beta-2 sympathomimetics.

Drug information website (n.d.). Terbutaline. Available at: https://www.drugs.com/pro/terbutaline.html

Peck, T.E. and Hill, S.A. *Pharmacology for Anaesthesia and Intensive Care*, 4th edition. Cambridge University Press, 2014: Chapter 13, Sympathomimetics: pp. 119–120.

Question 45:   Answer

A. True. Prednisolone is a glucocorticoid, and a permissive effect is to increase fat formation and deposition.

B. True. This is an immunosuppressive effect of prednisolone.

C. False. Protein synthesis is inhibited, and catabolism is stimulated by glucocorticoids.

D. True. Glucocorticoids cause insulin resistance in muscle but sensitization to insulin is seen in adipocytes.

E. True. Bone formation is reduced, and bone reabsorption increased by prednisolone.

Barrett, K.E. et al. *Ganong's Review of Physiology 25th Edition (E-Book)*. McGraw Hill Education, 2015: Section III, Chapter 20, The adrenal medulla and the adrenal cortex: pp. 363–365.

Peck, T.E. and Hill, S.A. *Pharmacology for Anaesthesia and Intensive Care*, 4th edition. Cambridge University Press, 2014: Chapter 26: pp. 336–337.

1. **Regarding the anatomy of the orbit and the eye**
   - **A.** the inferior orbital fissure contains the zygomatic branch of the maxillary nerve
   - **B.** limiting the needle length to 25 mm completely avoids the risk of globe perforation during peribulbar block
   - **C.** from an approximate orbital volume of 30 ml more than 70% is occupied by the globe
   - **D.** a retrobulbar injection may lead to brainstem anaesthesia
   - **E.** the supraorbital nerve block prevents movement of the upper eyelid

2. **With regards to the anatomy of the spinal cord and pain pathways**
   - **A.** the artery of Adamkiewicz arises from a left-sided segmental thoracolumbar artery in more than 80% of people
   - **B.** hemisection of the spinal cord causes ipsilateral hemiplegia and anaesthesia
   - **C.** pain and temperature are transmitted mainly in the lateral spinothalamic tract
   - **D.** sensory fibres from first-order neurons go to the thalamus
   - **E.** the spinothalamic tract includes anterior, lateral, and posterior parts

3. **Brachial plexus**
   - **A.** block may be associated with ptosis, miosis, enophthalmos, and hoarseness
   - **B.** block by the interscalene approach using a volume of fewer than 10 ml of local anaesthetic reduces the incidence of diaphragm paralysis
   - **C.** block by the interscalene approach is suitable for hand surgery
   - **D.** lies between superficial and deep cervical fascia
   - **E.** is mainly formed by the rami of C4–C7

4. **With regards to the innervation of the larynx**
   - **A.** anaesthesia of the larynx above the level of the vocal cords can be achieved by a local anaesthetic injection below the lesser cornu of the hyoid bone
   - **B.** left-side chest surgical procedures may result in postoperative hoarseness
   - **C.** the recurrent laryngeal nerves provide sensory supply to the laryngeal mucosa inferior to the vocal cords
   - **D.** the superior laryngeal nerve is a terminal branch of the glossopharyngeal nerve
   - **E.** topical application of local anaesthetic in the piriform fossa provides supplemental anaesthesia for laryngoscopy and bronchoscopy

5. **Regarding the anatomy of the thoracic inlet and the first rib**
   A. both inferior and middle trunks of the brachial plexus are located in the thoracic inlet
   B. major vascular trunks, cranial, and spinal nerves pass through the thoracic inlet
   C. for a successful ultrasound-guided supraclavicular nerve block, the local anaesthetic should be injected between the first rib and the pleura
   D. the sympathetic trunk is an anterior relation to the neck of the first rib
   E. the thoracic inlet is limited by T1 posteriorly, the first rib, and the coracoid process laterally

6. **Regarding the anatomy of the myocardial vasculature**
   A. there are no direct anastomoses between the coronary arteries supplying the myocardium
   B. a cardioplegic agent can be injected retrogradely through the coronary sinus to induce myocardial arrest
   C. coronary artery dominance is determined by the vessel that supplies the left ventricle
   D. the right coronary artery supplies mainly the right ventricle, and originates from the proximal pulmonary trunk
   E. more than 75% of the venous return from the myocardium drains directly into the four chambers of the heart

7. **Regarding the blood supply to the liver**
   A. the biliary system and connective tissue receive mostly venous blood
   B. the liver is supplied only by the common hepatic artery
   C. the microcirculation formed by the anastomosis of hepatic arterioles and portal venules is characterized by low pressure and low flow velocity
   D. portosystemic shunts are abnormal vascular connections that divert a portion or all of the hepatic portal blood into the systemic venous system
   E. a transjugular intrahepatic portosystemic shunt procedure decreases portal hypertension

8. **Regarding the anatomy of the cerebral circulation**
   A. global aphasia will result from occlusion of the anterior branch of the dominant hemisphere middle cerebral artery
   B. venous blood from deep regions of the brain drain via the great cerebral vein to the straight sinus
   C. the cavernous sinus drains venous blood from intracranial structures
   D. the circle of Willis provides collateral circulation for the brain, compensating for reduced flow through individual segments of the arterial circle
   E. the posterior cerebral artery supplies the pontine brainstem

9. **In the femoral triangle**
   A. there is access for performing an analgesic block for patients with fractured neck of femur
   B. the boundaries are the inguinal ligament, medial border of the adductor longus muscle and medial border of the sartorius muscle
   C. within the femoral sheath, the femoral artery lies lateral to the femoral nerve
   D. the femoral vein lies medial and anterior to the femoral artery
   E. the ilio-inguinal nerve can be blocked

10. Regarding the lumbar and sacral plexuses and their nerves

A. the lumbar plexus includes the ventral rami of T12–L5

B. the posterior cutaneous nerve of the thigh is a branch of the sciatic nerve

C. the sacral plexus is formed from the S1–S3 ventral rami

D. a sciatic nerve block in the popliteal fossa is suitable for foot surgery

E. a surgical tourniquet for knee arthroscopy may result in persistent foot drop

Question 1: Answer

A. True. The inferior orbital fissure between the maxilla and the greater wing of the sphenoid bone separates the lateral wall and the floor of the orbit, it contains the zygomatic branch of cranial nerve (CN) V2, pterygopalatine branches, and emissary veins. It communicates with the pterygopalatine fossa.

B. False. The average distance from the orbital rim to the optic nerve is 42–54 mm, with a normal axial length of 20–25 mm. In myopic patients, the globe may be longer, and its surface may present staphylomata (surface herniation). The risk of globe perforation is therefore increased with axial lengths greater than 26 mm; limiting needle length may reduce this risk but not avoid it completely.

C. False. Pyramidal in shape, with the base situated anteriorly and the apex pointing posteriorly, the orbit contains the eyeball, orbital muscles and vessels, the optic and orbital nerves, the lacrimal apparatus, fat, and connective tissue. Loose connective tissue occupies approximately 75% of the orbit volume, and 5% (about 7 ml) is occupied by the globe and muscle cone.

D. True. Brainstem anaesthesia is caused by the direct spread of local anaesthetic to the brainstem from the orbit. A retrobulbar block is a block where the tip of the needle is placed close to the optic nerve. The optic nerve is essentially a continuation of the brain and is covered by dura hence, during a retrobulbar block, puncture of the dural covering of the optic nerve is possible causing brain stem anaesthesia.

E. False. The eyelid's closing is controlled by CN–VII. The supraorbital nerve provides sensory innervation to the skin of the lateral forehead and upper eyelid, as well as the conjunctiva of the upper eyelid.

Georgiou, A., Thompson, C., and Nickells, J. *Applied Anatomy for Anaesthesia and Intensive Care.* Cambridge University Press, 2014: pp. 48–55.

Wakeman, B. et al. Recognizing and mitigating risk of ophthalmic regional anesthesia. In: B.T. Finucane, B.C.H. Tsui (eds.). *Complications of Regional Anaesthesia*, 3rd edition. Springer, 2007: p. 371.

Question 2: Answer

A. True. The artery of Adamkiewicz (arteria radicularis magna) arises in the lower thoracic and upper lumbar region (on the left in 80% of people) and may be responsible for the circulation to the lower two-thirds of the spinal cord.

B. False. Hemisection of the spinal cord will result in Brown–Séquard syndrome: ipsilateral paralysis and proprioception loss associated with contralateral loss of pain and temperature sensation beginning one or two segments below the lesion.

C. True. The lateral spinothalamic tract carries information about pain and temperature. The anterior spinothalamic tract carries sensory information regarding light, poorly localized touch.

D. False. First-order neurons (signals from the peripheral pain receptors to the spinal cord) synapse with second-order neurons in the posterior horn of the spinal cord. The second-order neurons cross over through the ventral white commissure ascending on the opposite side of the spinal cord and form the lateral (pain and temperature) or anterior (touch and pressure) spinothalamic tracts.

E. False. The spinothalamic tract is an afferent pathway to the thalamus, located anterolaterally within the peripheral white matter of the spinal cord, and contains anterior and lateral parts.

Georgiou, A., Thompson, C., and Nickells, J. *Applied Anatomy for Anaesthesia and Intensive Care.* Cambridge University Press, 2014: p. 24.

Yentis, S., Hirsch, N., and Ip, J. *Anaesthesia and Intensive Care A–Z*, 5th edition. Churchill Livingstone, 2013: pp. 446, 518–519, 538.

Question 3: Answer

A. True. Ptosis, miosis, and enophthalmos (Horner's syndrome) due to ipsilateral stellate ganglion block is a common condition after supraclavicular brachial plexus blocks. The stellate ganglion is a fusion of the inferior cervical ganglion and first thoracic ganglion, is present in approximately 80% of the population, and often shares the same prevertebral fascia sheath with the brachial plexus. A prevertebral sheath defect due to unintended perforation/puncture may lead to local anaesthetic spread toward the anterior area and subsequently paralyse the recurrent laryngeal nerve.

B. True. Diaphragm paralysis following interscalene brachial plexus block occurs due to phrenic nerve block. The phrenic nerve is formed at the lateral borders of the anterior scalene muscles mainly from the C4 nerve with contributions from C3 and C5, corresponding to the superior trunk of the brachial plexus in the interscalene groove. Injected at this level, volumes greater than 10 ml result in 100% ipsilateral phrenic nerve block, while volumes as low as 5 ml—still producing reliable analgesia—reduce the incidence of phrenic nerve block by about 50%.

C. False. An interscalene brachial plexus block targets the nerve roots of the brachial plexus and is appropriate for shoulder/proximal arm procedures. Local anaesthetic diffusion toward C8 and T1 roots may be inconsistent, making the technique unsuitable for hand surgery.

D. False. A sheath derived from the prevertebral fascia covers the roots, trunks, and divisions of the brachial plexus. All these structures lie behind the deep cervical fascia.

E. False. The roots forming the brachial plexus emerge from the intervertebral foramina with the anterior primary rami of the 5 to 8 cervical and first thoracic nerves.

Choi, S. et al. Complications of regional anesthesia: upper and lower extremity blockade. In: B.T. Finucane and B.C.H. Tsui (eds.). *Complications of Regional Anaesthesia*, 3rd edition. Springer, 2007: p. 192.

Hewson, D. and Hardman, J. Regional anaesthetic techniques. In: J. Thompson, I. Moppett, and M. Wiles (eds.). *Smith and Aitkenhead's Textbook of Anaesthesia*, 7th edition. Elsevier, 2019: pp. 547–549.

Question 4: Answer

A. False. To provide anaesthesia of the larynx above the level of the vocal cords one should block the superior laryngeal nerve by injecting a local anaesthetic below and anterior to the greater cornu of the hyoid bone (not lesser cornu).

B. True. The left recurrent nerve passes under the arch of the aorta in the thorax. In its thoracic course, it may be affected by malignant tumours of the lung or oesophagus, malignant or inflamed nodes, by an aneurysm of the aortic arch or even, in mitral stenosis, by compression between the left pulmonary artery (pushed upwards by the greatly enlarged left atrium) and the aortic arch. Therefore, the left recurrent nerve, whose intrathoracic course brings it into relationship with many additional structures, may be damaged following surgery, leading to partial or full paralysis of the corresponding vocal cord. Unilateral paralysis produces a slight hoarseness that usually disappears because of compensatory overadduction of the opposite normal cord. The right recurrent laryngeal nerve passes under the subclavian artery in the neck (at the thoracic inlet), and it never actually reaches the thorax.

C. True. The recurrent laryngeal nerves provide the sensory supply to the laryngeal mucosa inferior to the vocal cords, as well as the motor supply to the intrinsic muscles of the larynx apart from the cricothyroid.

D. False. The superior laryngeal nerve is a terminal branch of the vagus nerve (CN X). The glossopharyngeal nerve is a branch of CN IX, providing the sensory supply of the pharynx, middle ear, posterior one-third of the tongue, and the carotid body and sinus.

E. True. The sensory supply of the mucosa from the epiglottis to the level above the vocal cords is provided by the internal laryngeal nerve, which runs beneath the mucosa of the piriform fossa. In this position, it can easily be blocked by the topical application of local anaesthetic.

Bowness, J. and Taylor, A. *Anatomy for the FRCA*. Cambridge University Press, 2019: pp. 90–91.

Georgiou, A., Thompson, C., and Nickells, J. *Applied Anatomy for Anaesthesia and Intensive Care*. Cambridge University Press, 2014: pp. 87–92.

Question 5: Answer

A. False. The thoracic inlet contains neither roots nor trunks of the brachial plexus, only the ventral ramus of T1.

B. True. The thoracic inlet contains major vascular structures such as the brachiocephalic artery and vein (on the right), the left carotid, and the left subclavian artery, the thoracic duct, together with the n. vagus (CN X), the cervical sympathetic chains, and the phrenic nerves (C3–C5).

C. False. The supraclavicular part of the brachial plexus is situated superficially and posterolaterally to the subclavian artery, lying on the first rib. Successful anaesthesia is obtained when the needle is placed within the brachial plexus sheath posterior to the subclavian artery and above the first rib. The pleura is located medially and below the first rib.

D. True. The sympathetic trunk (stellate/cervicothoracic ganglion) lies on the anterior surface of the neck of the first rib.

E. False. The thoracic inlet is a kidney-shaped superior (cranial) opening of the thorax, bounded by the superior border of the manubrium sternum anteriorly, first thoracic vertebra posteriorly, and the first ribs laterally.

Ellis, H., Feldman, S., and Harrop-Griffiths, W. *Anatomy for Anaesthetists*, 8th edition. Blackwell Publishing, 2004: pp. 229–304.

Georgiou, A., Thompson, C., and Nickells, J. *Applied Anatomy for Anaesthesia and Intensive Care*. Cambridge University Press, 2014: pp. 71–74.

Question 6: Answer

A. False. There are anastomoses between the circumflex and right coronary arteries and between the anterior and posterior interventricular arteries, and at the arteriolar level as well. In the normal heart, these anastomoses are non-functional. A collateral circulation in chronic ischaemic heart disease is possible through these anastomoses, but in the event of an acute occlusion, it fails to prevent ischaemia.

B. True. The coronary sinus has no anatomical valves. Up to 90% of the coronary circulation drains into the coronary sinus. Therefore, retrograde infusion of cardioplegic solution is possible. The junction of the great cardiac vein and coronary sinus (sometimes called the 'valve of Vieussens') may prevent the passage of catheters into the coronary sinus but does not obstruct the flow of cardioplegic solution.

C. False. Coronary artery dominance is defined by the vessel that gives rise to the posterior interventricular artery (right coronary artery in 80–85% of hearts), which supplies the myocardium of the inferior third of the interventricular septum and atrioventricular (AV) node. A precise anatomic definition of dominance would be the artery supplying the AV node.

D. False. The right coronary artery arises from the proximal ascending aorta, above the right cusp of the aortic valve. It supplies the right side of the heart (the right atrium, the right ventricle), the posterior third, and the inferior end of the interventricular septum.

E. False. One-third of the venous return drains directly into the four chambers of the heart (but mostly into the right atrium) through the venae cordis minimae or Thebesian veins. These veins contribute to the shunt fraction of arterial blood.

Bowness, J. and Taylor, A. *Anatomy for the FRCA*. Cambridge University Press, 2019: pp. 81–83.

Georgiou, A., Thompson, C., and Nickells, J. *Applied Anatomy for Anaesthesia and Intensive Care*. Cambridge University Press, 2014: pp. 125–127.

Question 7: Answer

A. False. The hepatic artery alone supplies the biliary system and connective tissue whereas the rest of the liver receives a dual supply. This is the reason for biliary necrosis following hepatic artery thrombosis or an intraoperative section.

B. False. The liver has a dual blood supply: the hepatic artery supplies about 45% to 50% of the liver's oxygen requirements, and the portal vein supplies the remaining 50% to 55%.

C. True. A unique feature of the hepatic microcirculation is low pressure to prevent retrograde flow in the valveless portal system, and low flow velocity, to enhance the extraction of oxygen and other molecules of interest.

D. True. Portosystemic shunts develop in portal hypertension through several sites of anastomosis: lower oesophagus, retroperitoneal veins, bare area of the liver, periumbilical veins, upper anal canal, and ductus venosus. Venous dilatation of these anastomoses leads to oesophageal/anal varices, caput medusae, and telangiectasia.

E. True. A transjugular, intrahepatic portosystemic shunt procedure (TIPSS) establishes communication between the inflow portal vein and the outflow hepatic vein, therefore reducing pressure in the portal system.

Bowness, J. and Taylor, A. *Anatomy for the FRCA*. Cambridge University Press, 2019: pp. 81–83.

Ramsay, M. Hepatic physiology and anesthesia. In: J.F. Butterworth, D.C. Mackey, and J.D. Wasnick (eds.). *Morgan & Mikhail's Clinical Anesthesiology*, 5th edition. McGraw Hill Education, 2013: pp. 692–694.

Question 8: Answer

A. False. The dominant hemisphere's middle cerebral artery anterior branch supplies the anterior speech area and will result in expressive dysphasia (Broca's aphasia). Comprehension generally remains intact. Conversely, a middle cerebral artery posterior branch occlusion will result in receptive dysphasia (Wernicke, difficulty understanding written and spoken language), and global aphasia will result from occlusion of the dominant hemisphere middle cerebral artery.

B. True. Blood from superficial and deep veins enters the dural venous sinuses. The sinuses drain to the internal jugular veins, which leave the skull via the jugular foramen.

C. False. The cavernous sinus receives blood from the middle and inferior cerebral veins, but also from superior and inferior ophthalmic veins (a potential route of ingress for tracking infection). A unique feature of the cavernous sinus is the internal carotid artery passing through. With aneurysms of the intracavernous carotid artery, cavernous sinus syndrome (ophthalmoplegia, ophthalmic, and maxillary sensory loss) may occur due to adjacent cranial nerves' compression.

D. True. The circle of Willis is fed by both left and right internal carotid arteries and the basilar artery (junction of the left and right vertebral arteries). The anterior part of the circle is formed by the anterior communicating artery along with the left and right anterior cerebral arteries. The posterior part is formed by the posterior left and right cerebral and communicating arteries and the basilar artery.

E. False. The posterior cerebral artery supplies oxygenated blood to the occipital lobe. The pontine brainstem is supplied by the perforating branches of the basilar artery.

Bowness, J. and Taylor, A. *Anatomy for the FRCA*. Cambridge University Press, 2019: pp. 81–83.

Chandra, A. et al. The cerebral circulation and cerebrovascular disease I: anatomy. *Brain Circulation* 2017;3:45–56.

Question 9:   Answer

A. True. Pre- and postoperative analgesia for patients with fractured neck of femur can be performed using a fascia iliaca compartment block with access through the femoral triangle. The fascia iliaca compartment is a potential space between the deep fascia overlying the iliacus muscle, where femoral nerve and lateral cutaneous nerves are found. A large volume of local anaesthetic is required.

B. True. The femoral triangle (Scarpa's triangle) is a triangular fascial space in the proximal thigh. The floor is formed by iliopsoas, pectineus, adductor longus muscles, and covered by fascia lata; laterally it is limited by the medial border of sartorius, medially by the medial border of adductor longus, and superiorly by the inguinal ligament.

C. False. In Scarpa's triangle, from lateral to medial, the content is organized as follows: nerves (lateral cutaneous, femoral branch of the genitofemoral nerve and femoral nerve), femoral artery, and femoral veins. The femoral sheath encloses the proximal parts of the femoral vessels, but not the femoral nerve.

D. False. Emerging in the femoral sheath beneath the inguinal ligament, initially medial to the femoral artery, the femoral vein leaves the sheath before the femoral artery bifurcation and lies posteriorly to it at the apex of the femoral triangle.

E. False. The ilioinguinal nerve travels between internal and external oblique muscles, superior to the inguinal ligament, and then enters the superficial inguinal ring. Therefore, it cannot be anaesthetized in the femoral triangle.

Bowness, J. and Taylor, A. *Anatomy for the FRCA*. Cambridge University Press, 2019: pp. 48–50.

Georgiou, A., Thompson, C., and Nickells, J. *Applied Anatomy for Anaesthesia and Intensive Care*. Cambridge University Press, 2014: pp. 183–184.

Question 10: Answer

A. True. The lumbar plexus is derived from the anterior rami of the first to fourth lumbar nerve roots. About 50% of subjects receive an additional contribution from T12 and L5.

B. False. The posterior cutaneous nerve of the thigh arises from the collateral branches of the sacral plexus, S1–S2. It emerges through the greater sciatic foramen below piriformis, on the medial side of the sciatic nerve.

C. False. The sacral plexus is formed from a contribution of L4, from the entire L5, S1, 2, and 3 anterior primary rami, and from a part of S4.

D. False. The medial aspect of the foot, including the first metatarsal phalangeal joint, receives innervation from the saphenous nerve, originating from the femoral nerve.

E. True. Tourniquet-induced common peroneal nerve palsy is a well-documented complication of orthopaedic surgery (knee arthroscopy or arthroplasty) because of its anatomical location. The common peroneal (lateral popliteal) nerve descends from its origin at the apex of the popliteal fossa, and winds around the neck of the fibula. A surgical tourniquet (depending on its pressure, duration, cuff size/fit), positioning of the operative extremity, joint overextension, or malposition—alone or combined, may induce mechanical damage to the nerve resulting in temporary or permanent injury.

Ellis, H., Feldman, S., and Harrop-Griffiths, W. *Anatomy for Anaesthetists*, 8th edition. Blackwell Publishing, 2004: pp. 183–203.

1. **The correct SI unit for**
   A. force is the pascal
   B. mass is the gram
   C. time is the second
   D. length is the metre
   E. energy is the watt

2. **According to the laws of physics**
   A. Boyle's law assumes that molecular size is unimportant
   B. Boyle's law states that the volume of a gas varies inversely with pressure
   C. Charles' law predicts that as the temperature of a mass of gas is raised from 10°C to 20°C, its volume will double
   D. Dalton's law states that a gas dissolves in proportion to its partial pressure
   E. Laplace's law suggests that large alveoli should collapse

3. **The following are true of critical temperature**
   A. critical temperature is the temperature above which a substance cannot be liquefied however much pressure is applied
   B. the critical temperature of oxygen is –139°C
   C. nitrous oxide cylinders always contain liquid nitrous oxide
   D. the critical temperature of nitrous oxide is 44°C
   E. critical pressure is the vapour pressure of a substance at its critical temperature

4. **A liquid inhalational anaesthetic agent is allowed to come into equilibrium with a mixture of gases. Under these conditions, the partial pressure of the agent in the resulting gas mixture depends on**
   A. the atmospheric pressure
   B. the surface area of the liquid
   C. the volume of the liquid
   D. the temperature of the liquid
   E. the composition of the gas mixture

5. **Assuming gas flow is laminar through an endotracheal tube**

   A. the flow rate doubles if the pressure gradient across the tube doubles

   B. the flow rate doubles if the length of the tube doubles

   C. the flow rate doubles if the radius of the tube doubles

   D. the flow rate doubles if the viscosity doubles

   E. the resistance to the flow doubles if the radius halves

6. **When thinking of the heat loss from the human body during open abdominal surgery**

   A. convection represents the largest proportion compared with other forms of heat loss

   B. radiation increases with an increase in the rate of the theatre air exchange system

   C. conduction requires body contact with a cooler object

   D. the degree of evaporation depends on the area of body surface exposed

   E. respiration represents up to 30% of the total heat loss

7. **How long will an oxygen cylinder with a physical volume of 5 litres reading 120 Bar on the pressure gauge last if opened at 10 litres per min?**

   A. 24 min

   B. 50 min

   C. 60 min

   D. 60.5 min

   E. 120 min

8. **Humidity**

   A. is defined as the amount of water vapour in the air

   B. is usually presented as absolute humidity in mg/l or g/m^3

   C. requires estimation of the dew point for its measurement

   D. in the operating theatre should be kept between 70 and 80% to reduce the risk of explosion

   E. of the inspired gases when using heat and moisture exchange filters can achieve up to 40%

9. **With regards to the flow through a Venturi system**

   A. the Bernoulli principle states that the pressure of fluid as it flows through the narrowest point is higher than elsewhere

   B. the pressure at the narrowest point is often below atmospheric pressure

   C. at the narrowest point there is a considerable drop in velocity

   D. a Venturi oxygen mask uses the flow of air to entrain more oxygen for delivery to the patient

   E. an entrainment ratio of 5:1 means that a flow of 5 l/min of oxygen entrains 1 l/min of air

10. Flowmeters on the anaesthetic machine

A. are universally calibrated regardless of the type of gas
B. provide laminar flow across the range of flows available
C. are read from the bottom of the bobbin
D. use a rubber band around the bobbin to prevent it from sticking to the sides of the tube
E. use glass tubes of cylindrical shape

11. The Clark (polarographic) electrode

A. requires an external power source for its function
B. contains a lead anode and a gold mesh cathode
C. has a quick response time of less than 10 seconds
D. over-reads PO_2 in the presence of nitrous oxide
E. provides a reliable reading across a wide range of temperatures

12. Soda lime used in the anaesthetic circle system

A. contains 80% sodium hydroxide (NaOH)
B. will become more acidic as the reaction proceeds
C. requires the presence of water for absorption of carbon dioxide
D. cools down as the reaction proceeds
E. absorbs approximately 25 litres of carbon dioxide per 1 kg

13. A variable bypass plenum vaporizer

A. acts as a flow restrictor
B. contains a vaporizing chamber that is above atmospheric pressure
C. requires an electrical supply to operate the temperature compensation mechanism
D. contains a splitting mechanism dividing the flow entering the vaporizer approximately 50/50 between bypass and vaporizing chambers
E. produces the required output of anaesthetic independent of the gas flow

14. Regarding ultrasound

A. waves used in medical scanning are usually between 2 and 20 kHz
B. a probe produces ultrasound waves by the piezoelectric effect
C. frequency needs to be increased in order to see deeper anatomical structures
D. waves reflected from the blood in a vessel produce an acoustic shadow below that vessel
E. M-mode (motion mode) is the mainstay of conventional imaging

15. In a circle breathing system

A. a unidirectional valve must be located between the patient and reservoir bag only on the expiratory limb
B. fresh gas flow enters between the patient and the expiratory valve
C. an adjustable pressure limiting (APL) valve is located between the patient and the inspiratory valve
D. soda lime is an essential component for its use
E. there is better conservation of heat and moisture compared with a Bain circuit

16. In measuring cardiac output (CO)

A. a pulmonary artery catheter (PAC) thermodilution technique always requires the use of cold saline

B. using Fick's principle, CO is given by oxygen consumption divided by arterial blood tension of oxygen

C. using oesophageal Doppler, the measured value is the Doppler shift

D. the lithium dilution method requires lithium to be injected directly into arterial blood

E. using a dye dilution technique, the taller the peak of the wash-out curve the higher the CO

17. In arterial blood gas analysis

A. the Severinghaus carbon dioxide electrode is a modification of the pH electrode

B. a pH electrode needs pH-sensitive glass for its function

C. actual bicarbonate is a calculated parameter

D. an excess volume of heparin in the blood sample will cause an abnormally high PaO_2 reading

E. alpha-stat means adjusting the temperature of a blood sample to 37°C

18. The risk of operating room staff receiving an electric shock from contact with theatre equipment is reduced using

A. bipolar diathermy

B. multiple earthing points for the equipment

C. relative humidity over 50%

D. conductive shoes

E. floating circuits

19. The anaesthetic scavenging system

A. uses a standard 15 mm connector for attachment to the APL valve

B. ensures the maximum permitted limit of nitrous oxide (N_2O) in eight hours does not exceed two parts per million (ppm)

C. incorporates a pressure relief valve set at 30 cmH_2O

D. can utilize charcoal to absorb all wasted anaesthetic gases and vapours

E. is designed only to deal with a range of gas flows between 0–15 l/min

20. In a defibrillator

A. an in-built step-up transformer is used to isolate the patient from the mains voltage

B. a diode is required to convert direct current (DC) to alternating current (AC)

C. a capacitor is used which consists of two inductors wound around the same former

D. an inductor's function is to convert monophasic to biphasic current

E. in the absence of mains current the internal batteries will produce AC current

21. Concerning diathermy

A. in monopolar diathermy, the electrical frequencies used are in the region of 50–60 Hz

B. current density refers to the current per cross-sectional area

C. in monopolar diathermy, the highest current density is produced between the tips of the forceps

D. a bipolar diathermy circuit is earth-free

E. bipolar diathermy produces the same power output as monopolar diathermy

22. The Wheatstone bridge circuit

A. is an essential element of invasive blood pressure measuring equipment

B. requires a direct current voltage source

C. detects changes in the electrical resistance of the strain gauge

D. contains three resistors

E. requires a rectifier for its function

23. Regarding lasers

A. the Nd-YAG laser contains gas as a lasing substance

B. optical pumping can be achieved using another laser

C. all staff should wear universal protective glasses when lasers are in use

D. monochromatic light means that the phase difference between photons is constant

E. avoiding the use of N_2O and 100% O_2 intraoperatively is advisable when lasers are used

24. The emergency oxygen flush on the anaesthetic machine

A. bypasses the flowmeter block

B. provides an oxygen flow of at least 15 l/min

C. incorporates a lock-in mechanism to maintain it in the switched-on position

D. incorporates a pressure relief valve to prevent barotrauma

E. use may lead to awareness under anaesthesia

25. Regarding the electrocardiogram

A. typical voltages recorded at the skin are in the range of 5–10 mV

B. the P wave is associated with atrial depolarization

C. the QRS complex coincides with ventricular contraction

D. when an electrode detects depolarization moving towards it, a positive wave is produced

E. lead II is the best for detecting left-ventricular ischaemia

Question 1: Answer

A. False. The pascal is an SI unit of pressure. 1 Pa = 1 N/m^2. Force is expressed in newton. 1 N = 1 kg.m/s^2. A force of 1 N will give a mass of 1 kg an acceleration of 1 metre per sec per sec.

B. False. The SI unit of mass is the kilogram.

C. True. The correct SI unit for time is the second.

D. True. The correct SI unit for length is the metre.

E. False. The watt is a derived unit of power. The unit of energy is the Joule. 1 J = 1 Nm. One Joule is the energy expended when the point of application of a force of 1 N moves 1 m in the direction of the force.

Ebrahim, H. and Ashton-Cleary, D. *Maths, Physics and Clinical Measurement for Anaesthesia and Intensive Care.* Cambridge University Press, 2019: pp. 25–28.

Question 2: Answer

A. True. Boyle's law is an ideal gas law and assumes among other things that molecular size is unimportant.

B. True. This is the definition of Boyle's law.

C. False. Charles' law states that at a constant pressure, the volume of a given mass of gas varies directly with its absolute temperature. Absolute temperature is measured in kelvin. 0°C = 273 K. Hence, 10°C = 10 + 273 = 283 K and 20°C = 20 + 273 = 293 K. So, when temperature rises from 10 to 20°C, the pressure only goes up by 3.5% not doubles as the temperature change in kelvin is only 10 K (10 K is 3.5% of the initial 283 K).

D. False. Dalton's law states that in a mixture of gases the pressure exerted by each gas is equal to the pressure that would be exerted if that gas alone were present. Hence, the total pressure exerted by a mixture of gases is equal to the sum of the partial pressures of the individual gases.

E. False. Laplace's law for spheres is P = 2 T/R, where P is the pressure gradient across the wall, T is the tangential force acting along the length of the wall, and R is the radius. So, in large alveoli, the radius will be larger and consequently, the resultant pressure gradient across the wall will be smaller. That is why large alveoli do not collapse and there is a tendency for small alveoli to empty into large alveoli. But in normal lungs, it does not occur due to the presence of surfactant lining the alveoli.

Ebrahim, H. and Ashton-Cleary, D. *Maths, Physics and Clinical Measurement for Anaesthesia and Intensive Care.* Cambridge University Press, 2019: pp. 61–67.

Question 3: Answer

A. True. This is the definition of critical temperature.

B. False. The critical temperature of oxygen is –119°C.

C. False. At the very end of its use, there is no liquid left in the cylinder, only gas, and this is when the pressure in the cylinder starts to drop rapidly. At temperatures above its critical temperature, a cylinder of nitrous oxide will contain only gas.

D. False. The critical temperature of nitrous oxide is 36.5°C; 44 is the molecular weight of nitrous oxide.

E. False. The critical pressure of a substance is the pressure required to liquefy a gas at its critical temperature.

Smith, T., Pinnock, C., and Lin, T. *Fundamentals of Anaesthesia*. Cambridge University Press, 2009: pp. 736–737.

Question 4: Answer

At this point, an inhalational agent will be at its saturated vapour pressure (SVP). It is only the temperature of the liquid that influences the SVP. The higher the temperature the higher the SVP. Hence, the only correct answer is D.

A. False. The atmospheric pressure does not influence the SVP.

B. False. The surface area of the liquid does not influence the SVP.

C. False. The volume of the liquid does not influence the SVP.

D. True. The temperature of the liquid influences the SVP.

E. False. The composition of the gas mixture does not influence the SVP.

Ebrahim, H. and Ashton-Cleary, D. *Maths, Physics and Clinical Measurement for Anaesthesia and Intensive Care*. Cambridge University Press, 2019: p.115.

Question 5: Answer

A. True. According to the Hagen–Poiseuille equation (Fig 8.1) the flow is directly proportional to the pressure gradient (PG). Hence, if the PG doubles the flow will double as well.

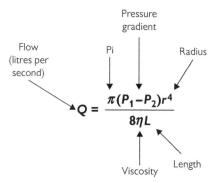

$$Q = \frac{\pi(P_1 - P_2)r^4}{8\eta L}$$

Fig 8.1 The Hagen–Poiseuille equation.

B. False. According to the same equation doubling the length of the tube will halve the flow as the flow is inversely proportional to the length of the tube.

C. False. Doubling the radius will increase the flow 16 times.

D. False. The flow will halve if viscosity doubles.

E. False. The resistance to the flow (R) is the PG divided by the flow. Using the Hagen–Poiseuille equation:

$$R = 8\eta L/\pi r^4$$

So, if the radius halves the resistance will increase 16 times.

Ebrahim, H. and Ashton-Cleary, D. *Maths, Physics and Clinical Measurement for Anaesthesia and Intensive Care.* Cambridge University Press, 2019: pp. 54–55.

Question 6: Answer

A. False. The largest amount of energy is lost through radiation (40%), followed by convection (30%), and evaporation from the skin (20%), so respiration accounts for approximately 10%.

B. False. Any object is capable of transferring and receiving heat in the form of infrared electromagnetic waves. Energy is transferred from a warm to a cold object without the need for direct contact. In the operating theatre heat loss by radiation will be increased if the ambient temperature drops. Increasing the flow rate of the air exchange system will influence heat loss by convection.

C. True. Heat energy is transferred from one molecule to another by an increase in kinetic energy of these molecules from the hotter to the colder substance. A cold operating table will receive heat from a warm body.

D. True. The larger the wet surface of an open abdomen exposed to the environment, the greater the energy required to turn it from liquid to vapour and this energy comes from the body tissues. Hence, cooling of the body increases.

E. False. Respiration accounts only for 10% of the heat losses. Heat and moisture exchange (HME) filters can significantly decrease this type of heat loss.

Ebrahim, H. and Ashton-Cleary, D. *Maths, Physics and Clinical Measurement for Anaesthesia and Intensive Care.* Cambridge University Press, 2019: Chapter 3, pp. 38–41.

Question 7: Answer

A. False.

B. False.

C. True.

D. False.

E. False.

Firstly, we need to calculate the absolute pressure in the cylinder (P1) from atmospheric pressure (P2, 1 atm) and gauge pressure (P3).

P1 = P2 + P3, which is 1 Bar + 120 Bar = 121 Bar

If V1 = physical volume of the cylinder, V2 = the volume of gas stored in the cylinder then V1 is 5 L, V2 is unknown.

We use Boyle's law to calculate the amount of oxygen left in the cylinder.

P1 x V1 = P2 x V2, so V2 = (P1 x V1) ÷ P2

So V2 = (121 x 5) ÷ 1, and V2 = 605 litres

Of course, the final 5 litres could not be discharged from the cylinder as at this point the pressure in the cylinder will be equal to the atmospheric pressure. Hence, we subtract 5 litres from 605 litres, giving 600 litres. This cylinder opened at 10 l/min flow will be used in 60 min.

Ebrahim, H. and Ashton-Cleary, D. *Maths, Physics and Clinical Measurement for Anaesthesia and Intensive Care.* Cambridge University Press, 2019: Chapter 4, p. 64.

Question 8: **Answer**

A. True. This is the definition of humidity.

B. False. The value given is usually relative humidity, as a percentage, reflecting the ratio of the mass of water vapour in a given volume of air to the mass needed to fully saturate the given volume of air at the specific temperature.

C. True. This is the principle behind the function of Regnault's hygrometer.

D. False. Relative humidity should be kept between 50 and 70%. Optimal humidity is 45–50% but the risk of static electricity built-up is higher at these levels, hence 50–70% as a safety/comfort compromise.

E. False. Under optimum conditions a relative humidity of 60–70% may be achieved.

Ebrahim, H. and Ashton-Cleary, D. *Maths, Physics and Clinical Measurement for Anaesthesia and Intensive Care.* Cambridge University Press, 2019: p. 115.

Question 9: **Answer**

A. False. Lower than elsewhere.

B. True. This is the principle of entrainment of air or fluid at the narrowest point.

C. False. Increase in velocity and gain of kinetic energy.

D. False. It uses the flow of oxygen to entrain air.

E. False. Entrainment ratio = entrainment flow/driving flow. Hence ER = 5/1 means that 1 l/min of oxygen entrains 5 l/min of air.

Ebrahim, H. and Ashton-Cleary, D. *Maths, Physics and Clinical Measurement for Anaesthesia and Intensive Care.* Cambridge University Press, 2019: Chapter 9, pp. 130–131.

Question 10: **Answer**

A. False. Rotameters are calibrated individually for different gases.

B. False. There is a mixture of turbulent and laminar flow. Laminar flow is at low flow rates and turbulent at higher flow rates.

C. False. The reading is taken from the top of the bobbin.

D. False. A conductive strip coating the inside of the tube is used to decrease electrostatic charges.

E. False. The rotameter tubes are of conical shape: narrower at the bottom and wider at the top.

Ebrahim, H. and Ashton-Cleary, D. *Maths, Physics and Clinical Measurement for Anaesthesia and Intensive Care.* Cambridge University Press, 2019: Chapter 5, pp. 76–77.

Question 11: **Answer**

A. True. The Clark electrode is battery powered, unlike a fuel cell that acts as a battery itself.

B. False. These are the anode and cathode in a fuel cell. The Clark electrode contains a silver/silver chloride anode and a platinum cathode.

C. False. The Clark electrode has a relatively slow response time of 30 seconds and although it is capable of measuring oxygen concentration in gases, it is mainly used in measuring oxygen tension in blood as a part of blood gas analysis.

D. True. A polarographic electrode over-reads PO_2 in the presence of strong oxidizing substances (such as halothane or nitrous oxide) as they are also reduced at the cathode.

E. False. One of the disadvantages of the Clark electrode is that it must be maintained at a constant temperature of 37 °C.

Ebrahim, H. and Ashton-Cleary, D. *Maths, Physics and Clinical Measurement for Anaesthesia and Intensive Care.* Cambridge University Press, 2019: Chapter 7, pp. 104–105.

Question 12: **Answer**

A. False. The most common soda lime composition is 80% calcium hydroxide ($Ca(OH)_2$), 4% sodium hydroxide ($NaOH$) and 16% water.

B. False. The pH of the reagents increases as the reaction proceeds, and this activates an indicator, which is used to show when the calcium hydroxide is exhausted.

C. True. 15% of soda lime is water, which is essential for the absorption of carbon dioxide:

$$CO_2 + H_2O = H_2CO_3 = H^+ + HCO^-_3$$

$$Ca(OH)_2 + H^+ + HCO^-_3 = CaCO^-_3 + 2H_2O$$

D. False. The reaction is exothermic, hence soda lime becomes hot during the reaction.

E. False. Soda lime absorbs approximately 250 litres of carbon dioxide per 1 kg.

Smith, T., Pinnock, C., and Lin, T. *Fundamentals of Anaesthesia*. Cambridge University Press, 2009: Chapter 3, pp. 845–846.

Question 13: **Answer**

A. True. Plenum vaporizers have relatively high resistance and, for a spontaneously breathing patient, require a circuit with a reservoir bag to ensure peak inspiratory flow rates can be maintained.

B. True. As gases enter a plenum vaporizer at a higher than atmospheric pressure, they pressurize the vaporizing chamber.

C. False. Temperature compensation in plenum vaporizers is achieved by incorporating dense metals, such as copper, with a high thermal capacity to act as a heat sink and by using a bimetallic strip to regulate the splitting ratio. Neither method requires any electrical supply to function.

D. False. About 75–80% of the flow entering the vaporizer is directed into the bypass chamber with only about 20–25% entering the vaporizing chamber.

E. False. The output is calibrated only between 0.5 and 15 l/min.

Ebrahim, H. and Ashton-Cleary, D. *Maths, Physics and Clinical Measurement for Anaesthesia and Intensive Care*. Cambridge University Press, 2019: Chapter 8, pp. 119–126.

Smith, T., Pinnock, C., and Lin, T. *Fundamentals of Anaesthesia*. Cambridge University Press, 2009: Chapter 3, pp. 838–841.

Question 14: **Answer**

A. False. Ultrasound frequencies used in medical scanning are usually between 2 and 20 MHz.

B. True. The piezoelectric effect is the production of an electric charge in response to an applied mechanical strain. Piezoelectric crystals within the ultrasound probe produce the *inverse* piezoelectric effect, which is the expansion and contraction of their structure as they convert the received electrical energy to mechanical energy which is released in the form of a sound wave.

C. False. Increasing frequency will obtain more detail in the scan and decreasing frequency will give more depth of penetration.

D. False. Fluids tend to be poor reflectors of ultrasound waves and produce so-called post-cystic enhancement of the structures beneath. Bones tend to be strong reflectors and produce an acoustic shadow so in order to see the structures beneath them the angle of the probe needs to be changed.

E. False. B-mode (brightness mode) is the mainstay of conventional imaging.

Ebrahim, H. and Ashton-Cleary, D. *Maths, Physics and Clinical Measurement for Anaesthesia and Intensive Care*. Cambridge University Press, 2019: Chapter 14, pp. 207–224.

Smith, T., Pinnock, C., and Lin, T. *Fundamentals of Anaesthesia*. Cambridge University Press, 2009: Section 4, Chapter 1, pp.762–770.

Question 15: Answer

A. False. A unidirectional valve must be located not only on the expiratory limb between the patient and reservoir bag but also on the inspiratory limb to provide unidirectional flow of the gas mixture.

B. False. Fresh gas flow should always enter the inspiratory limb and never the expiratory limb otherwise it will be wasted through the APL valve into the scavenging system.

C. False. The APL valve is located between the patient and expiratory valve; if positioned between the patient and the inspiratory valve, no fresh gas flow will be delivered to the patient when the valve is fully closed.

D. False. Soda lime is a desirable component for absorption of carbon dioxide particularly if low flows are used. However, in the absence of soda lime increasing the fresh gas flow rate will allow carbon dioxide elimination.

E. True. Conservation of heat and moisture is just one of the advantages of the circle system. Other advantages include low gas flow anaesthesia, reduction of atmospheric pollution, and economic use of inhalational agents.

Ebrahim, H. and Ashton-Cleary, D. *Maths, Physics and Clinical Measurement for Anaesthesia and Intensive Care*. Cambridge University Press, 2019: Chapter 9, pp. 136–137.

Smith, T., Pinnock, C., and Lin, T. *Fundamentals of Anaesthesia*. Cambridge University Press, 2009: Section 4, Chapter 3, pp. 844–845.

Question 16: Answer

A. False. Traditionally cold saline was used in thermodilution techniques. However, as it is quite cumbersome, modern PACs have an in-built heating element a few centimetres above the thermistor to warm the blood in the right atrium. A temperature change is then detected by the thermistor at the tip of the PAC.

B. False. The Fick principle relates CO through the whole body or an individual organ to the consumption of a substance (e.g., oxygen) by an organ divided by the arteriovenous difference of the substance going through an organ.

C. True. The Doppler principle of measuring velocity states that the shift in frequency of a reflected wave is proportional to the velocity of the moving object. In measuring CO, an ultrasound wave from the probe in the mid-oesophagus is reflected from moving red blood cells in the descending aorta and the shift of frequency is detected. The degree of this shift reflects the velocity of blood in the descending aorta which, together with a measure of the cross-sectional area of the aorta, gives the CO.

D. False. Although the lithium dilution technique is widely used for measuring CO, lithium is injected into a central vein and measured in arterial blood.

E. False. If the CO is high then any dye (e.g., saline, lithium) will be washed out faster producing a flat and short wash-out curve.

Ebrahim, H. and Ashton-Cleary, D. *Maths, Physics and Clinical Measurement for Anaesthesia and Intensive Care.* Cambridge University Press, 2019: Chapter 12, pp. 174–186.

Question 17: Answer

A. True. The Severinghaus carbon dioxide electrode is essentially a modification of the pH electrode. The same silver/silver chloride electrodes are used in both devices, but a thin layer of bicarbonate solution is added between the pH electrode and its covering in the carbon dioxide electrode. CO_2 from the blood sample will cross the permeable membrane and react with water in the bicarbonate solution producing H^+ ions that are detected by the pH electrode.

B. True. A pH electrode needs pH-sensitive glass for its function which is a complex framework of silicon oxides with Ca^{2+} and Na^+ ions embedded in it. Hydrogen ions from the blood sample displace sodium ions from within the glass but do not cross it. This draws chloride ions from the buffer solution to the internal surface of the glass. An electrical potential difference is therefore generated across the glass which can be measured and calibrated to determine the pH of the sample.

C. True. Standard and actual bicarbonate as well as base excess are the values calculated using the Siggard-Anderson nomogram. pH, pCO_2, and pO_2 are values that are directly measured by different electrodes in a blood gas analyser.

D. True. An excess volume of heparin in the blood sample will cause an abnormally high PaO_2 reading decrease the level of $PaCO_2$ and induce a slight reduction in the pH mainly due to a dilutional effect that becomes noticeable if there is more than 10% heparin present in the sample.

E. True. Alpha-stat means adjusting the temperature of a blood sample to a normal body temperature of 37°C and pH-stat means using the actual core body temperature. These adjustments are mainly relevant in cardiac anaesthesia where patients are deeply cooled during the bypass phase. There is no good-quality evidence to support either strategy but there is a suggestion for improved outcomes using a pH-stat approach in paediatric deep hypothermic cardiac arrest cases and an alpha-stat approach for adults (pH for paediatrics, alpha for adults).

Ebrahim, H. and Ashton-Cleary, D. *Maths, Physics and Clinical Measurement for Anaesthesia and Intensive Care.* Cambridge University Press, 2019: Chapter 7, pp. 105–108.

Question 18: Answer

A. True. In bipolar diathermy, the current flows between the tips of the forceps used to coagulate the tissues, unlike in monopolar diathermy where current flows across the body between an active electrode (cutting/coagulating) to the passive plate attached to a remote part of the body (e.g., thigh). Poor contact of the plate with the skin can cause burns and escape of the current with tissue damage.

B. False. Poor design of earth circuits can generate leakage currents, which can act as a source of microshock. This occurs where multiple earth connections are used, each connection being at a slightly different potential, causing small currents to flow through earth circuits or the patient. The optimum earth circuit connects all earth circuits to earth at a *single point* via a good-quality contact.

C. True. The optimal relative humidity in the operating theatre is between 50 and 70% to prevent the build-up of static electricity (see answer to Q 8D).

D. True. Suitable footwear is designed with an optimal impedance which should be high enough to prevent a large current from passing to earth (avoiding electric shock) if in contact with a high-voltage source, but low enough to allow a leakage current passing to earth to prevent staff and their clothing from accumulating a static charge. The optimal impedance of such shoes is usually between 100 kω and 1 Mω.

E. True. A floating circuit is where the mains electricity supply is separated from the patient circuits by an isolating transformer. The best example is a defibrillator.

Ebrahim, H. and Ashton-Cleary, D. *Maths, Physics and Clinical Measurement for Anaesthesia and Intensive Care.* Cambridge University Press, 2019: Chapter 10, pp. 148–158.

Smith, T., Pinnock, C., and Lin, T. *Fundamentals of Anaesthesia.* Cambridge University Press, 2009: Section 4, Chapter 1, pp. 755–761.

Question 19: Answer

A. False. The collecting part of the scavenging system uses a 30 mm connector in order to avoid inadvertent connection with the standard 15 mm connections used throughout breathing systems.

B. False. Acceptable levels of anaesthetic gases in the theatre environment are regulated by the Control of Substances Hazardous to Health (COSHH), part of UK law. Similar laws exist elsewhere, such as the Occupational Health and Safety Act (OHSA) in the USA. The maximum permitted limit for nitrous oxide in the UK is 100 ppm and 25 ppm in the USA.

C. False. The transfer part of the scavenging system incorporates a pressure relief valve set at 10 cmH$_2$O to allow expiratory flow even if the system becomes blocked.

D. False. Charcoal canisters (e.g., Cardiff Aldabsorber) can be used to absorb volatile anaesthetics (although *NOT* nitrous oxide). However, they are inefficient, and the charcoal needs to be changed after 12 hours of use.

E. False. The receiving part of the scavenging system protects the patient from both high and low pressures (–0.05 kPa to +5 kPa) and contains a reservoir to maximize efficiency in the presence of variable gas flow (between 0 l/min and 130 l/min).

Ebrahim, H. and Ashton-Cleary, D. *Maths, Physics and Clinical Measurement for Anaesthesia and Intensive Care.* Cambridge University Press, 2019: Chapter 10, pp. 146–147.

Question 20: Answer

A. True. A transformer consists of two inductors wound around the same former. A transformer can thus be used to step up or step down AC voltages in circuits. In a defibrillator, the step-up transformer is used to increase the mains voltage from 240 V AC to 5000 V AC.

B. False. A rectifier, which is a diode (semiconductor), in the capacitor charging circuit, converts AC voltage into DC voltage (5000 V AC to 5000 V DC). DC energy is used rather than AC because it is more effective, causes less myocardial damage, and is less arrhythmogenic.

C. False. A capacitor is indeed used in a defibrillator, but it consists of two plates separated by a thin layer of insulating material (or dielectric).

D. False. The function of an inductor is to slow down and spread out the delivered pulse of energy to the myocardium, which makes it more effective than the shorter sharper spike waveform that would be delivered without the inductor present.

E. False. Most defibrillators contain internal rechargeable batteries, but they produce DC current that needs to be converted to AC current by the invertor and after that, the step-up transformer increases the current to 5000 V AC. Subsequently, the rectifier converts it to 5000 V DC as explained in B above.

Ebrahim, H. and Ashton-Cleary, D. *Maths, Physics and Clinical Measurement for Anaesthesia and Intensive Care*. Cambridge University Press, 2019: Chapter 10, pp. 152–155.

Smith, T., Pinnock, C., and Lin, T. *Fundamentals of Anaesthesia*. Cambridge University Press, 2009: Section 4, Chapter 1, pp. 750–754.

Question 21:   Answer

A. False. These frequencies are characteristic of mains electricity. Surgical diathermy typically uses frequencies in the region of 0.4–1.5 MHz as human tissues are markedly less sensitive to electricity at very high frequencies.

B. True. This is the definition of current density. At the active small electrode, the current density is high to achieve cutting or coagulation but at the large plate (indifferent electrode) the current density is low, and tissue damage does not occur.

C. False. This is true of **bipolar** diathermy where the high-density current passes only between the tips of the forceps and then back to the generator and not through the rest of the body, unlike monopolar diathermy where a single probe (but occasionally forceps) is used to apply electrical energy to the target tissue for the desired surgical effect. The current then passes through the patient to a return pad and then back to the generator to complete the circuit. In monopolar diathermy using forceps, rather than a single probe, the two tips of the forceps act as a single electrode and are at the same potential so no current flows directly between the tips; the highest current density is between each tip and the tissue contacted. There is a much lower current density at the patient plate, which has a much larger surface area than the tissue being burned.

D. True. As no current passes through the body, no earthing of bipolar diathermy equipment is needed and a so-called floating circuit is used instead.

E. False. The power output produced by bipolar diathermy is much smaller and therefore it is mainly suitable for coagulation of small pieces of tissue and blood vessels.

Davey, A.J. and Diba, A. *Ward's Anaesthetic Equipment*, 6th edition. Elsevier, 2011: Chapter 24.

Question 22:   Answer

A. True. A Wheatstone bridge is normally used for invasive blood pressure measurement and its primary benefit is to provide extremely accurate measurement in contrast to a simple voltage divider.

B. True. It contains an in-built battery producing DC current.

C. True. The primary function of the Wheatstone bridge circuit is to detect any changes in the electrical resistance of the strain gauge in a pressure transducer.

D. False. It contains three known resistors (one of which is variable) and one unknown variable resistor (the strain gauge, in the case of a pressure transducer).

E. False. A rectifier is an element that is used in a defibrillator. The Wheatstone bridge requires a galvanometer for its accurate function to measure the electrical current.

Ebrahim, H. and Ashton-Cleary, D. *Maths, Physics and Clinical Measurement for Anaesthesia and Intensive Care*. Cambridge University Press, 2019: Chapter 11, pp. 166–167.

Smith, T., Pinnock, C., and Lin, T. *Fundamentals of Anaesthesia*. Cambridge University Press, 2009: Section 4, Chapter 1, pp. 750.

Questions 23: Answer

A. False. Nd-YAG is an example of a laser with a solid lasing substance. Helium, argon, and carbon dioxide are examples of gas lasers.

B. True. A source of energy is required to raise the electrons from the ground state to an excited one (a process known as optical pumping). Most often, a light from a flash tube is used for this purpose but alternatives include another laser, a heat source, a current, and a chemical reaction.

C. False. All staff must wear laser goggles specific to the wavelength of the laser in use.

D. False. This is the definition of coherence. Monochromatic means that the light is of a single wavelength.

E. True. A source of oxygen must be present for a fire to propagate. In the medical setting, this may be from air, concentrated oxygen, or nitrous oxide. In the presence of heat, nitrous oxide breaks down as follows: $2N_2O \rightarrow 2N_2 + O_2$ + Energy. This gives a 33% oxygen mixture and produces additional thermal energy. Therefore, nitrous oxide is both a fuel and an oxygen source.

Ebrahim, H. and Ashton-Cleary, D. *Maths, Physics and Clinical Measurement for Anaesthesia and Intensive Care*. Cambridge University Press, 2019: Chapter 10, pp. 148–149 and Chapter 15, pp. 239–245.

Smith, T., Pinnock, C., and Lin, T. *Fundamentals of Anaesthesia*. Cambridge University Press, 2009: Section 4, Chapter 1, pp. 781–782.

Question 24: Answer

A. True. In all modern anaesthetic machines, the bypass oxygen flow joins the back bar just before the common gas outlet from the intermediate pressure system (at 2 Bar) avoiding the flowmeter block.

B. False. It provides oxygen at a minimum flow rate of 30 l/min.

C. False. The emergency oxygen button cannot be locked to ensure that excessive pressure cannot build up within the patient's airway.

D. False. The pressure relief valve is situated at the outlet end of the back bar (threshold set to 30–40 kPa). This protects the rotameter block and vaporizers from overpressure damage, and to a very limited degree protects the patient from barotrauma.

E. True. During inhalational anaesthesia use of the oxygen bypass flow also bypasses the vaporizer so that awareness is possible.

Davey, A.J. and Diba, A. *Ward's Anaesthetic Equipment*, 6th edition. Elsevier, 2011: Chapter 4.

Smith, T., Pinnock, C., and Lin, T. *Fundamentals of Anaesthesia*. Cambridge University Press, 2009: Section 4, Chapter 3, p. 836.

Question 25: Answer

A. False. Typical voltages recorded at the skin are in the range of 1–2 mV.

B. True. The P wave is associated with atrial depolarization and contraction.

C. False. The QRS complex reflects ventricular depolarization and precedes ventricular contraction.

D. True. When an electrode detects depolarization of the atria or the ventricle moving towards it, a positive deflection/wave on the electrocardiogram (ECG) is produced. Alternatively, if depolarization is moving away from the electrode, it produces a negative deflection.

E. False. Lead II is best for detecting arrhythmias. To detect left-ventricular ischaemia, the CM5 configuration (clavicle–manubrium-V5) is recommended.

Ebrahim, H. and Ashton-Cleary, D. *Maths, Physics and Clinical Measurement for Anaesthesia and Intensive Care*. Cambridge University Press, 2019: Chapter 16, pp. 247–252.

Smith, T., Pinnock, C., and Lin, T. *Fundamentals of Anaesthesia*. Cambridge University Press, 2009: Section 2, Chapter 5, pp. 273–279.

1. **Features of a Normal (Gaussian) distribution**
    A. the Normal distribution is continuous
    B. the median is lower than the mean
    C. approximately 68% of observations lie within one standard deviation on either side of the mean
    D. approximately 2.5% of observations are expected to be greater than two positive standard deviations from the mean
    E. the values of the variance and mean are equal

2. **Variance**
    A. is the squared value of the standard deviation for a Normal (Gaussian) distribution
    B. of a sample taken from a defined population is a true (unbiased) estimate for the mean of that population
    C. describes the spread of values in a defined distribution
    D. in a Poisson distribution has an equal value to the mean
    E. is independent of the mean value in a Normal (Gaussian) distribution

3. **The standard error of the mean**
    A. is used to determine a confidence interval around a sample mean
    B. is inversely related to the sample size
    C. is smaller than the sample variance
    D. is preferred to the standard deviation when drawing error bars on charts
    E. is used to estimate the variance of the population from which the sample was taken

4. **In a double-blind, randomized, controlled trial**
    A. the patient does not know which treatment group they belong to
    B. the clinician looking after the patient will know to which treatment group the patient has been allocated
    C. The observer, who records results from the patient's treatment, does not know to which treatment group the patient has been allocated
    D. one of the treatment groups always receives a placebo
    E. interim analysis is not permitted

5. **A 95% confidence interval**
   A. around a sample mean always contains the true value of the population mean
   B. around a sample mean is narrower for a large compared with a small sample taken from the same population
   C. around a sample mean depends on the variance of the sample values
   D. is wider than a 90% confidence interval
   E. can only be calculated if the sample data come from a Normal (Gaussian) distribution

6. **Regarding types of data for statistical analysis**
   A. systolic blood pressure readings are continuous data
   B. Glasgow Coma Scale (GCS) scores are nominal data
   C. blood group data are ordinal data
   D. the number of cans of fizzy drink opened per person per day is categorical data
   E. the results of rolling dice are discrete data

7. **In a sample of 51 observations taken from a population that has a Normal distribution**
   A. the standard deviation is the square root of the sum of all the observations
   B. the median value is the average of the 25th and 26th ranked observations
   C. the interquartile range (IQR) lies between the 13th and 39th ranked observations
   D. a confidence interval around the mean will be greater than that for a sample of size 102
   E. the sample mean and median will be exactly the same

8. **Regarding data distribution**
   A. the standard deviation of the standard Normal distribution is one
   B. the Poisson distribution is defined by two parameters, the mean and variance
   C. the range of values in a Normal distribution is infinite
   D. the binomial distribution defined by $p = 0.25$ is positively skewed
   E. a t-distribution on five degrees of freedom describes the distribution of the means of samples size 6 taken from the same population

9. **When interpreting statistical test results**
   A. the sensitivity of a test is the false positive rate
   B. the power of the test is the same as the beta (β) error
   C. the probability of a type I error is determined by the investigator
   D. the probability of a false negative result is a type II error
   E. specificity is the same as the true negative rate

10. In a clinical trial

A. the placebo effect can be eliminated by randomization

B. tossing an unbiased coin is an acceptable method of randomization when equal numbers are required in two small study groups

C. randomization is used only when a new treatment is compared with a placebo control group

D. the type of statistical analysis of results is decided after the collection of data is complete

E. A Latin square method of randomization is used to minimize the effects of two possible confounding variables such as time and order of treatments

Question 1: Answer

A. True. A continuous distribution is one where any value is possible such as measuring length as opposed to discrete, where only specific values are possible such as integers when counting the number of objects.

B. False. The Normal distribution is symmetrical and bell-shaped so the mean, median, and mode are the same.

C. True. Approximately 34% within one positive and 34% within one negative standard deviation from the mean.

D. True. Approximately 95% of observations will fall within two standard deviations of the mean, 2.5% above and 2.5% below these values.

E. False. In a Normal distribution, the mean and the variance take different values.

Altman, D.G. *Practical Statistics for Medical Research*. Chapman & Hall, 1992: Chapter 4, Theoretical distributions: pp. 51–60.

Question 2: Answer

A. True. The standard deviation is the square root of the variance, so can be positive or negative, whereas variance is always positive.

B. False. The size of any sample is generally much smaller than that of the population from which it is taken, so probability tells us that the sample is less likely to contain extreme values than the population; as a result, the variance of the sample is smaller than that of the population; the sample variance is therefore biased and needs correcting before it can estimate the population variance.

C. True. The spread of values determines the variance.

D. True. One of the characteristics of a Poisson distribution is that the mean and variance are identical.

E. True. Although variance is calculated using the mean, the mean value itself only acts to place the position of the peak of the distribution along a line of all possible means; for example, the variance in height of adult males may well be the same as the variance in height of adult females but the mean value for each population (adult males and adult females) is different.

Altman, D.G. *Practical Statistics for Medical Research*. Chapman & Hall, 1992: Chapter 3, Describing data: pp. 33–36; Chapter 4, Theoretical distributions: pp. 66–67.

Question 3: Answer

A. True. A 95% confidence interval is the sample mean plus or minus the standard error of the mean (SEM) multiplied by 1.96.

B. True. SEM is defined as the standard deviation divided by the square root of the sample size.

C. True. This can be implied from the definition of SEM: the sample standard deviation is smaller than the variance and this is then divided by the sample size.

D. True. Error bars using SEM will be smaller than standard deviation and give a better measure of how reliable those values are.

E. False. The SEM is not an estimate for the population variance; it provides an estimate for the variability expected in sample means for samples of the same size taken from the same population.

Altman, D.G. *Practical Statistics for Medical Research.* Chapman & Hall, 1992: Chapter 8, Principles of Statistical Analysis: pp. 155–160.

Question 4: Answer

A. True. This is one of the two aspects of double-blinding a trial: it prevents bias from the patient when reporting symptoms.

B. False. This is the second of the two aspects of double-blinding: the clinician will not know to which group the patient is allocated, it avoids bias from the clinician.

C. True. This is important: usually the observer is the clinician looking after the patient and reporting back to the trial organizer.

D. False. The use of a placebo is not mandatory and can be detrimental to a patient's health: the 'control' part of the trial may be the standard treatment used for the particular condition being investigated.

E. False. If the design of the trial, particularly one that is long and has potentially dangerous outcomes, is such that interim analysis is included in the design then interim analysis is allowed by the statistician (but they will often inform the trial organizer only if there are issues identified such as an unexpected increase in mortality or significant morbidity).

Altman, D.G. *Practical Statistics for Medical Research.* Chapman & Hall, 1992: Chapter 15, Clinical Trials: pp. 440–455.

Question 5: Answer

A. False. Only on 95% of occasions will the 95% confidence interval (CI) for a sample mean contain the true population value.

B. True. The CI is calculated from the SEM, so a larger sample will have a smaller SEM, making the CI narrower the larger the sample. This is only true for samples taken from the same population.

C. True. The CI is calculated from the SEM, which uses the standard deviation—the square root of the variance.

D. True. For a CI to contain the true population value 95 times out of 100 the range of possible values must be greater than if it contains the true value only 90 times out of 100.

E. False. CIs can be constructed for parameters, including the mean, from many distributions as well as the Normal distribution.

Altman, D.G. *Practical Statistics for Medical Research.* Chapman & Hall, 1992: Chapter 16, Principles of Statistical Analysis: pp. 162–165.

Question 6: Answer

A. True. Any numerical value is possible, the accuracy depends on the type of machine.

B. False. GCS scores are numbers and range from 3 to 15 but each number represents a clinical state, not a value, so they should be considered categorical data. However, we would all write the possible scores in the same order, so they are ordinal categorical data.

C. False. There is no good reason to list blood groups in any particular order, so they are nominal categorical data.

D. False. These are discrete numerical data.

E. True. These are discrete data.

Altman, D.G. *Practical Statistics for Medical Research*. Chapman & Hall, 1992: Chapter 2, Types of data: pp. 10–13.

Question 7:   Answer

A. False. The standard deviation (s.d.) is the square root of the variance, which is the sum of the squared differences between each observation and the mean (m) divided by the number of observations (n) minus 1 (variance = $\Sigma(x-m)^2/(n-1)$).

B. False. The median value is the middle value of the observations when ranked from lowest to highest. When there is an odd number of observations, it is the central observation—the 26th value, with 25 values on either side.

C. True. The lower quartile is the $(n + 1)/4$th value and the upper quartile is the $3(n + 1)/4$th value: the 13th and 39th values.

D. True. The larger the sample, the smaller the SEM. The confidence interval around the mean is calculated using the SEM.

E. False. The *sample* mean and median will be close, but it is unlikely that in a small sample such as this that they will be exactly the same. The mean and the median will be the same in the *population* from which the sample was drawn.

Altman, D.G. *Practical Statistics for Medical Research*. Chapman & Hall, 1992: Chapter 3, Describing data: pp. 31–36; Chapter 8, Principles of statistical analysis: p. 154.

Question 8:   Answer

A. True. The standard Normal distribution has a mean of zero and a variance of one, so the s.d. is also one. This is sometimes written as N (0, 1).

B. False. The Poisson distribution is defined by a single parameter, λ; the mean and variance are equal. λ is the mean number of events in a given time period.

C. True. the Normal distribution is a theoretical distribution symmetric about its mean with a range of $-\infty$ to $+\infty$

D. True. A binomial distribution with a probability of success less than 0.5 is positively skewed—the lower the probability the more skewed the distribution. If the probability of success is greater than 0.5 then the distribution is negatively skewed.

E. True. A t-distribution on n degrees of freedom describes the distribution of means of sample size (n + 1) taken from a single population.

Altman, D.G. *Practical Statistics for Medical Research*. Chapman & Hall, 1992: Chapter 4, Theoretical distributions: pp. 51–68; Chapter 8, Comparing groups—continuous data: p. 181.

Question 9:   Answer

A. False. The sensitivity of a test is the true positive rate—the probability that a positive result is actually correct.

B. False. The power of a test is $(1-\beta)$, where β is the beta error.

C. True. The alpha or type I error is the probability of a false-positive result, which is set by the investigator.

D. True. A false-negative result is a type II error, usually due to insufficient data—the sample size was too small.

E. True. Specificity is the true negative rate—the probability that a negative result is actually correct.

Altman, D.G. *Practical Statistics for Medical Research.* Chapman & Hall, 1992: Chapter 14, Some common problems in medical research: p. 410; Chapter 8, Hypothesis testing: p. 169.

Question 10: Answer

A. False. The placebo effect refers to a small positive response in the control group that receives no active treatment. It is thought to be due to the patient responding to increased attention by medical staff and therefore psychologically feeling improved. This cannot be eliminated by blinding the patient to treatment.

B. False. In studies with small numbers of participants, coin-tossing is very unlikely to provide equal numbers in each of two groups. Block randomization should be used.

C. False. Some form of randomization should be used in **all** clinical trials; the control group is not necessarily a placebo treatment.

D. False. The type of data analysis should be decided before the trial is started as this will decide the number of patients to recruit. Data analysis that was not agreed before the trial is sometimes performed, but the results of this *post-hoc* analysis are not necessarily valid.

E. True. This method is used in designing trials with cross-over treatments where time might influence outcomes.

Altman, D.G. *Practical Statistics for Medical Research.* Chapman & Hall, 1992: Chapter 15, Clinical trials: pp. 450–451; Chapter 5, Designing research: pp. 85–88.

Rao, P.V. *Statistical Research Methods in the Life Sciences.* Duxbury Press, 1998: pp. 720–722.

PRACTICE FOR PART I: PAPER B

1. **When assessing a patient's airway to identify difficult intubation**
   A. Mallampati Class 3 is when the soft palate is not visible
   B. the Mallampati test shows high sensitivity
   C. the Mallampati test shows high specificity
   D. the thyro-mental distance test is more sensitive than the Mallampati test
   E. the upper lip bite test shows high specificity and sensitivity

2. **In the modified Cormack and Lehane grading of direct laryngoscopy**
   A. Grade 1 is the most frequently occurring view
   B. Grade 2a usually requires the use of another intubation aid
   C. Grade 2b means that the glottis is visible
   D. Grade 3 means that the posterior arytenoids are visible
   E. Grade 4 means that only the epiglottis is visible

3. **Minimum standards of monitoring during anaesthesia require**
   A. a depth of anaesthesia monitor in all cases of general anaesthesia
   B. temperature measurement in all cases lasting more than one hour
   C. capnography use for all patients in the recovery unit
   D. the same standards of monitoring for regional as for general anaesthesia
   E. a peripheral nerve stimulator for all cases when neuromuscular blocking agents are used

4. **Malignant hyperthermia**
   A. is a rare disease with an incidence of about 1 in 1,000,000 anaesthetics
   B. is more prevalent in the paediatric population
   C. can be triggered by thiopental
   D. initial dantrolene treatment dose is 1 mg/kg
   E. follow-up requires muscle biopsy as the first, immediate step to confirm the diagnosis

5. **To prevent adrenal crisis in patients with primary and secondary adrenal insufficiency presenting for a major elective operation**
   A. hydrocortisone 50 mg should be given intravenously at induction
   B. an infusion of hydrocortisone should be started after the initial dose at a rate of 200 mg over 24 h
   C. intramuscular administration of hydrocortisone is an acceptable alternative
   D. when oral intake resumes, the usual dose of hydrocortisone is administered orally
   E. dexamethasone could be used in place of hydrocortisone

6. **When anaesthetising a patient with morbid obesity**
   A. drug dosing should be based on total body weight
   B. obstructive sleep apnoea develops when body mass index (BMI) is over 40 kg/m²
   C. ondansetron is the agent of choice as an anti-emetic
   D. a single induction dose of propofol based on lean body mass will result in quicker wakening up compared with the non-obese patient
   E. succinylcholine is the neuromuscular blocking drug of choice during rapid sequence induction

7. **When dealing with an unexpected difficult airway**
   A. the total number of laryngoscopy attempts should be limited to three
   B. cricoid pressure should be maintained until successful intubation
   C. blind intubation through an intubating laryngeal mask airway is recommended when intubation still fails despite using all laryngoscopy attempts
   D. if facemask ventilation with the two-person technique is difficult, muscle relaxant should be given
   E. a size 5 uncuffed endotracheal tube should be used when a 'can't intubate can't oxygenate' situation has been declared

8. **When administering general anaesthesia to a patient with sickle cell disease, sickle cell crisis can be provoked by**
   A. hypothermia
   B. hypocarbia
   C. hypotension
   D. alkalosis
   E. the use of an arterial tourniquet

9. **When testing patients' pseudocholinesterase activity using dibucaine**
   A. more than 90% of patients will have a dibucaine number of 80 or higher
   B. a dibucaine number of 80 means that 80% of the patient's plasma cholinesterase is inhibited by dibucaine
   C. a dibucaine number of 20 means that patients can be paralysed for up to 4 to 8 hours after receiving succinylcholine
   D. a dibucaine number of 60 means that the patient is of a heterozygous genotype
   E. can distinguish between acquired and inherited causes of succinylcholine apnoea

10. Accidental awareness under general anaesthesia

A. is reported with an incidence of 1 in 100,000 administered anaesthetics

B. occurs more often in obese patients

C. occurs more frequently in men compared with women

D. is less likely under total intravenous anaesthesia

E. increases more than 10-fold using neuromuscular blocking drugs

11. Minimum alveolar concentration (MAC)

A. prevents reflex response to a surgical incision in 95% of the population

B. is reduced in the elderly

C. is reduced during pregnancy

D. is close to the concentration of the anaesthetic agent at the end of inspiration

E. of desflurane is 6.35% making it the most potent volatile anaesthetic

12. Following anaesthesia consisting of a propofol infusion, fentanyl, and rocuronium, a patient did not regain spontaneous breathing. Suitable treatment includes

A. administration of flumazenil

B. administration of naloxone

C. train-of-four (TOF) ratio measurement using a peripheral nerve stimulator

D. administration of neostigmine

E. hypoventilation to increase the level of CO_2 to stimulate the patient's breathing

13. Regarding capnography during general anaesthesia

A. acute haemorrhage increases end-tidal CO_2 concentration

B. pulmonary embolism leads to a gradual decrease in end-tidal CO_2 concentration

C. it confirms the position of the endotracheal tube above the carina

D. the response time of a side-stream sampling method is quicker than that of a mainstream one

E. end-tidal CO_2 is usually slightly higher than arterial CO_2

14. Contraindications for day-case surgery include

A. BMI over 35 kg/m^2

B. age over 70

C. non-elective procedures

D. insulin dependent diabetes mellitus

E. obstructive sleep apnoea

15. **When providing anaesthesia for head and neck surgery, airway conduits may include**

A. naso-tracheal tube

B. supraglottic airway device

C. jet ventilation catheter

D. tracheostomy tube

E. no airway device

16. **Transurethral resection of prostate (TURP) syndrome is characterized by**

A. high serum osmolality

B. hypernatraemia

C. hypovolaemia

D. early hypertension

E. visual loss

17. **Features of thyroid storm under general anaesthesia include**

A. body temperature above 38°C

B. heart rate more than 100 beats per minute

C. hypercalcaemia

D. atrial fibrillation

E. a high plasma level of thyroid stimulating hormone (TSH)

18. **Acute intermittent porphyria (AIP)**

A. is more common in elderly men

B. can cause severe muscle weakness leading to respiratory failure

C. treatment includes hemin solution

D. can be precipitated by benzodiazepines

E. can be diagnosed by estimating the plasma level of porphobilinogen

19. **Regarding the provision of anaesthesia away from the operating theatre**

A. usually requires only the application of a pulse oximeter

B. cardiovascular instability is the main complication due to oversedation

C. most complications occur during gastroenterological procedures

D. conscious sedation means that no airway manipulation should be needed

E. barbiturates are an acceptable choice of sedation for children undergoing CT scan

20. **Permanent visual loss after general anaesthesia occurs as a recognized complication of**

A. cardiac surgery

B. transurethral resection of the prostate

C. cataract excision

D. spinal surgery

E. head and neck surgery

21. **When providing general anaesthesia for surgery involving a laser**
    A. the long wavelength of a CO_2 laser means that eye protection is unnecessary
    B. the most common hazard is an airway fire
    C. nitrous oxide should be used to reduce the oxygen concentration when volatile anaesthesia is used for laser surgery of the airway
    D. use of the neodymium:yttrium-aluminium-garnet (Nd:YAG) laser has been associated with venous gas embolism
    E. all windows into the operating room must be covered when using lasers

22. **When assessing the risk for postoperative nausea and vomiting (PONV) using the Apfel simplified risk score**
    A. female gender scores one point
    B. use of a volatile anaesthetic scores one point
    C. duration of anaesthesia is not included in the simplified risk score
    D. the maximum score is four points
    E. a score of two points is associated with a 50% risk of PONV

23. **During general anaesthesia for intra-abdominal laparoscopic surgery in a patient with normal cardiac and respiratory function**
    A. urine output is maintained at baseline level during pneumoperitoneum
    B. left-ventricular ejection fraction is reduced by 30% when intra-abdominal pressure increases to 15 mmHg
    C. endobronchial intubation can occur during laparoscopic cholecystectomy
    D. the incidence of fatal gas embolism during laparoscopic surgery is between 0.01% and 0.05%
    E. initial treatment of capnothorax is the insertion of a chest drain

24. **Regarding preoperative assessment of an adult patient undergoing non-cardiac surgery**
    A. a well-designed, standardized questionnaire that is completed by the patient in advance of surgery is recommended as a screening tool
    B. there is good evidence that abstaining from alcohol for one week prior to surgery reduces morbidity
    C. routine chest radiography in patients over 60 years of age is recommended
    D. the recommended period for smoking cessation prior to surgery is a minimum of four weeks
    E. a calculated glomerular filtration rate (cGFR) is a better predictor of renal impairment than serum creatinine

25. Recommended coagulation management during severe perioperative bleeding includes

A. intravenous fibrinogen concentrate should be used if the plasma fibrinogen level is below 1.5 g/l

B. cryoprecipitate should be the first-line treatment for patients who were on oral anticoagulant therapy preoperatively

C. desmopressin is recommended in the treatment of hypothermic coagulopathy

D. there is no place for the use of vitamin K for any patient experiencing perioperative bleeding

E. in the presence of adequate fibrinogen levels and low clot strength, factor XIII concentrate should be administered

Question 1: Answer

A. False. Modified Mallampati Class 3 is when the soft palate is visible but only the base of the uvula can be seen.

B. False. The original Mallampati test has a sensitivity of 0.42 and the modified test has a sensitivity of 0.51.

C. True. The original Mallampati test has a specificity of 0.93; that of the modified test is 0.87.

D. False. The thyro-mental distance test has a sensitivity of 0.24 in predicting difficult intubation.

E. True. Several studies have shown a sensitivity of > 0.7 and specificity of > 0.85.

Faramarzi, E. et al. Upper lip bite test for prediction of difficult airway: a systematic review. *Pak J Med Sci*, 2018;34(4):1019–1023.

Roth, D. et al. Bedside tests for predicting difficult airways: an abridged Cochrane diagnostic test accuracy systematic review. *Anaesthesia*, 2019;74:915–928.

Samsoon, G.L.T. and Young, J.R.B. Difficult tracheal intubation: a retrospective study. *Anaesthesia*, 1987;42:487–490.

Question 2: Answer

A. True. Up to 68% of all laryngoscopies are of Grade 1 view.

B. False. Grade 2a usually does not require any additional intubation aids with only a small proportion of the upper part of the glottis not visible.

C. True. In Grade 2b most of the glottis is obscured from view but still visible. However, this usually means that an additional intubation aid (e.g., bougie) is required.

D. False. In Grade 3 only the epiglottis is visible.

E. False. In Grade 4 neither epiglottis nor glottis are visible.

Yentis, S.M. and Lee, D.J. Evaluation of an improved scoring system for the grading of direct laryngoscopy. *Anaesthesia*, 1998;53:1041–1044.

Question 3: Answer

A. False. Depth of anaesthesia monitoring is recommended when using total intravenous anaesthesia with neuromuscular blockade.

B. False. Temperature measurement should be used for any procedure of more than 30 min duration.

C. False. Capnography in the recovery unit is required if the patient has a tracheal tube, supraglottic airway device in situ, or is deeply sedated.

D. True. The same standards of monitoring apply when the anaesthetist is responsible for local/regional anaesthesia or sedation techniques.

E. True. A peripheral nerve stimulator must be used whenever neuromuscular blocking drugs are given. A quantitative peripheral nerve stimulator is recommended.

Checketts, M.R. et al. Recommendations for standards of monitoring during anaesthesia and recovery 2015: Association of Anaesthetists of Great Britain and Ireland. *Anaesthesia*, 2016;71:85–93.

Question 4: Answer

A. False. Malignant hyperthermia (MH) is a rare disease, but the incidence is between 1 in 10,000 and 1 in 150,000 anaesthetics.

B. True. The highest reported incidence of MH occurs in paediatric populations and there is also a consistently higher incidence of MH in men compared with women.

C. False. The causative agents are succinylcholine and volatile anaesthetic agents.

D. False. The initial dantrolene treatment dose is 2–3 mg/kg. Subsequent doses of 1 mg/kg are recommended until the treatment goals are achieved.

E. False. The first follow-up step is DNA screening. If a genetic change associated with MH is not found, the patient will then undergo a muscle biopsy if they are old enough (over 10 y). For index cases who are younger than 10, with a negative genetic test, both parents will be offered muscle biopsy tests. It should be noted that the muscle biopsy will not be done within 4 months of an acute reaction as the response of previously damaged muscle is unreliable.

Hopkins, P.M. et al. Malignant hyperthermia 2020. *Anaesthesia*, 2021;76(5):655–664.

Question 5: Answer

A. False. 100 mg intravenously at induction is recommended.

B. True. The initial dose is followed by an intravenous infusion of 200 mg over 24 h.

C. True. Alternatively, hydrocortisone 50 mg could be given every 6 h by intramuscular injection.

D. False. When oral intake is resumed, hydrocortisone doses are doubled for 48 h or for up to a week following major surgery.

E. False. Dexamethasone is not adequate for treatment in primary adrenal insufficiency as it has no mineralocorticoid activity.

Woodcock, T. et al. Guidelines for the management of glucocorticoids during the peri-operative period for patients with adrenal insufficiency: Guidelines from the Association of Anaesthetists, the Royal College of Physicians and the Society for Endocrinology UK. *Anaesthesia*, 2020;75(5):654–663.

Question 6: Answer

A. False. Drug dosing should generally be based upon lean body weight and titrated to effect, rather than on total body weight.

B. False. Severe obstructive sleep apnoea (OSA) occurs in 10–20% of patients with BMI > 35 kg/m^2 and is often undiagnosed.

C. False. There is evidence of an increased incidence of prolonged QT interval with increasing BMI and therefore a potential increased risk with drugs such as ondansetron.

D. True. In the obese patient, after a bolus of an anaesthetic induction agent, anaesthesia will occur before redistribution from the central compartment, and the induction dose required to produce unconsciousness correlates well with lean body weight. However, more rapid redistribution of induction agents into the larger fat mass means that patients wake up more quickly than non-obese patients after a single bolus dose.

E. False. Succinylcholine-associated fasciculations increase oxygen consumption and have been shown to shorten the safe apnoea time. Consequently, it is unlikely to wear off before profound hypoxia occurs, and so may not be the drug of choice for obese patients. With the advent of sugammadex, aminosteroids (e.g. rocuronium) could instead be considered the neuromuscular blocking drugs of choice.

Nightingale, C.E. et al. Peri-operative management of the obese surgical patient 2015. *Anaesthesia*, 2015;70:859–876.

Question 7: Answer

A. False. The number of attempts at laryngoscopy should be limited to three by the original operator. However, a fourth attempt could be undertaken by a more experienced colleague. Hence, the total number of attempts is 3 plus 1.

B. False. Cricoid pressure should be removed during Plan A if laryngoscopy was difficult and (in the absence of regurgitation) should remain off during insertion of a supraglottic airway device.

C. False. First-attempt success rates are higher using fibreoptic guidance; a guided technique has been shown to be of benefit in patients with difficult airways. There is potential for serious adverse outcomes with blind techniques: with repeated insertion attempts to achieve success and a low first-time success rate even with second-generation devices, the blind technique is redundant.

D. True. If it is not possible to maintain oxygenation using a face mask, ensuring full paralysis before critical hypoxia develops offers a final chance of rescuing the airway without recourse to Plan D.

E. False. A size 6 cuffed endotracheal tube is recommended in Plan D when a 'can't intubate, can't oxygenate' scenario has been declared.

Frerk, C. et al. Difficult Airway Society 2015 guidelines for management of unanticipated difficult intubation in adults. *Br J Anaesthesia, 115*(6):827–848.

Question 8: Answer

A. True.

B. False. Hypercarbia can precipitate a sickle cell crisis (SCC), not hypocarbia.

C. True. Hypotension and hypovolaemia may precipitate SCC.

D. False. Acidosis can precipitate SCC.

E. True. The use of an arterial tourniquet is contraindicated in patients with sickle cell disease.

Miller, R.D. et al. *Miller's Anesthesia*, 8th edition. Elsevier, 2015: Chapter 39, p. 1211.

Smith, T., Pinnock, C., and Lin, T. *Fundamentals of Anaesthesia*. Cambridge University Press, 2009: Section 1, Chapter 1, p.18.

Question 9: Answer

A. True. Up to 94% of patients have a normal homozygous genotype and will metabolize succinylcholine within 1–5 min.

B. True. The dibucaine number represents the percentage inhibition of the enzyme by the local anaesthetic dibucaine. Normal individuals, who are homozygous for the wild-type gene, have a dibucaine number of 80 because their plasma cholinesterase is 80% inhibited by dibucaine.

C. True. Individuals who are homozygous for the atypical genes have a dibucaine number of 20 (corresponding to 20% inhibition) and can be paralysed for up to 4 to 8 hours after receiving succinylcholine.

D. True. A dibucaine number of 60 means that the patient is heterozygous and may have a prolonged reaction to succinylcholine for up to 10 min.

E. True. Patients with acquired causes of reduced efficiency of plasma cholinesterase will have a normal dibucaine number of 80 and the action of succinylcholine will only be prolonged by few minutes.

Miller, R.D. et al. *Miller's Anesthesia*, 8th edition. Elsevier, 2015: Part IV, Chapter 38, pp. 1135–1136.

Question 10: Answer

A. False. Accidental awareness under general anaesthesia (AAGA) is reported with an incidence of 1 in 19,600 according to the largest patient-centred report, the 5th National Audit Project (NAP5) of the Royal College of Anaesthetists.

B. True. Obese patients were three times more likely to experience AAGA.

C. False. 74% of claims of AAGA are from women.

D. False. AAGA occurred in 18% of cases when total intravenous anaesthesia was used vs. 8% overall.

E. True. The incidence of AAGA increased from 1 in 135,000 to 1 in 8200 general anaesthetics when neuromuscular blocking drugs were used.

Pandit, J.J. et al. The 5th National Audit Project (NAP5) on accidental awareness during general anaesthesia: summary of main findings and risk factors. *Anaesthesia*, 2014;69:1089–1101.

Question 11: Answer

A. False. MAC is defined as that concentration of anaesthetic agent that will prevent reflex response to a skin incision in 50% of a population.

B. True. MAC is reduced in the elderly, with pregnancy, the addition of opioids, local anaesthetics, intravenous anaesthetics, hypothermia, anaemia, hypercarbia, hypoxia, and hypotension.

C. True. See above.

D. False. The MAC of the agent is measured at the end of exhalation, it is an end-tidal concentration.

E. False. The lower the MAC value the more potent the inhalational anaesthetic. Desflurane is the least potent compared with halothane, enflurane, isoflurane, and sevoflurane.

Smith, T., Pinnock, C., and Lin, T. *Fundamentals of Anaesthesia*. Cambridge University Press, 2009: Section 3, Chapter 5, pp. 559–561.

Question 12: Answer

A. False. Flumazenil is a competitive benzodiazepine receptor antagonist. It will reverse the action of benzodiazepines only.

B. True. Naloxone will reverse the action of fentanyl that could have been administered in an excessive dose.

C. True. TOF ratio measurement may show that this patient is still deeply paralysed and requires reversal using either neostigmine or sugammadex.

D. True. Administration of neostigmine will reverse the residual action of rocuronium. However, the depth of the neuro-muscular blockade needs to be assessed by using the TOF ratio beforehand.

E. False. This method may work if a patient is adequately reversed, and no excessive dose of opioids was given. Otherwise, this approach leads to hypercapnia and respiratory acidosis further compromising the level of consciousness.

Peck T.E. and Hill S.A. *Pharmacology for Anaesthesia and Intensive Care*, 4th edition. Cambridge University Press, 2014.

Question 13: Answer

A. False. Acute haemorrhage leads to hypoperfusion of all tissues hence less CO_2 will be produced and exhaled.

B. False. Pulmonary embolism leads to a very rapid drop in end-tidal CO_2 concentration due to sudden hypoperfusion of the lungs.

C. False. Capnography confirms that the endotracheal tube is sited in the trachea but cannot distinguish between bilateral or unilateral lung ventilation. The former is confirmed by auscultation, fibreoptic, or imaging techniques.

D. True. The response time is quicker using a mainstream sampling method.

E. False. End-tidal CO_2 is usually slightly lower than arterial CO_2 since a pressure gradient is essential for diffusion.

Miller, R.D. et al. *Miller's Anesthesia*, 8th edition. Elsevier, 2015: Chapter 51, pp. 1551–1555.

Question 14: Answer

A. False. Fitness for a procedure should relate to the patient's functional status as determined at pre-anaesthetic assessment, and not by ASA physical status, age, or BMI. The only patients routinely not included in day surgery are those with unstable medical conditions.

B. False. See above.

C. False. Patients presenting with acute conditions requiring urgent surgery can be efficiently and effectively treated as day cases via a semi-elective pathway.

D. False. Patients with a stable chronic disease such as diabetes are often better managed as day cases because there is minimal disruption to their daily routine.

E. False. See explanations above in answer to option A.

Bailey, C.R. et al. Guidelines for day-case surgery 2019: guidelines from the Association of Anaesthetists and the British Association of Day Surgery. *Anaesthesia*, 2019;74(6):778–792.

Question 15: Answer

A. True. All these devices could be used depending on the duration of the operation and nature of the disease process.

B. True.

C. True.

D. True.

E. True. Open airway surgery could be performed using high-flow nasal oxygen apnoeic oxygenation and carbon dioxide elimination for short-lasting procedures.

Charters, P. et al. Anaesthesia for head and neck surgery: United Kingdom National Multidisciplinary Guidelines. *J Laryngol Otol*, 2016;*130*(S2):S23–S27.

Patel, A. and Nouraei, S.A.R. Transnasal Humidified Rapid-Insufflation Ventilatory Exchange (THRIVE): a physiological method of increasing apnoea time in patients with difficult airways. *Anaesthesia*, 2015;70:323–329.

Question 16: Answer

A. False. The TURP syndrome presents within 15 min to 24 hours after the operation and is characterized by cardiovascular, respiratory, neurological, and metabolic features. Serum osmolality usually drops due to hyponatraemia.

B. False. See answer A.

C. False. Hypervolaemia usually develops due to increased absorption of irrigation fluid.

D. True. Initially, hypertension develops due to increased irrigation fluid absorption followed by hypotension due to heart failure leading to pulmonary oedema.

E. True. Possible mechanisms underlying visual changes include cerebral oedema, glycine toxicity involving the retina and cerebral cortex, ammonia toxicity, and increased intraocular pressure (IOP).

Miller, R.D. et al. *Miller's Anesthesia*, 8th edition. Elsevier, 2015: Chapter 72, pp. 2229–2235, Chapter 100, pp. 3028–3029.

Question 17: Answer

A. True. The Burch-Wartofsky Point Scale for diagnosis of thyroid storm includes increase in temperature above 38°C, tachycardia more than 130 beats per minute, atrial fibrillation, symptoms of congestive heart failure, gastrointestinal-hepatic dysfunction (nausea, vomiting, diarrhoea) and central nervous system (CNS) disturbance (less than 14 on the Glasgow Coma Scale).

B. False. See answer A.

C. False. Hypercalcaemia is one of the features of hyperparathyroidism.

D. True. See answer A.

E. False. In the presence of thyrotoxicosis, a reduced plasma level of TSH will be observed with elevated levels of free triiodothyronine (FT3) or free thyroxine (FT4).

Miller, R.D. et al. *Miller's Anesthesia*, 8th edition. Elsevier, 2015: Chapter 39, p. 1116, 1173–1175.

Satoh, T. et al. 2016 Guidelines for the management of thyroid storm from The Japan Thyroid Association and Japan Endocrine Society (First edition). *Endocr J*, 2016;63(12):1025–1064.

Question 18: Answer

A. False. AIP typically occurs in young adults and is more common in women.

B. True. Muscle weakness can be so severe that respiratory failure ensues.

C. True. Specific therapy for an acute attack is the infusion of hemin solution that inhibits 5-aminolevulinic acid synthase and decreases the production of toxic intermediates. Liver transplantation has been effective for some patients with AIP.

D. True. AIP can be precipitated by many drugs including sedatives: benzodiazepines, etomidate, and barbiturates.

E. True. Urinary porphobilinogen is the first test to consider as it is markedly elevated during an acute attack and can be detected with a rapid test kit within 5 minutes. However, a raised level of porphobilinogen in plasma can also be diagnostic.

Barash, P.G. et al. *Clinical Anesthesia*, 8th edition. Wolters Kluwer, 2017: Chapter 24, pp. 1573–1577.

Question 19: Answer

A. False. In all cases, the standards of anaesthesia care and monitoring should be no different from those provided in the conventional operating room.

B. False. Respiratory depression secondary to oversedation was the most common type of adverse event in a closed claims study.

C. False. Adverse events appear to occur more frequently in patients undergoing radiology procedures and in cardiology.

D. True. Conscious sedation usually means that no airway manipulation is required, adequate spontaneous ventilation is preserved, cardiovascular stability is maintained, and the patient has a purposeful response to verbal and tactile stimulation.

E. False. Older sedation practices in paediatric patients included the use of oral chloral hydrate, 'lytic cocktails', and barbiturates. These techniques, however, are being superseded by the use of short-acting agents including propofol, remifentanil, and dexmedetomidine, which provide more reliable pharmacologic profiles and have preferable track records for adverse events.

Barash, P.G. et al. *Clinical Anesthesia*, 8th edition. Wolters Kluwer, 2017: Chapter 33, pp. 2183–2226.

Question 20: Answer

A. True. Open heart cardiac surgery is associated with the formation of emboli that may occlude the retinal arteries.

B. False. Only transient visual loss may occur after transurethral resection of the prostate (TURP) due to cerebral oedema, glycine toxicity involving the retina and cerebral cortex, ammonia toxicity, and increased IOP in case of TURP syndrome development.

C. False. There is no evidence that cataract excision causes permanent visual loss. However, if performed under peribulbar or sub-Tenon blockade temporary visual loss occurs lasting for the duration of the blockade.

D. True. Patients who undergo prolonged spinal operative procedures in the prone position with large blood loss are at high risk for development of ischaemic optic neuropathy (ION) due to excessive compression of the eyeballs.

E. True. Central retinal artery (CRA) occlusion has occurred after neck and nasal or sinus surgery, although most cases of visual loss in neck dissection are from ION. The incidence of orbital complications after endoscopic sinus surgery is 0.12%. Orbital haemorrhage from blunt trauma during the procedure can result in orbital compartment syndrome. Indirect damage to the CRA from intra-arterial injections of 1% lidocaine with adrenaline has also been described; the mechanism of action is thought to be arterial spasm or embolism.

Miller, R.D. et al. *Miller's Anesthesia*, 8th edition. Elsevier, 2015: Chapter 100, pp. 3011–3030.

Question 21: Answer

A. False. Carbon dioxide lasers have the longest wavelength but can still cause eye damage, so plain plastic or glass goggles must be worn.

B. False. Airway fires may occur, especially during airway procedures using lasers, but in general the most common hazards are gas embolism and vascular- or organ-perforation.

C. False. Nitrous oxide supports combustion as it will dissociate when exposed to fire releasing heat and free oxygen, so it should not be used with volatile agents. Medical air should be used instead.

D. True. The Nd:YAG laser penetrates more deeply than the CO_2 laser and vessels that are not clearly visible can be damaged and gas embolism is a recognized complication.

E. True. Energy beams from lasers, apart from CO_2 lasers, can pass through glass so all OR windows must be covered, and a warning sign posted outside all doors to the OR.

Miller, R.D. et al. *Miller's Anesthesia*, 8th edition. Elsevier, 2015: Chapter 88, pp. 2601–2607.

Question 22: Answer

A. True. The Apfel simplified risk score for PONV scores one point for each of: female gender; non-smoking status; a history of previous PONV or motion sickness and finally the use of postoperative opioid analgesics.

B. False. Although there is good evidence that the incidence of PONV is higher following a volatile anaesthetic than total intravenous anaesthesia, this is not part of the Apfel score as described above.

C. True. See answer A.

D. True. See answer A.

E. False. The risk of PONV with a score of two points is 40%. The risk for scores of 0, 1, 2, 3, 4 are 10%, 20%, 40%, 60%, and 80%, respectively.

Miller, R.D. et al. *Miller's Anesthesia*, 8th edition. Elsevier, 2015: Chapter 97, p. 2947.

Question 23: Answer

A. False. The increase in intra-abdominal pressure (IAP) reduces the glomerular filtration rate and urine output falls to 50% of the preoperative baseline level.

B. False. In a patient without cardiovascular disease, left-ventricular ejection fraction does not decrease significantly during pneumoperitoneum despite an increase in afterload.

C. True. There is a risk of the endotracheal tube being displaced into one of the main bronchi during pneumoperitoneum, whether in the head-up or head-down position. This is related to the cephalad movement of the diaphragm and carina.

D. False. The risk of fatal gas embolism is lower than 0.01% (1 in 10,000 cases). The quoted incidence is around 1.4 in 100,000 or 0.0014%.

E. False. Initial treatment of capnothorax is decompression of the abdomen, application of positive end-expiratory pressure (PEEP) and hyperventilation to encourage and treat hypercapnia. In most incidences, capnothorax can be treated conservatively.

Barash, P.G. et al. *Clinical Anesthesia*, 8th edition. Wolters Kluwer, 2017: Chapter 44 p 3150–3156; 3165–3157.

Question 24: Answer

A. True. The most important feature of a preoperative questionnaire is that it is well-designed and allows screening for co-morbidities that might need further evaluation. The questionnaire should be computerized wherever possible.

B. False. There is little evidence that a short period of abstention from alcohol is of any benefit preoperatively.

C. False. Chest radiography rarely identifies features that predict perioperative morbidity and is not recommended for routine use.

D. True. Ideally 6–8 weeks is the recommended period for smoking cessation, but the minimum time recommended in the European Society of Anaesthesiology and Intensive Care (ESAIC) guidelines is four weeks.

E. True. Although serum creatinine is commonly used to identify preoperative renal impairment, a calculated glomerular filtration rate (GFR) is superior. There are several methods that are used but all predict impaired renal function better than serum creatinine alone.

De Hert, S. et al. Task Force on Preoperative Evaluation of the Adult Noncardiac Surgery Patient of the European Society of Anaesthesiology. Preoperative evaluation of the adult patient undergoing non-cardiac surgery: guidelines from the European Society of Anaesthesiology. *Eur J Anaesthesiol*, 2011;28(10):684–722.

Question 25: Answer

A. True. The ESAIC guidelines suggest that a trigger for fibrinogen concentrate administration should be < 1.5–2 g/l, when an initial dose of 20–50 mg/kg should be administered.

B. False. The first-line treatment recommended for patients on preoperative anticoagulants is prothrombin complex and vitamin K. Cryoprecipitate is recommended for management of hypofibrinogenaemia, but only if fibrinogen concentrate is not available.

C. False. The recommended treatment for hypothermic coagulopathy is recombinant Factor VIIa. Desmopressin (DDAVP) is recommended only for acquired von Willebrand syndrome.

D. False. Vitamin K is recommended for patients on preoperative anticoagulants, particularly warfarin and coumarins.

E. True. In the presence of a normal fibrinogen level but low clot strength, it is likely that factor XIII fibrin (stabilizing factor) activity is significantly low. If FXIII activity is < 60%, then 30 IU/kg FXIII concentrate can be administered.

Kozek-Langenecker, S.A. et al. Management of severe perioperative bleeding: guidelines from the European Society of Anaesthesiology. *Eur J Anaesthesiol*, 2013;30(6):270–382.

1. **The following regional anaesthesia and analgesia components are recognized as part of an enhanced recovery pathway for total knee arthroplasty**
   A. opioid-free spinal anaesthesia
   B. single-injection adductor canal block
   C. continuous adductor canal block
   D. local infiltration analgesia (LIA)
   E. perineural dexamethasone

2. **Compared with general anaesthesia, neuraxial anaesthesia for primary total hip arthroplasty is associated with a reduced incidence of the following postoperative events**
   A. surgical site infection
   B. pneumonia
   C. the need for blood product transfusion
   D. urinary retention
   E. 30 (thirty) day mortality

3. **Regarding intercostal nerve block (ICNB)**
   A. it is indicated for postoperative pain relief after lower abdominal surgery
   B. it is a useful adjunct to multimodal analgesia for the management of abdominal visceral pain
   C. it is considered to be safe in patients with mild coagulation disorders
   D. for a multiple-injection ICNB 10 ml of 0.25% bupivacaine is injected at each level to provide adequate block
   E. bilateral ICNB is an appropriate choice of regional analgesia for bilateral multiple rib fractures

4. **Regarding intravenous regional anaesthesia (IVRA)**
   A. IVRA can be used for surgical procedures or manipulations for both upper and lower extremities, with lower limbs requiring greater volumes of local anaesthetic solution
   B. 30–50 ml of 0.5% lidocaine is an appropriate dose and volume for a 3-hour upper limb procedure in a 70 kg adult
   C. an absolute contraindication to IVRA is anticoagulation
   D. mepivacaine is a suitable local anaesthetic for IVRA
   E. both proximal and distal cuffs are inflated at the same time, with the proximal cuff deflated 25–30 min after the onset of anaesthesia

5. **Regarding risks associated with abdominal blocks**
    A. inadvertent femoral nerve block is a recognized complication of ilioinguinal and iliohypogastric blocks in adult but not paediatric patients
    B. neurological injury due to needle trauma is a common complication
    C. rectus sheath block is not associated with the inadvertent spread of local anaesthetic to the lumbar plexus
    D. the risk of local anaesthetic (LA) systemic toxicity following abdominal wall blocks is generally low due to poor vascularization of intermuscular tissue planes
    E. following transversus abdominis plane (TAP) block, the average time to peak plasma concentration is 15 min

6. **Regarding contraindications to central neuraxial blockade (CNB)**
    A. patient refusal is an absolute contraindication
    B. increased intracranial pressure is an absolute contraindication to both spinal and epidural CNB
    C. CNB is used safely in patients with mild coagulation disorders
    D. sepsis is a relative contraindication for the administration of epidural analgesia
    E. significant spinal deformity such as scoliosis is an absolute contraindication

7. **The following information can be obtained during ultrasound imaging of the lumbar spine in adults**
    A. location of the midline in morbidly obese patients
    B. identification of the optimal interspace
    C. identification of the angle of approach
    D. estimation of the depth to the ligamentum flavum/dura complex
    E. spinal cord termination level

8. **Regarding spinal blockade**
    A. the spinal cord terminates at L1/2 in 90% of the population and in 10% at L2/3 or lower
    B. Tuffier's line joins the iliac crests and reliably passes through the body of L4
    C. with the midline approach the needle passes through supraspinous and interspinous ligaments, and ligamentum flavum before passing through the dura and adjacent arachnoid mater meninges
    D. spinal stenosis may cause a very slow cerebrospinal fluid (CSF) flow or 'dry' tap
    E. a Sprotte type spinal needle is associated with a higher risk of incomplete or short duration block

9. **Regarding epidural blockade**
    A. the tip of the scapula usually corresponds to T8
    B. mid-thoracic epidural insertion often requires a paramedian approach
    C. severe itching caused by epidural opioids can respond to ondansetron
    D. following observed accidental dural puncture with an epidural needle, inserting an epidural catheter intrathecally and running continuous spinal anaesthesia has been shown to reduce the incidence of post-dural puncture headache (PDPH)
    E. the last dose of prophylactic low molecular weight heparin (LMWH) should not be administered within 12 hours of attempted CNB

10. **A 70 kg elderly patient with normal BMI (body mass index) and a history of mild aortic stenosis and pulmonary fibrosis with significantly decreased respiratory reserve requires an open reduction and external fixation of an open fractured ankle. The following regional anaesthesia and analgesia techniques are appropriate**

   A. a single-shot spinal block with 2.75 ml of 0.5% hyperbaric bupivacaine and popliteal and adductor canal peripheral nerve blocks for postoperative pain relief

   B. a combination of a single-shot spinal block with 3 ml of 2% hyperbaric prilocaine for surgical anaesthesia and popliteal and adductor canal peripheral nerve blocks for postoperative pain relief

   C. a combination of distal sciatic (popliteal) and adductor canal peripheral nerve blocks and sedation

   D. a single-shot spinal block with 3 ml of 5% hyperbaric lidocaine and patient-controlled analgesia postoperatively

   E. a single-shot spinal block with 2.5 ml of 0.5% hyperbaric bupivacaine with 0.5 mcg of preservative-free morphine

11. **The following statements are true regarding local and regional anaesthesia for ophthalmic surgery**

   A. sub-Tenon's block is associated with a high incidence of the oculo-cardiac reflex

   B. topical anaesthesia is a recognized technique for cataract surgery using phacoemulsification

   C. topical lidocaine causes corneal epithelial toxicity

   D. modern retrobulbar blocks are performed with the eye in the neutral position to minimize the risk of optic nerve injury

   E. a high degree of myopia decreases the risk of unintentional eye globe perforation during eye blocks

12. **The following statements are correct regarding cervical plexus blocks**

   A. cervical plexus blocks are divided into superficial, intermediate, and deep cervical

   B. deep cervical plexus block is recommended for carotid endarterectomy

   C. superficial cervical plexus block is likely to cause hemi-diaphragmatic paralysis

   D. deep cervical plexus block can cause Horner's syndrome

   E. superficial cervical plexus block can be used for analgesia after thyroid surgery

13. **The following statements are correct regarding proximal upper limb blocks**

   A. a curved ultrasound probe is required for axillary brachial plexus block in obese patients

   B. in patients with mild anticoagulation abnormalities axillary block is preferred over the infraclavicular approach

   C. at the level of the axilla, the musculocutaneous, median, ulnar, and radial nerves always lie in four quadrants around the axillary artery

   D. ultrasound guidance decreases complications compared with a multiple-nerve stimulation technique

   E. a successful axillary block results in anaesthesia of the entire proximal arm

14. **The following statements are correct regarding sciatic nerve block at different levels**

    A. in the popliteal fossa, a curved ultrasound probe is required in obese patients
    B. the in-plane approach in the popliteal fossa is preferable to the out-of-plane approach
    C. for continuous popliteal sciatic nerve blockade, placement of a catheter using the lateral approach is advantageous compared to the prone or the supine position with the leg raised
    D. if nerve stimulator guidance is used for anterior sciatic nerve block, a patellar twitch is sought to locate the nerve
    E. successful blockade of the sciatic nerve using the posterior approach results in complete sensory loss in the lower leg

15. **Regarding regional anaesthesia and analgesia in patients with pre-existing neurological conditions**

    A. multiple sclerosis is a contraindication to epidural analgesia in labour
    B. undiagnosed spinal stenosis is a risk factor for cauda equina syndrome following epidural anaesthesia
    C. peripheral blocks do not exacerbate the symptoms of amyotrophic lateral sclerosis
    D. neuraxial anaesthesia is considered safe and effective in preventing intraoperative autonomic dysreflexia in patients with spinal cord injury
    E. addition of adrenaline (epinephrine) to LA is considered safe in patients with diabetic polyneuropathy

Question 1: Answer

A. True. Recent large population-based studies showed that neuraxial anaesthesia is associated with superior results for most but not all outcomes compared with general anaesthesia (GA). When spinal anaesthesia is used as part of the enhanced recovery pathway, opioids should be avoided to minimize the risk of urinary retention, pruritis, PONV, etc. Also, it should be noted that some studies provide evidence of good outcomes for GA in combination with peripheral blocks and/or LIA.

B. True. Both single and continuous adductor canal blocks (ACBs) induce less quadriceps weakness compared to single-shot or continuous femoral block. It is not proven that femoral nerve blocks provide superior analgesia.

C. True. As above.

D. True. Many randomized controlled trials (RCTs) have shown that LIA is associated with better pain scores and lower opioid requirements up to 72 h after surgery.

E. False. There is no consistent data showing that perineural administration of dexamethasone is superior to intravenous.

Kopp, S. et al. Anaesthesia and analgesia practice pathway options for total knee arthroplasty: an evidence-based review by the American and European Societies of Regional Anaesthesia and Pain Medicine. *Reg Anesth Pain Med*, 2017;42 (6):683–697.

Memtsoudis, S.G. et al. Anaesthetic care of patients undergoing primary hip and knee arthroplasty: consensus recommendations from the International Consensus on Anaesthesia-Related Outcomes after Surgery group (ICAROS) based on a systematic review and meta-analysis. *Br J Anaesth*, 2019;123(3):269–287.

Question 2: Answer

A. True. Recent systematic reviews and meta-analysis showed that among all hip arthroplasties neuraxial anaesthesia (NA) was associated with fewer complications in most categories, except for urinary retention, when compared with patients who received GA. Therefore, in the absence of contraindications and with the patient's agreement, NA can be advocated as a preferred anaesthetic technique for total hip arthroplasty.

B. True. As above.

C. True. As above.

D. False. As above.

E. True. As above.

Memtsoudis, S.G. et al. Anaesthetic care of patients undergoing primary hip and knee arthroplasty: consensus recommendations from the International Consensus on Anaesthesia-Related Outcomes after Surgery group (ICAROS) based on a systematic review and meta-analysis. *Br J Anaesth*, 2019;123(3):269–287.

Perlas, A., Chan, V.W.S., and Beattie, S. Anesthesia technique and mortality after total hip or knee arthroplasty: a retrospective, propensity score–matched cohort study. *Anesthesiology*, 2016;125(4):724–731.

Question 3: Answer

A. False. The intercostal nerves innervate most of the skin and musculature of the chest and abdominal wall. Intercostal nerve block (ICNB) is used in a variety of acute and chronic conditions affecting the thorax and upper abdomen, including breast and chest wall surgery. It is not suitable for lower abdominal surgery.

B. False. ICNB does not provide analgesia for visceral pain.

C. True. A disorder of coagulation is not an absolute contraindication and the benefits need to be weighed against the risks.

D. False. 3–5 ml of LA is required at each level to provide adequate block, this—in conjunction with a high absorption rate—makes this block a high risk for systemic LA toxicity (LAST).

E. False. ICNB provides excellent analgesia for rib fractures. However, if applied bilaterally, there is a high risk of LAST and risk of bilateral pneumothorax with devastating consequences.

Hadzic, A. *Textbook of Regional Anesthesia and Acute Pain Management,* 2nd edition. McGraw Hill, 2017: pp. 1374–1379.

Question 4: Answer

A. True. A bigger volume for lower extremities is required to fill the larger vascular compartment.

B. False. IVRA is recommended for procedures for up to an hour.

C. False. Patient refusal is the only absolute contraindication.

D. False. Lidocaine and prilocaine are preferred in the USA and Europe, respectively. The potent vasoconstrictive properties of mepivacaine detract from its overall attractiveness as an agent for IVRA.

E. False. The distal cuff is inflated 25–30 min after the onset of anaesthesia or when the patient complains of tourniquet pain; after its inflation, the proximal cuff can be deflated.

Hadzic, A. *Textbook of Regional Anesthesia and Acute Pain Management,* 2nd edition. McGraw Hill, 2017: pp. 301–316.

Question 5: Answer

A. False. This complication is possible in both groups of patients.

B. False. Up to the time of writing, this has not been reported, most likely because the nerves are small.

C. True. This is correct.

D. False. The intermuscular tissue plane presents a large well-vascularized surface for LA absorption.

E. False. It is 30–45 min.

Chin K.J., McDonnell J.G., Carvalho B., Sharkey A., Pawa A., Gadsden J.: Essentials of Our Current Understanding: Abdominal Wall Blocks. *Reg Anesth Pain Med* 2017; 42:133–183.

Question 6: Answer

A. True. While an uncooperative patient is a relative contraindication and valid consent needs to be obtained if the patient lacks mental capacity, refusal of a patient with full mental capacity is an absolute contraindication and performing the procedure can lead to litigation.

B. True. Spinal CNB is contraindicated. If an epidural block is complicated by inadvertent dural puncture, devastating consequences may follow.

C. True. In patients with deranged coagulation, CNB is justified with an international normalized ratio (INR) up to 1.5, especially if there are significant perceived benefits of CNB over GA.

D. True. Epidural abscess—spontaneous or in association with CNB—is a very rare occurrence. It is perceived that appropriate antibiotics in a patient with general sepsis or other infection (e.g., osteomyelitis) —will decrease the risk of an epidural abscess to 'normal' incidence.

E. False. In patients with scoliosis, both rotational and lateral ultrasound assistance can be very useful in overcoming technical challenges and finding a space with the least asymmetrical anatomy and the best insertion angle. Aim to angle the probe during the transverse imaging to achieve the most symmetrical image and note the angle. CNB can be very beneficial for opioid-sparing postoperative pain relief and restoration of respiratory function in this subgroup of patients. Preoperative MRI can also be useful.

Butterworth, J.F., Mackey, D.C., and Wasnick, J.D. *Morgan and Mikhail's Clinical Anesthesiology*, 6th edition. Mackey McGraw Hill Education, 2018: pp. 959–996.

Warman, P. et al. *Regional Anaesthesia, Stimulation, and Ultrasound Techniques (Oxford Specialist Handbooks in Anaesthesia)*. Oxford University Press, 2014; pp. 500–529.

Question 7: Answer

A. True. Pre-procedural US scanning is an easy and safe technique facilitating central neuraxial procedures and is particularly useful in 'difficult' patients including those in whom bony structures are difficult to palpate such as morbidly obese patients. Spinous processes can be easily identified using transverse interspinal views. A curvilinear probe is normally used.

B. True. A paramedian sagittal oblique scan is helpful in counting the spaces, usually from the sacrum in the cephalad direction (L5/S1, L5/4, etc.). Transverse interspinous scanning allows choosing the 'best' lower lumbar level based on the images of articular and transverse processes, ligamentum flavum/(posterior) dura complex, and the deeper complex comprising anterior dura, posterior longitudinal ligament, and posterior surface of the vertebral body; the spinal canal is between the latter two complexes. Pattern recognition ('flying bat') is the key to success and comes with practice in straightforward patients.

C. True. Angulation of the curvilinear probe allows for identifying the best 'window' and angle of future needle insertion. This is particularly useful in pathology affecting symmetry such as scoliosis.

D. True. The measurement from the skin (over the middle of the spinous process shadow) to the ligamentum flavum/dura complex allows a reliable estimate of depth. Care needs to be taken not to insert too much pressure with the probe in obese patients, which would lead to underestimation of the depth.

E. False. The termination of the spinal cord can normally be visible only in young paediatric patients (neonates and infants).

Warman, P. et al. *Regional Anaesthesia, Stimulation, and Ultrasound Techniques (Oxford Specialist Handbooks in Anaesthesia)*. Oxford University Press, 2014; pp. 531–544.

Question 8: Answer

A. True. This has been shown in MRI studies. The intercristal (Tuffier's) line is unreliable and mistakes are common; when the operator thinks they are palpating L3/4, the level may be L2/3 or even higher. Therefore, it is advisable to aim lower and use imaging, especially in anatomically difficult cases. Spinals should not be performed higher than L2/3.

B. False. As above.

C. True. Two approaches are widely used: midline and paramedian. The paramedian approach allows bypassing the supraspinous ligament which can be ossified in 'older' backs.

D. True. A narrowed spinal canal and decreased CSF volume may lead to slow CSF flow or inability to aspirate and mistaken primary 'failure' and/or multiple attempts. Choosing the best safe intervertebral space using MRI and US imaging is recommended. There is also a risk of higher block for any given volume of injectate. Severe spinal stenosis is a relative contraindication to spinals.

E. True. A Sprotte needle is a side-injection needle with a long opening which may be responsible for a possible leak of LA during injection with subsequent incomplete or short duration block. A Whitacre type pencil-point needle is associated with a lower risk of PDPH than a cutting Quincke needle with an end-injection opening.

Butterworth, J.F., Mackey, D.C., and Wasnick, J.D. *Morgan and Mikhail's Clinical Anesthesiology*, 6th edition. Mackey McGraw Hill Education, 2018: pp. 959–996 (specifically 977 onwards).

Warman, P. et al. *Regional Anaesthesia, Stimulation, and Ultrasound Techniques (Oxford Specialist Handbooks in Anaesthesia)*. Oxford University Press, 2014; p. 502, 504.

Question 9: Answer

A. True. Other useful bony landmarks—the lowest rib is attached to T12; Tuffier's (intercristal) line often passes through the body of L4 but see Answers 8A and B above; sacral hiatus (apex of equilateral triangle with posterior superior iliac spines, PSIS) corresponds to S5.

B. True. The paramedian approach is easier and more reliable, especially in the mid-thoracic region (suitable for an epidural for thoracotomy, upper gastrointestinal (GI), open nephrectomy, AAA repair).

C. True. Other options include naloxone; chlorphenamine (chlorpheniramine); remove opiate.

D. True. This is a particularly valuable option in the obstetric population.

E. True. Patients should have received their last dose of prophylactic LMWH > 12 h before performing CNB; the first postoperative dose should be at least 4 h after any manipulation of the spinal canal, i.e., CNB administration, removal of an epidural or spinal catheter.

Heesen, M. et al. Intrathecal catheterisation after observed accidental dural puncture in labouring women: update of a meta-analysis and a trial-sequential analysis. *Int J Obstet Anesth*, 2020;41:71–82.

Warman, P. et al. *Regional Anaesthesia, Stimulation, and Ultrasound Techniques (Oxford Specialist Handbooks in Anaesthesia)*. Oxford University Press, 2014; p. 502, 504.

Question 10: Answer

A. True. On balance, regional anaesthesia (RA) would be better for the above patient than GA. Mild aortic stenosis is not a crucial consideration, while a well-conducted CNB represents a very good option for respiratory-compromised patients with a positive impact on outcome. Choice of the best technique can be difficult, depending on the operator, surgeon, and patient agreement. CNB encroaching on thoracic levels will reduce FEV1 and forced vital capacity (FVC) and may lead to decompensation. Both anaesthetist and surgeon need to be experienced. The ankle washout and open reduction and internal fixation (ORIF) should not take more than 2–2.5 h in quick hands. It will require a tourniquet. Therefore, a single spinal with 2.5–3 ml of 0.5% hyperbaric bupivacaine will give reliable surgical anaesthesia and peripheral nerve blocks will provide opiate-sparing postoperative pain relief for the first 24–48 h. Continuous epidural anaesthesia is a possible option but is associated with its own risks for a respiratory-compromised patient.

B. False. 3 ml of 2% hyperbaric prilocaine is an excellent recipe for spinal anaesthesia for surgery up to 90 min, which may not be enough.

C. False. Not enough surgical anaesthesia, especially to cover for tourniquet pain.

D. False. 5% hyperbaric lidocaine is associated with transient neurological symptoms.

E. False. 0.1–0.2 mcg of preservative-free morphine or short-acting fentanyl are safer in relation to the risk of delayed respiratory depression. Admission to a high-dependency unit may be prudent for this subgroup of patients.

Butterworth, J.F. et al. *Regional Anaesthesia, Stimulation, and Ultrasound Techniques (Oxford Specialist Handbooks in Anaesthesia)*. Oxford University Press, 2014: pp. 521–525.

Hadzic, A. *Textbook of Regional Anesthesia and Acute Pain Management*, 2nd edition. McGraw Hill, 2017: pp. 896–900.

Question 11: Answer

A. False. Sub-Tenon's (Episcleral) block is one of the most popular choices for RA as it can generally achieve akinesia and has a good safety profile. LA is placed into the potential space between Tenon's capsule and the sclera. The oculo-cardiac reflex (bradycardia or other arrhythmias including ventricular tachycardia and asystole) can be caused by traction on the extraocular muscles, pressure on the globe, retrobulbar block, ocular trauma, and other stimuli. Sub-Tenon's block reduces the incidence of the oculo-cardiac reflex.

B. True. Instillation of LA eye drops provides corneal anaesthesia and thus can allow minimally invasive cataract surgery by phacoemulsification 'without needles' in cooperative patients. Additional intracameral injection of LA can substantially enhance analgesia with the topical approach.

C. True. All topical LAs can cause some degree of transient corneal epithelial toxicity including reversible corneal thickening and opacification.

D. True. The classical approach of injecting 2–4 ml of LA inside the muscular cone with 'up-and-in' gaze position is not recommended due to the increased risk of optic nerve injury. Even with an improved approach, the popularity of retrobulbar anaesthesia (RBA) has largely decreased.

E. False. A highly myopic eye (i.e., a long eyeball) and inadequate experience of the operator are the main risk factors for unintentional globe perforation, a devastating complication of eye blocks.

Hadzic, A. *Textbook of Regional Anesthesia and Acute Pain Management*, 2nd edition. McGraw Hill, 2017: pp. 683–698.

Question 12: Answer

A. True. Recent cadaveric studies suggest three types of blocks are possible: superficial (subcutaneous) cervical plexus block (CPB); intermediate (subfascial, requiring an injection deep to the investing fascia of the neck); and deep, requiring an injection beneath the deep cervical fascia close to the transverse process of the vertebra.

B. False. All three blocks have been used, alone or in combination. However, deep cervical plexus block is more likely to require conversion to general anaesthetic and is more likely to cause life-threatening complications compared with a superficial CPB.

C. False. Deep and intermediate CPBs can cause hemi-diaphragmatic paralysis due to phrenic nerve blockade.

D. True. Deep CPB can cause Horner's syndrome due to stellate ganglion blockade. Inadvertent intrathecal or epidural injection, vertebral artery puncture, and spinal cord damage have all been described.

E. True. Superficial CPB can be used for analgesia after thyroid, carotid, mastoid, and ear surgery.

Warman, P. et al. *Regional Anaesthesia, Stimulation, and Ultrasound Techniques (Oxford Specialist Handbooks in Anaesthesia)*. Oxford University Press, 2014; pp. 235–244.

Question 13: Answer

A. False. The nerves in the axilla are relatively superficial, even in obese patients, hence a linear transducer probe is appropriate.

B. True. This is due to the compressible nature of vessels in the axilla, compared with the subclavian artery behind the clavicle.

C. False. Interindividual variability in nerve arrangement is common, therefore dynamic scanning is very useful.

D. False. This has not been reliably demonstrated.

E. False. A successful axillary block will anaesthetise the arm from mid-humerus down to the hand but a separate blockade of the musculocutaneous nerve is required to provide anaesthesia of the antero-lateral skin at the level of the forearm.

Hadzic, A. *Textbook of Regional Anesthesia and Acute Pain Management*, 2nd edition. McGraw Hill, 2017: pp. 580–585.

Warman, P. et al. *Regional Anaesthesia, Stimulation, and Ultrasound Techniques (Oxford Specialist Handbooks in Anaesthesia)*. Oxford University Press, 2014; pp. 303–310.

Question 14: Answer

A. False. The nerves in the popliteal fossa are relatively superficial even in obese patients; a linear transducer probe is appropriate. It is important to identify the bifurcation of the sciatic nerve into the tibial and common peroneal nerves.

B. False. The best approach depends on the configuration of tibial and common peroneal branches at the site of injection. Using hydrodissection is often very helpful.

C. True. Several reasons combine to make this the best approach: biceps femoris tends to stabilize the catheter; during catheter placement, the side of the thigh is less mobile; access to the catheter site is easier.

D. False. The operator should seek a motor response of the calf muscles and plantar flexion of the toes and foot (tibial nerve component stimulation) and dorsiflexion (common peroneal nerve component). A patellar twitch is a response to stimulating the femoral nerve.

E. False. A combination of both sciatic and femoral (or its saphenous branch) nerves is required for complete sensory block of the lower leg.

Hadzic, A. *Textbook of Regional Anesthesia and Acute Pain Management*, 2nd edition. McGraw Hill, 2017: pp. 620–635.

Question 15: Answer

A. False. There is no evidence of a higher incidence of relapse in multiple sclerosis patients who have received epidural analgesia in labour compared to those who have not.

B. True. The possible mechanism is ischaemia due to compression of the already narrowed spinal canal with LA in the epidural space.

C. True. There is no evidence that amyotrophic lateral sclerosis is exacerbated by neuraxial or peripheral blocks, while avoidance of airway manipulation and the use of relaxants and opioids is beneficial.

D. True. NA helps prevent autonomic dysreflexia while GA does not.

E. False. Diabetic polyneuropathy puts patients at risk of neural ischaemia due to changes within the endoneural microvasculature. Avoiding adrenaline (epinephrine) and reducing the dose and concentration of LA are recommended.

Hadzic, A. *Textbook of Regional Anesthesia and Acute Pain Management*, 2nd edition. McGraw Hill, 2017: pp. 910–920.

1. **Regarding amniotic fluid embolism (AFE)**
    A. cardiac arrest is one of the main diagnostic criteria of AFE
    B. identification of squamous cells in the maternal pulmonary circulation is pathognomonic of AFE
    C. coagulopathy usually occurs after 4 hours
    D. the American Heart Association recommends that delivery of the foetus should occur within 10 minutes in patients with AFE
    E. patients show a biphasic cardiovascular response to AFE

2. **In obstetric patients with depression**
    A. those treated with antidepressants may have higher postoperative pain scores
    B. lithium should be discontinued during the first trimester due to its high teratogenic effect
    C. ketamine improves a postoperative depressive state
    D. postoperative transfusion requirements in patients on serotonergic antidepressants are increased
    E. those on fluoxetine needing epidural anaesthesia require a higher dose of ropivacaine than normal patients

3. **In patients with pre-eclampsia**
    A. symptoms can manifest within 48 hours postpartum
    B. during treatment, the target therapeutic range for magnesium is 4-8 mEq/l
    C. regional anaesthesia is a preferable choice of anaesthesia
    D. the number and function of platelets are both adversely affected
    E. failure of cerebral autoregulation most commonly occurs in the anterior circulation

4. **In patients with peripartum cardiomyopathy**
    A. cardiomyopathy in most cases has a viral aetiology
    B. there is an increased risk of recurrence during subsequent pregnancies
    C. wall motion abnormalities are typically seen on transoesophageal echocardiography (TOE)
    D. onset of heart failure during the last month of pregnancy or within 5 months of delivery is one of the traditional diagnostic criteria of peripartum cardiomyopathy
    E. angiotensin-converting enzyme (ACE) inhibitor therapy should be used only in the postpartum period

5. **In postpartum haemorrhage**
   A. significant blood loss is equal to or more than 500 ml
   B. secondary postpartum haemorrhage is more likely to result in maternal morbidity or mortality
   C. absence of vaginal bleeding excludes the diagnosis of uterine atony
   D. methergine cannot be administered intravenously
   E. intraoperative blood salvage strategy can be used

6. **In paediatric airway management**
   A. more than two attempts at intubation significantly increases the risk of critical respiratory events
   B. in a 'cannot intubate, cannot oxygenate' (CICO) situation a surgical airway is the first choice for children between 1 and 8 years old
   C. blind intubation through a laryngeal mask airway (LMA) is often successful
   D. obstruction of the airway might occur during dilation of the oesophagus by a gastroenterologist
   E. the risk of cervical spinal cord compression should be taken into consideration in patients with Down's syndrome

7. **The Jackson-Rees breathing circuit**
   A. cannot be used with modern anaesthesia machines
   B. due to absence of valves allows rapid change of inspiratory gases
   C. represents a modification of a Mapleson A system
   D. demands a minimal fresh gas flow of 120 ml/kg/min for controlled ventilation
   E. is easier to use during controlled ventilation than a Mapleson E circuit

8. **In paediatric regional anaesthesia**
   A. perforation of the rectum during caudal anaesthesia is a recognized complication
   B. it is important to remember that the tibial nerve runs behind the lateral malleolus
   C. transversus abdominis plane block (TAP block) involves an injection of local anaesthetic between the internal oblique and transversus abdominis muscles
   D. the C8 spinal nerve is easy to visualize during an interscalene approach in an ultrasound-guided block of the brachial plexus
   E. the distance to the epidural space in the lumbar region is 1 mm/kg of body weight

9. **According to the American Heart Association (AHA) and European resuscitation guidelines for children**
   A. in supraventricular tachycardia (SVT) the recommended energy for the second attempt at cardioversion is 4 J/kg
   B. in resuscitation due to cardiac arrest with a shockable rhythm, amiodarone can be given as a bolus after the third shock
   C. torsade-de-pointes can present as a pulseless electrical activity (PEA) rhythm
   D. the ratio of chest compressions to ventilation of an intubated child with two providers should be 15:2
   E. equipment failure is not included in the DOPES acronym

10. In neonates

A. before repair of a diaphragmatic hernia an arterial line should be inserted in the left radial artery

B. metabolic acidosis is the typical finding before operative correction of congenital pyloric stenosis

C. the haemoglobin level that triggers transfusion is higher than in older children

D. the enzymes that metabolize remifentanil are fully active at birth

E. evaporation is responsible for the greatest proportion of heat loss

11. In patients on one-lung ventilation (OLV)

A. propofol anaesthesia decreases the level of inflammatory mediators

B. acute lung injury (ALI) is one of the most serious postoperative complications

C. a bronchopleural fistula is an absolute contraindication to the application of positive end-expiratory pressure (PEEP)

D. permissive hypercapnia up to 9.3 kPa (70 mmHg) is well tolerated for a short time

E. the goal of the anaesthesiologist is to minimize pulmonary vascular resistance (PVR) in the non-ventilated lung

12. In a patient who needs lung isolation

A. the initial depth of insertion of a double-lumen tube by a blind technique for patients with height 170 cm is 29 cm

B. a right-sided double-lumen tube (DLT) is the preferred first choice

C. a bronchial blocker is a better choice than a DLT in difficult airways

D. use of bronchial blockers is associated with difficulty in suctioning

E. an undersized left-sided DLT can cause pneumothorax

13. In Difficult Airway Society (DAS) algorithms

A. face mask ventilation is included in 'plan C' in unanticipated difficult intubation

B. one option during extubation of an 'at risk' patient is to have a remifentanil infusion running

C in obstetric patients only two intubation attempts are recommended

D. if emergency front of neck access (FONA) is needed then cannula cricothyroidotomy is the first choice

E. face mask ventilation during rapid sequence induction is appropriate

14. In awake fibreoptic intubation, it is important to remember that

A. proton pump inhibitors (PPIs) have been shown to be as effective as H_2-receptor antagonists at increasing gastric pH and decreasing gastric volume before the procedure

B. the superior laryngeal nerve provides sensory innervation for the area below the vocal cords

C. the sphenopalatine ganglion and anterior ethmoidal nerve are responsible for the majority of the sensory innervation of the nasal cavity

D. oxygenation of the patient is effective only if spontaneous breathing is present

E. atelectasis is a side effect of preoxygenation

15. In patients with bronchopleural fistula

A. awake fibreoptic intubation is recommended

B. a thoracic drain should be inserted after induction of general anaesthesia

C. lung function tests are important diagnostic tools

D. pleuritis is a possible complication

E. high-frequency ventilation can provide adequate gas exchange

16. In traumatic brain injury

A. coning can be predicted by intracranial pressure monitoring

B. cerebral perfusion pressure (CPP) should be maintained between 60 and 70 mmHg

C. barbiturates are recommended for prophylaxis against development of intracranial hypertension

D. the use of steroids is not recommended

E. if hyperventilation is applied, the minimal recommended $PaCO_2$ value is 25 mmHg (3.3 kPa)

17. Regarding tumours of the posterior fossa

A. in venous air embolism, the lethal volume of air is approximately 3–5 ml/kg

B. only Type I Chiari malformations may require posterior fossa decompression surgery

C. total intravenous anaesthesia (TIVA) is a better choice of anaesthesia if somatosensory-evoked potentials are going to be used for neuromonitoring

D. transoesophageal echocardiography (TOE) is more sensitive than pre-cordial Doppler as an indicator of air embolism

E. an increase in end-tidal CO_2 and a decrease in $PaCO_2$ are common signs of venous air embolism

18. In spinal cord injury

A. methylprednisolone is not recommended

B. a patient with spinal cord injury at the level of T6 scheduled for ureteroscopy does not need anaesthesia, except light sedation

C. vital capacity (VC) is greater in the upright compared with the supine position in tetraplegic patients

D. a patient with spinal cord injury may become poikilothermic

E. an intrathecal baclofen pump can contribute to delayed emergence from anaesthesia

19. Regarding the influence of drugs used in anaesthesia on the brain

A. nitrous oxide increases cerebral blood flow (CBF)

B. fentanyl has negligible effects on CBF and metabolism

C. sevoflurane does not change cerebral autoregulation below 1.5 MAC

D. isoflurane increases the volume of cerebrospinal fluid (CSF)

E. propofol maintains cerebrovascular autoregulation and coupling between $CMRO_2$ and CBF

20. Regarding intracranial aneurysm

A. aneurysms with diameter ≤ 5 mm have a 2% risk of rupture

B. in patients with subarachnoid haemorrhage (SAH) electrocardiogram (ECG) abnormalities are usually related to left ventricular dysfunction

C. a Glasgow Coma Scale score of 12 corresponds to Grade 3 of the World Federation of Neurological Surgeons (WFNS) grading scale

D. induced hypothermia is recommended during temporary clipping of an aneurysm

E. nimodipine reduces the risk of secondary ischaemia after aneurysmal SAH

21. In adult patients on extracorporeal membrane oxygenation (ECMO)

A. the veno-venous approach involves only gas exchange, without the use of haemodynamic support

B. sedation is necessary throughout all periods of ECMO support

C. the veno-venous approach improves cardiac functions

D. a minimal left ventricular ejection fraction (LVEF) of 20–25% is a prerequisite for weaning from veno-arterial ECMO

E. pneumothorax can be treated conservatively

22. In patients with uncorrected tetralogy of Fallot

A. the 'pink' variant is typically seen when there is a small ventricular-septal defect (VSD)

B. palliative repair is performed in the majority of surgical cases

C. increase in peripheral vascular resistance contributes to the 'tet spells'

D. risk of foetal loss is increased

E. inhalational anaesthesia induction is prolonged

23. In an adult patient undergoing surgery with cardiopulmonary bypass

A. the first dose of heparin is injected after cannulation of the ascending aorta

B. a roller pump is safer than a centrifugal pump

C. the effect of anterograde cardioplegia will be diminished by aortic insufficiency

D. pH-stat strategy is used by most medical centres

E. pulsatile arterial blood flow is lost

24. In cardiac intensive care unit (ICU) patients

A. insertion of an intra-aortic balloon pump increases systolic blood pressure

B. extravascular lung water measured by Pulse index Continuous Cardiac Output (PiCCO) correlates with pulmonary oedema

C. a reduction in mixed central venous saturation (SvO_2) indicates decreased oxygen consumption

D. the Doppler principle can be used to measure cardiac output

E. thermodilution using a small volume of injectate (< 5 ml) into a pulmonary artery flotation catheter overestimates cardiac output

25. **In a 65-year-old patient with two-vessel coronary artery disease and poorly controlled arterial hypertension presenting for coronary artery bypass surgery**
    A. preoperative functional status can be classified into four grades
    B. a septal–lateral E/e' ratio ≥ 15 measured by transoesophageal echocardiography is associated with increased postoperative mortality
    C. sternotomy could be avoided
    D. TIVA is the preferred choice
    E. an epicardial pacemaker should be set in VVI mode in case of atrial fibrillation

26. **Side effects and complications likely to occur after coeliac plexus block with 96% alcohol include**
    A. diarrhoea
    B. hypotension
    C. constipation
    D. paraplegia
    E. pneumothorax

27. **Drugs used to alleviate chronic pain in cancer patients include**
    A. meperidine
    B. transdermal fentanyl
    C. methadone
    D. oxycodone
    E. hydromorphone

28. **Characteristics of neuropathic pain include**
    A. burning pain
    B. pin-prick hypoaesthesia in the painful area
    C. erythema in the painful area
    D. swelling in the painful area
    E. itching in the painful area

29. **Pain related to neural oedema due to compression of the nerve root may be relieved by**
    A. intramuscular dexamethasone
    B. transforaminal dexamethasone injection
    C. diclofenac sodium
    D. paracetamol
    E. bed rest

30. **A patient with type 1 diabetes of 15 years' duration, who presents with burning foot pain, is more likely to have pain relief with**

A. pregabalin

B. paracetamol

C. aspirin

D. dexketoprofen

E. duloxetine

Question 1: Answer

A. True. According to the Society of Maternal-Fetal Medicine (SMFM) and Amniotic Fluid Foundation the symptoms of AFE are:

- Sudden onset of cardiorespiratory arrest, or both hypotension and respiratory compromise.
- Documentation of overt DIC, after the appearance of initial signs and symptoms.
- Clinical appearance during labour or within 30 minutes of delivery of the placenta.
- No fever (greater or equal to 38.0°C) during labour.

B. False. Identification of squamous cells in the maternal pulmonary circulation is not pathognomonic of AFE, since contamination with squamous cells during insertion of a pulmonary artery catheter may occur in pregnant as well as non-pregnant patients. Squamous cells coated with neutrophils or platelets, accompanied by foetal debris, or eosinophilic granular material with adherent leucocytes, are more suggestive of AFE.

C. False. Coagulopathy is associated with AFE in 83% of patients. The onset can occur as quickly as 10 to 30 minutes from the onset of symptoms or may be delayed by as many as 4 hours.

D. False. The American Heart Association (AHA) recommends that delivery of the foetus should occur within 5 minutes.

E. True. During the initial phase, acute pulmonary hypertension results in right ventricular dilation, a decrease in cardiac output and ventilation-perfusion (V/Q) mismatch resulting in oxygen desaturation. The release of endogenous catecholamines may produce a brief period of systemic hypertension. A second phase commences when right ventricular function improves, typically 15–30 minutes after the initial event. At this point left ventricular failure may persist as a result of ischaemic injury to the left ventricle or direct myocardial depression, and is accompanied by decreased systemic vascular resistance, decreased left ventricular stroke index, and pulmonary oedema.

Chestnut, D.H. et al. *Chestnut's Obstetric Anesthesia: Principle and Practice*, 6th edition. Elsevier, 2020.

Suresh, M.S. et al. *Schnider and Levinson's Anesthesia for Obstetrics*, 5th edition. Lippincott, Williams & Wilkins, 2013: pp. 342–343.

Question 2: Answer

A. True. A patient treated with antidepressants may have a high postoperative pain score.

B. False. The teratogenic risk of using lithium in the first trimester is small compared with the potential complication of relapse during pregnancy.

C. True. A small dose of ketamine (an NMDA antagonist) improves a postoperative depressive state and is a suitable anaesthetic in depressed patients.

D. False. Patients receiving a serotonergic antidepressant show significantly higher but clinically unimportant blood loss, without an increase in perioperative transfusion requirement.

E. False. The dose of LA should be decreased. Ropivacaine is metabolized primarily by cytochrome P450 CYP1A2 with CYP3A4 serving as a secondary enzyme for metabolism. Fluoxetine and its principal metabolite norfluoxetine are together significant inhibitors of both these enzymes. Inhibition of action of these enzymes results in a decreased rate of metabolism of ropivacaine.

Marcucci, C. et al. *A Case Approach to Perioperative Drug-Drug Interactions.* Springer, 2015: p. 2008

Suresh, M.S. et al. *Schnider and Levinson's Anesthesia for Obstetrics*, 5th edition. Lippincott, Williams & Wilkins, 2013: pp. 650–653.

Question 3: Answer

A. True. Postpartum preeclampsia usually manifests within 7 days of delivery.

B. True. A therapeutic range of 4.8 to 8.4 mg/dl (2.0 to 3.5 mmol/l) has been recommended based on retrospective data.

C. True. The major advantage is avoidance of GA and the risk of difficult airway management. Conventional epidural anaesthesia provides very good haemodynamic stability. In patients with pre-eclampsia undergoing spinal anaesthesia, the incidence of hypotension is significantly less compared with normotensive women.

D. True. In addition to thrombocytopenia, pre-eclampsia adversely affects platelet function. The presence of platelet dysfunction, independent of the number of platelets, is a unique problem in pre-eclampsia.

E. False. Failure of autoregulation occurs most commonly in the posterior circulation; these changes may result in posterior reversible leukoencephalopathy syndrome (PRES).

Chestnut, D.H. et al. *Chestnut's Obstetric Anesthesia: Principle and Practice*, 6th edition. Elsevier, 2020: Location 49291.

Suresh, M.S. et al. *Schnider and Levinson's Anesthesia for Obstetrics*, 5th edition. Lippincott, Williams & Wilkins, 2013: pp. 444, 452–453.

Question 4: Answer

A. False. Peripartum cardiomyopathy is a unique cardiomyopathy of unknown cause that occurs during pregnancy or the postpartum period. Many potential factors, including viruses, may contribute to it. Experimental research suggests a common final pathway with enhanced oxidative stress, cleavage of prolactin to an angiostatic N-terminal 16 kDA prolactin fragment, and impaired vascular endothelial growth factor (VEGF) signalling.

B. True. The risk associated with subsequent pregnancies is substantially higher in women who do not recover normal left ventricular function. Even in patients with normalized left ventricular function, careful counselling is advised due to the significant risk of recurrence of left ventricular dysfunction.

C. False. Ischaemic cardiomyopathy is typically accompanied by regional wall motion abnormalities, whereas peripartum or non-ischaemic cardiomyopathy typically results in a global decrease in contractility.

D. True. Diagnostic criteria for peripartum cardiomyopathy:

Traditional criteria:

- Onset of heart failure during the last month of pregnancy or within 5 months of delivery.
- No other identifiable cause of heart failure.
- No known heart disease before pregnancy.

Echocardiographic criteria:

- LVEF < 45%.
- Fractional shortening < 30%.
- Left ventricular end-diastolic dimension ≥ 27 mm/m^2.

E. True. ACE inhibitors are generally contraindicated in the antepartum period due to the risk of teratogenicity, neonatal anuria, neonatal renal failure, and neonatal death. ACE inhibitors are used effectively postpartum, even if the mother is breastfeeding.

Chestnut, D.H. et al. *Chestnut's Obstetric Anesthesia: Principle and Practice*, 6th edition. Elsevier, 2020: Location 59550, 59613, 59573,59593.

Suresh, M.S. et al. *Schnider and Levinson's Anesthesia for Obstetrics*, 5th edition. Lippincott, Williams & Wilkins, 2013: p. 506.

Question 5: Answer

A. True. WHO defines haemorrhage as blood loss greater or equal to 500 ml, or blood loss accompanied by signs or symptoms of hypovolaemia within 24 hours of birth.

B. False. Primary postpartum haemorrhage occurs within the first 24 hours of birth and secondary postpartum haemorrhage occurs between 24 hours and 6 weeks after delivery. Primary postpartum haemorrhage is more likely to result in maternal morbidity or mortality.

C. False. The absence of vaginal bleeding does not exclude a diagnosis of uterine atony, because the atonic engorged uterus may contain more than 1000 ml of blood. Unrecognized bleeding may manifest initially as tachycardia; worsening hypovolaemia eventually leads to hypotension.

D. False. Bolus intravenous administration of methergine is not recommended. It should not routinely be administered IV because of the possibility of inducing sudden hypertension and cerebrovascular accident. Intravenous administration should only be considered during life-threatening situations. Generally, if administered intravenously, it should be administered as a quick infusion (diluted in 100 ml of normal saline) over a 5–10-minute period.

E. True. The washing and use of leucocyte depletion filters have been shown to remove hazardous particles (foetal squamous cells, lamellar bodies, bacteria). The American College of Obstetricians and Gynecologists (ACOG), the Obstetric Anaesthetist Association of Great Britain and the British Confidential Enquiry into Maternal and Child Health (CEMACH) have advocated the use of blood salvage in obstetrics. There is a theoretical concern that reinfusing amniotic fluid may cause AFE, but it has been documented only once and may have been prevented with washing. The risk of bacterial contamination is also minimal. Salvaged blood may contain foetal erythrocytes, but this is not a major concern as Rh-D alloimmunization in an Rh-D-negative mother can be prevented by the administration of anti-D immune globulin. ABO incompatibility reactions cannot be prevented, but are unlikely to be serious.

Chestnut, D.H. et al. *Chestnut's Obstetric Anesthesia: Principle and Practice*, 6th edition. Elsevier, 2020: Locations 52906, 52952, 53066.

Suresh, M.S. et al. *Schnider and Levinson's Anesthesia for Obstetrics*, 5th edition. Lippincott, Williams & Wilkins, 2013: pp. 326–327.

World Health Organization (WHO). *WHO Recommendations for the Prevention and Treatment of Postpartum Haemorrhage.* World Health Organization, 2012. Available at: https://www.ncbi.nlm.nih.gov/books/NBK131942/

Question 6: Answer

A. True. The increase is twofold according to the APRICOT (Anaesthesia Practice in Children Observational Study: Epidemiology of Sever Critical Events) study.

B. False. The DAS guideline (in collaboration with the Association of Paediatric Anaesthetists) has stated that percutaneous cannula cricothyroidotomy is the first choice (if an ENT specialist is absent).

C. False. Blind intubation, though an LMA in paediatrics results in failure in most cases.

D. True. This complication is described in children and even in adults during percutaneous gastrostomy or transoesophageal echocardiography. The oesophagus runs immediately posterior to the trachea from the level of the cricoid cartilage down to the gastroesophageal junction. The posterior portion of the trachea is susceptible to external compression because of a lack of structural support from cartilage.

E. True. Approximately 20% of children with Down's syndrome have loose ligaments of the atlantoaxial joint. Intubation may predispose to cervical cord compression during induction if accompanied by hyperextension, hyperflexion, or extensive rotation of the head. The usefulness of preoperative screening of asymptomatic patients with Down's syndrome for atlantoaxial instability is a controversial topic. The usual recommended practice is to keep the head in neutral position.

DAC guidelines. Available at: https://das.uk.com/.

Habre, C.W. et al. Incidence of severe critical events in paediatric anaesthesia (APRICOT): a prospective multicentre observational study in 261 hospitals in Europe. *Lancet Respir Med*, 2017;5:412–425.

Hagberg, A. et al. *Hagberg and Benumof's Airway Management*, 4th edition. Elsevier. 2018: Chapter 36, Airway management in pediatric patients: congenital cervical spine instability.

Jöhr, M. *Managing Complication in Paediatric Anesthesia*. Cambridge University Press, 2018: Locations 978, 1061–1079.

Question 7: Answer

A. False. Semi-open systems, including Jackson-Rees, can be connected and are used in many modern anaesthesia machines.

B. True. The absence of valves is an advantage of the Jackson-Rees system and allows quick inhalation induction.

C. False. The Jackson-Rees system is a modification of the Mapleson F, see Fig 12.1.

D. False. A high fresh gas flow is necessary to prevent rebreathing and is a disadvantage of the Jackson-Rees circuit. The minimal fresh gas flow should be 200 ml/kg/min if the child is ventilated. The other disadvantages are lack of humidification and venting the scavenged gas directly into the theatre environment.

E. True. The Mapleson E system has no bag and to generate positive pressure, intermittent occlusion of the limb outlet is necessary. Mapleson E and F systems are mostly used for children under 20–25 kg, see Fig 12.1.

Jöhr, M. *Managing Complication in Paediatric Anesthesia*. Cambridge University Press, 2018: Locations 978, 1061–1079.

Sdrales, L.M. and Miller, R.D. *Miller's Anesthesia Review*, 2nd edition. Elsevier. 2013: Chapter 12, Anesthesia delivery systems: pp. 130–131.

Yentis, S.M. et al. *Anaesthesia and Intensive Care A–Z*, 5th edition. Churchill Livingstone, 2013: p. 33.

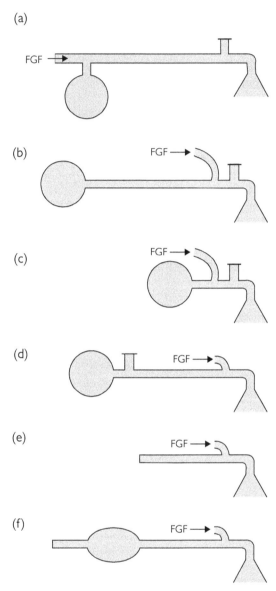

Fig 12.1 The Mapleson classification of breathing systems. Types A–F are shown in (a)–(f) respectively. Types E and F are used in paediatric anaesthesia.

Reproduced from S.M. Yentis at al. (2013) "Anaesthesia and Intensive Care A-Z". Churchill Livingstone. 5th edition pp. 33.

Question 8: Answer
   A. True. It is a rare complication, but a few cases have been described in the literature.
   B. False. The tibial nerve runs behind the medial malleolus under the flexor retinaculum and lies posterior to the pulsation of the posterior tibial artery.

C. True. This block is intended to stop the transmission of pain impulses from sensory roots of T6–T11 (intercostal nerves), T12 (subcostal nerve), and L1 (ilioinguinal and iliohypogastric nerve). These nerves run in a plane known as TAP, see Fig 12.2. It is situated between the internal oblique and transversus abdominis muscles.

D. False. Ultrasound imaging allows visualization of spinal nerves C5, C6, and C7. C8 is more difficult to visualize, especially in neonates. During interscalene block, the inferior trunk (C8–T1) is often spared.

E. True. This formula gives a good correlation for children between 6 months and 10 years of age.

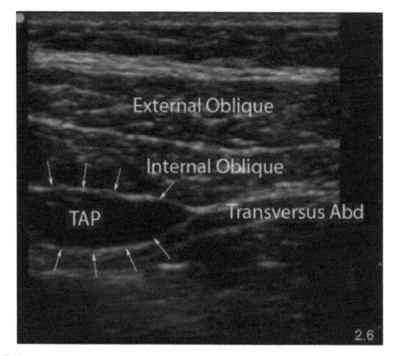

Fig 12.2 An annotated ultrasound image demonstrating the anatomy of a TAP block.

Hadzic, A. *Hadzic's Textbook of Regional Anesthesia and Acute Pain Management*, 2nd edition. McGraw-Hill Education, 2017: Location 20334.

Holzman, R.S. et al. *Pediatric Anesthesiology Review. Clinical Cases for Self-assessment.* Springer, 2010: Location 8582.

Jöhr, M. *Managing Complication in Paediatric Anesthesia.* Cambridge University Press, 2018: Location 4334.

Question 9: Answer

A. False. Narrow-QRS complex and wide-QRS complex stable (with good perfusion) tachycardia can be treated with vagal manoeuvres and adenosine (immediately followed by a bolus of normal saline). If two doses of adenosine are unsuccessful, proceed to synchronized cardioversion. The first energy dose is 0.5–1.0 J/kg, the second dose is 2 J/kg. For unstable wide-QRS complex tachycardia synchronized cardioversion is the treatment of choice. A wide-QRS complex is defined by a QRS duration > 90 milliseconds.

B. True. Amiodarone is given after the third shock during resuscitation with shockable rhythms (ventricular fibrillation and pulseless ventricular tachycardia).

C. False. PEA, formerly known as electromechanical dissociation (EMD), is the presence of electrical activity of the heart without a detectable cardiac output (palpable pulse or measurable blood pressure) during cardiac arrest. Ventricular fibrillation, torsade-de-pointes, and ventricular tachycardia cannot be described as PEA. PEA and asystole belong to non-shockable rhythms.

D. False. In cases of resuscitation with positive pressure ventilation via an endotracheal tube, the ventilations can be asynchronous and chest compressions continuous (only pausing every 2 min for rhythm check). Ventilation frequency should be adjusted to the lower limit of the normal rate for age.

E. False. DOPES is an acronym for the causes of sudden deterioration in an intubated child or failure to improve after intubation. Certain steps should be taken to assess the situation and rule out or confirm the possible causes:

- **D**isplacement of the tracheal tube (in the oesophagus, pharynx, or endobronchially)
- **O**bstruction of the tracheal tube, the heat and moisture exchanger (HME) or the circuit
- **P**neumothorax and other pulmonary disorders (bronchospasm, oedema, pulmonary hypertension, etc.)
- **E**quipment failure (source of gas, bag-mask, ventilator, etc.)
- **S**tomach (gastric distension may alter diaphragm mechanics)

Topjian, A.A. et al. Part 4: Pediatric Basic and Advanced Life Support: 2020 American Heart Association guidelines for cardiopulmonary resuscitation and emergency cardiovascular care. *Circulation*, 2020;142:S469–S523.

Van de Voorde, P. et al. European Resuscitation Council Guidelines 2021: paediatric life support. *Resuscitation*, 2021;161:327–387.

Question 10: Answer

A. False. An arterial line for blood sampling and monitoring of arterial blood pressure should preferably be inserted into the right radial artery. The right radial artery represents preductal (brain and heart) oxygenation. Targeting preductal arterial blood gas measurements may provide a more physiological approach to ventilator management.

B. False. The typical picture is hyperchloraemic and hypokalaemic metabolic alkalosis. Pyloric stenosis causes dehydration and hypovolaemia due to prolonged vomiting (with considerable loss of H^+, Na^+ and Cl^-). An overall extracellular volume deficit leads to compensatory fluid retention by the kidney triggered by aldosterone secretion. It results in the exchange of potassium and hydrogen ions for sodium in the distal tubule resulting in metabolic alkalosis. The loss of hydrogen ions in urine causes 'paradoxical aciduria' in the alkalotic patient. Metabolic alkalosis is compensated with respiratory hypoventilation.

C. True. The haemoglobin transfusion trigger is higher due to the presence of HbF. Regarding the threshold for blood transfusion, there is little consensus in the national societies.

According to the latest guidelines, the threshold for newborns with respiratory support within 1 week of life is 120 g/l (UK) or 115 g/l (Canada).

D. True. Remifentanil is metabolized by non-specific esterases in tissue and erythrocytes. These processes are mature, even in preterm infants, and are independent of liver and renal function.

E. False. The biggest part of heat loss is radiation (39%), followed by convection (34%). Evaporation is in third place at 24%. Conduction has the smallest contribution at 3%. The recommended temperature in the operating theatre before neonatal surgery is 25–28°C.

Lerman, J. *Neonatal Anesthesia*. Springer, 2015: pp. 73, 100, 226.

Sims, C. et al. *A Guide to Pediatric Anesthesia*, 2nd edition. Springer, 2020: Location 6623, 6681.

Slinger, P. et al. *Principle and Practice of Anesthesia for Thoracic Surgery*, 2nd edition. Springer Nature Switzerland, 2019: Location 50998.

Yentis, S.M. et al. *Anaesthesia and Intensive Care A–Z*, 5th edition. Churchill Livingstone, 2013: pp. 491–492.

Question 11: Answer

A. False. Inhalational anaesthesia with sevoflurane has been shown to have beneficial effects in comparison with propofol anaesthesia in terms of decreasing the level of pro-inflammatory mediators. Another positive effect of inhalational anaesthesia is minimizing reperfusion injury and glycocalyx breakdown.

B. True. Lung injury occurs in both lungs but the reasons for these injuries are different. The ventilated lung is affected mostly by hyperperfusion and ventilator-induced lung injury, whereas in the collapsed lung, ischaemia–reperfusion injury, and shear stress after starting re-ventilation play important roles. The diagnosis of acute lung injury (ALI) is based on an acute reduction in the PaO_2/FiO_2 ratio to < 300 in the presence of at least 5 cmH$_2$O PEEP or CPAP along with diffuse pulmonary infiltrates on the chest radiograph or CT (according to Berlin's ARDS criteria: 'mild ARDS'). One of the independent risk factors is the duration of one-lung ventilation (OLV > 100 minutes).

C. True. The presence of a bronchopleural fistula is the only real contraindication to the administration of PEEP. The level of PEEP should be adjusted according to the individual patient and respiratory mechanics. For example, in severe obstructive lung disease, a low level of PEEP is recommended (2–5 cmH$_2$O), in restrictive lung disease, or unchanged lung physiology the level of PEEP should be 5–10 cmH$_2$O.

D. True. It is not only well-tolerated but also helps to prevent lung ventilation injury. A higher level of CO_2 should be avoided in most patients due to the risk of cardiovascular instability (tachycardia, dysrhythmia, negative inotropic effect).

E. False. The goal of the anaesthesiologist is to maximize PVR in non-ventilated and minimize PVR in the ventilated lung in order to prevent hypoxaemia. Total PVR is at a minimum at the functional residual capacity (FRC). It reflects the optimal balance of vascular resistance in alveolar and extra-alveolar pulmonary vessels. If pulmonary volume increases, the capillaries become narrower and stretched and PVR will be increased. If pulmonary volume decreases some capillaries become kinked or bent. As a result, PVR is higher. That is why it is important to keep ventilated lung as close as possible to its FRC. In the non-ventilated lung, air volume should be kept close to residual volume (RV). See Fig 12.3.

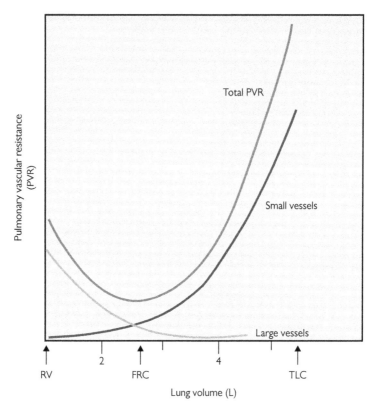

Fig 12.3 The relationship between PVR and lung volume.

Reproduced from 'Miller's Anesthesia'. Elsevier Saunders. 8th edition. 2015. Chapter 66 'Anesthesia for thoracic surgery' p. 1969 with permission from Elsevier.

Miller, R.D. et al. *Miller's Anesthesia*, 8th edition. Elsevier Saunders, 2015: p. 1969.

Slinger, P. et al. *Principle and Practice of Anesthesia for Thoracic Surgery*, 2nd edition. Springer Nature Switzerland, 2019: Location 4935–5023, 5009–5020, 5178, 5283.

Question 12: Answer

A. True. If a blind technique with direct laryngoscopy is used, the depth of insertion at the level of the teeth of the DLT is 29 cm for a patient of 170 cm height (both men and women) with a correction of 1 cm for each 10 cm height difference.

B. False. A left-sided DLT is easier to insert and is safer. This is due to a fundamental difference in lung anatomy. The left main bronchus is longer (length 4–5 cm) and bifurcates to the left upper lobe bronchus and left lower lobe bronchus. The right main bronchus is shorter (length 1.4–2.5 cm), bifurcating to the right upper lobe bronchus and intermediate bronchus. The right upper lobe bronchus is at risk of inadvertent occlusion by a right-sided DLT. But there are special situations when a right-sided DLT is indicated, for example, distorted anatomy of the entrance of the left mainstem bronchus, left-sided lung transplantation, and left-sided pneumonectomy.

C. True. Difficult airways, especially those involving awake fibreoptic intubation, are an indication for use of bronchial blockers.

D. True. Arndt, Cohen, Fuji, or EZ-blockers have a central channel that can be used for suction, but the diameter is small between 1.0 and 2.0 mm.

E. True. There are reports that an undersized DLT migrates too far into the left lower bronchus and the entire tidal volume is then delivered to the lower lobe.

Miller, R.D. et al. *Miller's Anesthesia*, 8th edition. Elsevier Saunders, 2015: p. 1961.

Slinger, P. et al. *Principle and Practice of Anesthesia for Thoracic Surgery*, 2nd edition. Springer Nature Switzerland, 2019: Location 13959, 13992, 14042, 14081, 14091, 14096, 14431, 14549.

Question 13: Answer

A. True. According to the DAS guidelines of 2015, in unanticipated difficult intubation 'plan C' is a final mask ventilation attempt before waking up the patient or announcing a 'cannot intubate cannot oxygenate' scenario.

B. True. This is one of the techniques in the DAS guidelines to facilitate difficult extubation. It should be considered for patients in whom adverse haemodynamic effects and coughing associated with extubation are undesirable (e.g., reactive airway disease, after ophthalmic procedures, or after neurosurgery). Before extubation, the rate of remifentanil infusion is adjusted depending on spontaneous respiration and the level of consciousness of the patient. The patient should obey commands and tolerate the tube. The remifentanil infusion is stopped after extubation.

C. False. Three intubation attempts are advocated in the obstetric difficult intubation algorithm. The third one must be performed by the most experienced colleague. Remember that a further dose of intravenous anaesthetic should be considered to prevent awareness.

D. False. In an emergency FONA situation, scalpel cricothyroidotomy is the first choice. All anaesthetists should be trained to perform a surgical airway and this training is to be repeated at regular intervals.

E. True. Currently, gentle facemask ventilation with maximal inflation pressure below 20 cmH$_2$O is recommended during rapid sequence induction. It is especially useful in patients with poor respiratory reserve or high metabolic requirements.

Frerk, C. et al. Difficult Airway Society 2015 guidelines for management of unanticipated difficult intubation in adults. *Br J Anaesth*, 2015;*115*, (6):827–848.

Mushambi, M.C. et al. Obstetric Anaesthetists Association and Difficult Airway Society guidelines for the management of difficult and failed tracheal intubation in obstetrics. *Anaesthesia*, 2015;*70*:1221–1225.

Popat, M. et al. Difficult Airway Society Guidelines for the management of tracheal extubation. *Anaesthesia*, 2012;*67*(3):318–340.

Question 14: Answer

A. False. PPIs have not been shown to be as effective as H$_2$-antagonists at increasing gastric pH and decreasing gastric volume before operation. This difference is especially true of oral administration.

B. False. The internal branch of the superior laryngeal nerve (a branch of the vagus nerve) provides sensory innervation to the area above the vocal cords: the base of the tongue; the posterior surface of the epiglottis; aryepiglottic folds; and arytenoids. The vocal cords and area below the vocal cords are innervated by the recurrent laryngeal nerve.

C. True. The two main sources of nasal cavity sensory innervation are the sphenopalatine ganglion and the anterior ethmoidal nerve. Both are branches of the trigeminal nerve (V).

D. False. Apnoeic oxygenation is effective if airways are patent. Oxygen consumption during apnoea is 230 ml/min. At the same time, the amount of CO_2 delivered to alveoli from the blood is only 20 ml/min. The remaining CO_2 produced is buffered. The negative gas exchange rate is therefore 210 ml/min. This difference creates a pressure gradient between the upper airway and alveoli and allows the movement of oxygen down the trachea.

E. True. Absorption atelectasis is the most common side effect of pre-oxygenation. Nitrogen, which is poorly soluble and maintains alveolar volume, is replaced with oxygen. The loss of this additional oxygen into the blood promotes the development of atelectasis. To prevent this, recruitment manoeuvres (PEEP, CPAP) should be implemented.

Hagberg, C. et al. *Hagberg and Benumof's Airway Management*, 4th edition. Elsevier, 2018: Chapter 14, Preoxygenation: complications of preoxygenation: pp. 219, 226–227, 229, 251, 264.

Smith, I. et al. Perioperative fasting in adults and children. Guidelines from the European Society of Anaesthesiology. *Eur J Anaesthesiol*, 2011;28(8):556–569.

Yentis, S.M. et al. *Anesthesia and Intensive Care A–Z*, 5th edition. Churchill Livingstone Elsevier, 2013: p. 352.

Question 15: Answer

A. False. One needs to assess the fistula size and amount of airflow through the fistula before induction. There is no sole method for this assessment. Bronchoscopy, CT (especially with 3D reconstruction), clinical evaluation (expansion or collapse of the lung in the presence of thoracic drainage, degree of bubbling, presence of leak during stages of the respiratory cycle) can be used. If the fistula's size and air leak are small, then conventional induction with intravenous anaesthetics, opioids, muscle relaxant, and subsequent airway management with mask ventilation and endotracheal intubation could be performed. If the fistula's size and air leak are large, it is important to avoid positive pressure ventilation until lung isolation has occurred. It can be implemented in two ways: inhalational induction with spontaneous breathing or awake fibreoptic intubation.

B. False. A thoracostomy tube should be inserted before induction to prevent tension pneumothorax and ensuing haemodynamic changes after initiation of positive pressure ventilation.

C. False. Lung function tests are not reliable in the presence of bronchopulmonary fistula.

D. True. Normally the pleural space is sterile but bacteria from the airway can be disseminated through the fistula into the pleural space, which could cause infection and further impede the closure of the fistula.

E. True. The advantage of high-frequency ventilation (HFV) is a lower peak and mean airway pressure and as a result lower bronchopleural fistula airflow.

Slinger, P. et al. *Principle and Practice of Anesthesia for Thoracic Surgery*, 2nd edition. Springer Nature Switzerland, 2019: Location 34077, 34095, 34115, 34137, 34170, 34192, 34367, 34210.

Question 16: Answer

A. False. Intracranial pressure monitoring has no relevance for emergency management. Coning is a clinical diagnosis that can occur at various levels of intracranial pressure (ICP) elevation and cannot be predicted by ICP values.

B. True. CPP is the difference between mean arterial blood pressure and ICP. The recommended target CPP for survival and a favourable outcome is between 60 and 70 mmHg (level of recommendation: IIB). Avoiding aggressive attempts to maintain CPP above 70 mmHg with fluids and pressors may be considered because of the risk of adult respiratory failure (level of recommendation: III).

C. False. Administration of barbiturates to induce burst suppression measured by electroencephalogram (EEG) as prophylaxis against the development of intracranial hypertension is not recommended (level of recommendations: IIB). High-dose barbiturate administration is recommended to control elevated ICP refractory to maximum standard medical and surgical treatment (level of recommendation: IIB).

D. True. The use of steroids is not recommended for improving outcome or reducing ICP. In patients with severe traumatic brain injury, high-dose methylprednisolone was associated with increased mortality and is contraindicated (level of recommendation: I). The body of evidence was updated in 2016 to include the 6-month outcomes of the CRASH (Corticosteroid Randomisation After Significant Head Injury) trial.

E. True. Prolonged prophylactic hyperventilation with $PaCO_2$ of 25 mmHg (3.3 kPa) or less is not recommended (level of evidence: IIB). Hyperventilation should be avoided during the first 24 hours after injury when CBF is often critically reduced (level of evidence: formal recommendation).

Carney, N. et al. *Guidelines for the Management of Severe Traumatic Brain Injury*, 4th edition. Brain Trauma Foundation, 2016: pp. 63,68, 76, 181–182.

Mashour, G.A. et al. *Oxford Textbook of Neuroscience and Anesthesiology*. Oxford University Press, 2019. p. 346.

Question 17: Answer

A. True. In adults, the lethal volume is thought to be between 200 and 300 ml, or 3-5 ml/kg. If the embolism is larger in volume, it will immediately cause cardiac arrest. Children are considered to be at lower risk for venous air embolism (VAE) because in children the dural venous pressure is higher than in adults.

B. False. Chiari malformations (CM) are represented by four classes of hindbrain disorders. Type I, II, and III CM may require surgery with decompression of posterior fossa structures.

C. True. Intraoperative neurophysiological monitoring is used to monitor brainstem integrity. Somatosensory-evoked potentials (SSEPs) monitor dorsal sensory pathways. Motor evoked potentials (MEPs) monitor anterior corticospinal tracts. Brainstem auditory evoked potentials (BAEPs) record the integrity of the auditory pathway. The use of evoked potentials provides additional safety, reduces the risk of iatrogenic damage to the nervous system, monitors for cerebral ischaemia, and enables completion of tumour resection. These modalities typically require TIVA because they are sensitive to the depressant effects of volatile anaesthetics. In particular, MEPs are very sensitive to inhalation agents, while somatosensory-evoked potentials (SSEPs) are less sensitive. The BAEPs are most resistant to the action of volatile anaesthetics. The effect on motor and sensory evoked potentials seen with volatile anaesthetics (decrease in amplitude and increase in latency) can be observed at concentrations as low as 0.3–0.5 MAC.

D. True. The most sensitive way to monitor for VAE is using TOE. It can detect as little as 0.02 ml/kg of air. Pre-cordial Doppler can detect 0.05 ml/kg air and is the most sensitive among non-invasive monitors. The major disadvantage of pre-cordial Doppler is interference with the use of cautery during surgery.

E. False. The common signs of VAE are tachypnoea, tachyarrhythmia, hypoxemia, hypotension, wheezes on auscultation, and a decrease in $EtCO_2$ with an increase in $PaCO_2$.

Mashour, G.A. and Engelhard, K. *Oxford Textbook of Neuroscience and Anaesthesiology*. Oxford University Press, 2019: pp. 467, 495–496.

Matta, B.F. et al. *Core Topics in Neuroanaesthesia and Neurointensive Care*. Cambridge University Press, 2011: Location 7541, 7590.

Soriano, S.G. and McClain, C.D. *Essentials of Pediatric Neuroanesthesia*. Cambridge University Press, 2019: p. 56.

Question 18: Answer

A. True. In 2013, the American Association of Neurological Surgeons and Congress of Neurological Surgeons issued guidelines for the management of acute cervical spine and spinal cord injuries where it has been stated that the use of glucocorticoids in acute spinal cord injury is not recommended (level of recommendations: I; level of evidence: I and II). High-dose methylprednisolone can be a treatment option (not a treatment standard) for non-penetrating spinal cord injury, except for polytrauma including brain injury (level of evidence: III). If used a bolus dose of 30 mg/kg (2.4 g for 80 kg patient), is infused over 30–45 minutes. This is followed by continuous infusion at 5.4 mg/kg/hour for 23 hours (total dose 10 g for 80 kg patient) commenced 45 minutes after the completion of the initial bolus.

B. False. Autonomic dysreflexia (AD) can occur as a result of mass sympathetic discharge, and is usually triggered by noxious pelvic visceral stimulation (e.g., colorectal or bladder distension) if the patient is not properly anaesthetised. It usually occurs during the chronic stage of injury. The stimulus from parasympathetic and sympathetic afferents and the lack of inhibitory descending signals from higher centres leads to profound vasoconstriction below the level of injury and a rapid rise in blood pressure. The intact baroreceptor reflex (cranial nerves IX and X) leads to bradycardia. The remaining functioning sympathetic system attempts to counteract the rise in blood pressure by dilatation of the remaining controlled vasculature. As a result, the patient will develop hypertension, sweating, headache, and blurred vision. The incidence of AD is higher in patients with lesions above T6–T7 but has been known to occur in patients with a lesion as low as T10. Mortality is rare with AD, but stroke, retinal haemorrhage, and pulmonary oedema can occur if the patient is not treated.

C. False. The tetraplegic patient experiences a drop in VC of up to 15% when moving from a supine to an upright position because their diaphragm is drawn down to a less mechanically efficient curvature by the abdominal contents, which are not supported due to the lack of abdominal wall tone.

D. True. High spinal cord injury disrupts hypothalamic efferent pathways controlling body temperature. Such patients lose the ability to sweat or vasoconstrict within affected dermatomes. Additionally, the disruption of afferent pathways from peripheral temperature receptors causes problems in the transmission of thermal information. As a result, patients become poikilothermic, with body temperature reflecting the environment, and their core temperature falls. The level of injury plays an important role. Patients with a higher level of injury have a more severe thermoregulatory disability. If the patient is hyperthermic other causes of fever should be ruled out.

E. True. Delayed emergence from anaesthesia related to the use of an intrathecal baclofen pump has been reported. However, discontinuation of a baclofen infusion before an operation is not recommended due to the risk of rebound spasticity.

Mashour, G.A. and Engelhard, K. *Oxford Textbook of Neuroscience and Anesthesiology*. Oxford University Press, 2019: pp. 659, 662, 665.

Matta, B.F. et al. *Core Topics in Neuroanesthesia and Neurointensive Care*. Cambridge University Press, 2011: Location 11938, 11986–12002.

Question 19: Answer

A. True. N_2O increases ICP and CBF by stimulating cerebral metabolism.

B. True. Fentanyl has negligible cerebral vascular effects. It is important to remember that fentanyl may have an indirect effect on CBF through induced hypercapnia due to respiratory depression.

C. True. Sevoflurane has been shown not to alter cerebral autoregulation below 1.5 MAC.

D. False. Isoflurane does not affect CSF production but facilitates CSF reabsorption.

E. True. Intravenous anaesthetic agents except for ketamine, decrease both $CMRO_2$ and CBF and maintain coupling between the two. Cerebrovascular autoregulation is not affected by propofol.

Flood, P. et al. *Stoelting's Pharmacology and Physiology in Anaesthetic Practice*, 5th edition. Wolters Kluwer, 2015: p. 164.

Matta, B.F. et al. *Core Topics in Neuroanesthesia and Neurointensive Care*. Cambridge University Press, 2011: Location 5745–5761.

Yao, F.-S.F. et al. *Yao & Artusio's Anesthesiology: Problem-oriented Patient Management*, 9th edition. Wolters Kluwer, 2020: Location 21869–21886.

Question 20: Answer

A. True. The risk of rupture is directly related to the size of the aneurysm according to Laplace's law (wall tension increases with an increase in the radius of the vessel).

B. False. ECG changes (tachycardia, bradycardia, ST-depression, T-inversions, QT-prolongation) after SAH are common and usually have neurogenic rather than cardiogenic origin. In haemodynamically stable patients if the level of Troponin I is not increased no further investigations are necessary.

C. False. A Glasgow Coma Scale score of 12 corresponds to Grade 4 of the WFNS grading scale (see Table 12.1).

Table 12.1 The World Federation of Neurological Surgeons (WFNS) grading scale for intracranial aneurysm

WFNS Grade	Glasgow Coma Scale Score	Presence of motor deficit
1	15	−
2	13–14	−
3	13–14	+
4	7–12	+/−
5	3–6	+/−

Reprinted from Mashour, G.A. and Engelhard, K. *Oxford Textbook of Neuroscience and Anesthesiology*. Oxford University Press, 2019, with permission from Oxford University Press.

D. False. A large study of 1001 patients ('Intraoperative hypothermia during surgery for intracranial aneurysm') with WFNS grades I–III randomized to intraoperative hypothermia (target temperature 33°C, with the use of a surface cooling technique) or normothermia (target temperature 36.5°C) showed no advantage of hypothermia in improving neurologic outcome. In fact, postoperative bacteraemia was documented in five patients in the hypothermic group and only three patients in the normothermic group (p-value 0.05). At the same time, one needs to remember that hyperthermia is detrimental and should be avoided.

E. True. Vasospasm usually occurs 72 hours after SAH. Cochrane analysis revealed a beneficial effect (reduced the risk of vasospasm and secondary ischaemia) of oral nimodipine in patients with aneurysmal SAH. It should be administered orally with a dose of 60 mg every 4 hours in adults (level of evidence: class I, level of recommendations: level A). Nimodipine can be used intravenously if necessary (level of recommendations: good clinical practice).

Mashour, G.A. and Engelhard, K. *Oxford Textbook of Neuroscience and Anaesthesiology.* Oxford University Press, 2019: p. 484, 502.

Matta, B.F. et al. *Core Topics in Neuroanaesthesia and Neurointensive Care.* Cambridge University Press, 2011: Location 10780–10796, 1262.

Steiner, T. et al. European Stroke Organization guidelines for the management of intracranial aneurysms and subarachnoid haemorrhage. *Cerebrovasc Dis*, 2013;35:93–112, p. 104.

Question 21: Answer

A. True. Veno-venous extracorporeal membrane oxygenation (ECMO) is used where respiratory failure is the main issue but the heart can provide adequate cardiac output (CO) to meet circulatory needs. The blood is extracted from the femoral or jugular vein, goes through an oxygenator and returns to the venous circulation. Veno-venous ECMO provides respiratory support, but the patient is dependent upon their own haemodynamic function. Appropriate medication is used to control CO and blood pressure.

B. False. Sedation or anaesthesia is definitely necessary for the period of cannulation and many patients do receive continuous infusions of analgesics and sedatives during the ECMO period. The concept of 'awake ECMO' has been developed more recently that avoids the negative effects of mechanical ventilation and sedation. Veno-venous (VV) ECMO is considered the most suitable technique for awake ECMO.

C. True. Oxygenated blood that enters the pulmonary circulation will reduce PVR and thereby improve right heart function. Moreover, the oxygenated blood that reaches the coronary arteries may also improve left ventricular function.

D. True. Weaning from veno-arterial ECMO is not an easy process and is not always associated with survival. Firstly, the aetiology of cardiac failure should be compatible with recovery. Secondly, few parameters that provide hemodynamic and pulmonary stability (including a mean arterial pressure (MAP) of at least 60 mmHg, on low catecholamine support, absence of metabolic disturbances) are incorporated into standardized weaning protocols. If all these issues are resolved, a weaning trial is initiated with a gradual decrease in ECMO support. Echocardiography is used to assess the right and left ventricles. An LVEF of 20–25% on minimal ECMO support (1.0–1.5 l/min for at least 15 minutes) suggests weaning is feasible.

E. True. Insertion of thoracic drainage constitutes a significant risk of bleeding. If the patient is haemodynamically stable and the pneumothorax is less than 20%, then conservative treatment is recommended.

ELSO General Guidelines. Version1.4. August 2017, pp. 13, 18–20. Available at: https://www.elso.org/Portals/0/ELSO%20Guidelines%20General%20All%20ECLS%20Version%201_4.pdf.

Kaplan, J.A. et al. *Kaplan's Cardiac Anesthesia*, 7th edition. Elsevier, 2017: pp. 1050, 1219, 1223–1224.

Question 22: Answer

A. False. 'Pink tetralogy' represents a situation with minimal right ventricle outflow tract (RVOT) obstruction with a large and unrestrictive VSD. These anatomical features result in predominantly left-to-right shunt through the VSD and the child does not develop cyanosis. But as time goes on, the clinical condition can change to classical symptoms of tetralogy of Fallot (TOF).

B. False. Complete intracardiac correction is performed in the majority of surgical cases in a one-stage operation (as long as the branches of the pulmonary artery are not very small) usually at the age of around 6 months. The goals of the operation are to close the VSD with a patch and enlarge the right ventricular outflow tract to relieve the obstruction (ideally with preservation of the pulmonary valve).

C. False. The spell is caused by a relatively sudden decrease in blood flow to the lungs due to transient near occlusion of the RVOT. 'Tet spells' are characterized by profound cyanosis. Actually, an increase in PVR is one of the treatment components of 'tet spells' (putting the child in the knee–chest position). It will decrease right-to-left shunt and diminish cyanosis. The other components of therapy are fluids (improve RV filling and pulmonary flow), oxygen (a pulmonary vasodilator and systemic vasoconstrictor), and calming the patient.

D. True. The risk of foetal loss is increased, especially in women with a haematocrit > 65%. Pregnancy in uncorrected TOF also brings significant risk for the mother, mostly due to progressive right ventricular failure.

E. True. The right-to-left intracardiac shunt and poor pulmonary blood flow prolong an inhalational induction (shunted blood with no volatile anaesthetic decreases arterial partial pressure of the inhalational anaesthetic). Poorly soluble inhalational anaesthetics are most affected. On the contrary, intravenous induction is faster.

Fleisher, L.A. *Anesthesia and Uncommon Diseases*, 6th edition. Saunders, 2012: Location 6419, 6397.

Kaplan, J.A. et al. *Kaplan's Cardiac Anesthesia*, 7th edition. Elsevier, 2017: pp. 819, 833, 834.

Question 23: Answer

A. False. Heparin is always injected before cannulation to ensure adequate anticoagulation, confirmed by an activated clotting time (ACT) > 400 seconds.

B. False. There are major differences between the two types of pumps. Roller pumps can generate unlimited pressure because of occlusion at the roller head. They are preload but not afterload dependent, and do not allow retrograde flow.

Centrifugal pumps are non-occlusive, and will not pump against any resistance. They are less likely to result in vessel dissection or pump tubing disconnection, are both preload and afterload dependent, and allow retrograde flow. In centrifugal pumps, risk of air embolism is diminished because the air will get trapped within the vortex of the pump head and so be less likely to be embolic. Other possible advantages of centrifugal pumps are reduced haemolysis, platelet preservation, and less effect on renal function, especially during prolonged cardiopulmonary bypass (CPB).

C. True. In anterograde cardioplegia, the cardioplegic solution is administered into the aorta at a flow of 200–300 ml/min and a pressure of 60–100 mmHg. In aortic insufficiency, there is a retrograde escape of cardioplegic solution across the aortic valve back to the ventricle, rather than anterograde perfusion of the coronary arteries. Hence, retrograde cardioplegia (via the coronary sinus) is administered instead of or in addition to the aortic infusion.

D. False. α-stat strategy is used by most medical centres in adult patients.

E. True. Loss of pulsatile blood flow is one of the major physiological changes under CPB. The theoretical advantages of pulsatile flow are improved microcirculation and tissue perfusion due to transmission of additional hydraulic energy, and decreased vasoconstriction as a result of decreased release of baroreceptor reflex hormones. Pulsatility during bypass can be achieved by using an intra-aortic balloon pump (IABP) or changing the speed of rotation of the pump. But it must be said that a pulsatile pressure waveform may not automatically guarantee effective pulsatile flow.

Kaplan, J.A. et al. *Kaplan's Cardiac Anesthesia*, 7th edition. Elsevier, 2017: pp. 1118–1119, 1167, 1184, 1199–1200.

Wahba, A. et al. 2019 EACTS/EACTA/EBCP. Guidelines on cardiopulmonary bypass in adult cardiac surgery. *Eur J Cardiothorac Surg*, 2020;57:210–251.

Question 24: Answer

A. False. An IABP decreases the systolic (by up to 10%) and increases the diastolic blood pressure. The balloon is deflated just before aortic valve opening (at the end of diastole) and creates an area of low pressure in the aorta. It reduces systolic blood pressure developed by the left ventricle, facilitates forward movement of blood, and increases stroke volume. Inflation of the balloon occurs immediately after aortic valve closure (in diastole), which displaces blood from the thoracic aorta, and increases diastolic and coronary perfusion pressures. This increase in diastolic pressure is called 'diastolic augmentation'.

B. True. Accumulation of extravascular lung water (EVLW) is the hallmark of pulmonary oedema of both cardiac and non-cardiac origin. EVLW includes water in the lung interstitium and alveolar space, the normal value is 4–5 ml/kg. EVLW > 10 ml/kg indicates lung oedema and EVLW > 15 ml/kg indicates severe oedema.

C. False. A reduction in SvO_2 can indicate either an increased oxygen demand or consumption (increase in the work of breathing, seizures, tremor, hyperthermia, pain) or decreased oxygen delivery (hypoxia, bleeding, hypovolaemia, decreased CO). Increased SvO_2 does not always reflect 'luxury perfusion' but can also indicate a decrease in oxygen consumption due to mitochondrial depression in critical areas (such as in septic shock or cyanide poisoning). The addition of fibreoptic technology to pulmonary artery flotation catheters now allows continuous monitoring of SvO_2.

D. True. Doppler technology has been incorporated into the oesophageal probe. The accuracy of measurement is dependent on the right position and alignment of the probe. It measures the velocity of blood flow in the descending thoracic aorta. When an ultrasonic wave meets a moving object, the shift in frequency of the reflected wave is proportional to the velocity of ejected blood. The device generates a velocity/time waveform to which is applied a calibration factor derived from the patient's height, weight, and age. The cross-sectional area of the aorta is calculated from a nomogram. The oesophageal Doppler monitor will display CO, stroke volume (SV), and the corrected systolic flow time (FTc). The FTc is normally between 330 and 360 msec and is an indicator of volaemic status. FTc is inversely related to afterload/resistance. One of the most common causes of increased afterload/resistance is hypovolaemia, so a low (short) FTc is associated with inadequate filling.

E. True. In adults 10 ml of normal saline at room temperature (in most cases) or at 4°C is injected as a rapid bolus over 2–4 seconds into a proximal lumen of the pulmonary artery flotation catheter (for children a volume of 0.15 ml/kg is recommended). The closer the temperature of the injectate to the temperature of the blood, the greater the degree of error introduced into the measurement. End-expiration is the best time for thermodilution measurement.

Kaplan, J.A. et al. *Kaplan's Cardiac Anesthesia*, 7th edition. Elsevier, 2017: pp. 411, 412–414, 1044.

Marcucci, C. et al. *Avoiding Common Anesthesia Errors*, 2nd edition. Wolters Kluwer, 2020: p. 119.

Question 25: Answer

A. True. The New York Heart Association (NYHA) classification places patients in one of four categories, based on how much they are limited during physical activity: Class I. No limitation of physical activity; Class II. Slight limitation of physical activity; Class III. Marked limitation of physical activity; Class IV. Inability to carry out any physical activity without discomfort.

B. True. Septal–lateral E/e' ratio is the ratio of the peak velocity of blood during early diastole (E), over the average of septal and lateral mitral annular diastolic peak velocities (e').

- E is the early diastolic flow of blood, recorded by pulse Doppler, between the tips of the mitral leaflets.
- e' is the movement of the mitral annulus in diastole towards the probe, recorded by pulse tissue Doppler.

The ratio E/e' is one of four important parameters measured by transoesophageal echocardiography for diagnosis of diastolic dysfunction (or heart failure with preserved ejection fraction). This ratio correlates with ventricular stiffness and values > 15 have high specificity for increased left ventricular filling pressures. Diastolic dysfunction is associated with increased postoperative mortality. The other echocardiographic parameters for diagnostic diastolic failure are:

- septal mitral e' velocity < 7.0 cm/s or lateral mitral e' velocity < 10.0 m/s (if the patient is < 75 years) and septal mitral e' velocity < 5.0 cm/s or lateral mitral e' velocity < 7.0 m/s (if the patient is > 75 years)
- tricuspid regurgitation velocity > 2.8 m/s
- Left atrial volume index > 34 ml/m^2

C. True. Sternotomy can be avoided if off-pump coronary artery bypass surgery (OPCAB) is chosen with minimally invasive direct coronary artery bypass (MIDCAB) or an endoscopically assisted approach. For the minimally invasive approach, a small thoracotomy is used and, in general, only the left internal mammary artery is grafted to the left anterior descending artery. These methods provide additional challenges for the surgical team and anaesthesiologist, including readiness for emergency conversion to on-pump, and a requirement for lung separation in some procedures.

D. False. Inhalational anaesthetics retain an important role in intraoperative cardiac anaesthesia. There is good evidence that inhalational anaesthetics provide long-lasting protective effects against myocardial ischaemia by eliciting cellular responses similar to those seen with ischaemic preconditioning, leading to reduced cardiac biomarker release. Another reason for preferring inhalational anaesthesia is the ability to monitor the end-expiratory concentration of anaesthetic, which allows the anaesthesiologist to adjust levels to minimize the risk of cardiovascular depression and intraoperative awareness. The introduction of target-controlled infusion pumps in recent years has improved the safe use of TIVA. The question as to which anaesthetic technique is better in coronary bypass surgery remains controversial. A major recent study (MYRIAD multicentre trial) did not show any significant difference in 1-year mortality in patients operated under volatile anaesthesia or TIVA (3% in TIVA group versus 2.8% in a volatile anaesthetic group).

E. True. Placement of temporary epicardial pacing wires after coronary artery bypass grafting, immediately before chest closure, is a routine procedure in many centres. Atrial and/or ventricular pacing wires are placed by the surgeon into the myocardium. Pacing helps to achieve an effective rhythm before weaning from CPB. In the presence of atrial fibrillation,

VVI mode is a reasonable choice (V –the pacing device is located in the ventricle, V-sensing for ventricular activity, I-the pacing device will inhibit itself from pacing when it senses intrinsic ventricular activity) although atrial-ventricular synchrony is not maintained in this mode.

Gravlee, G.P. et al. *Hensley's Practical Approach to Cardiothoracic Anesthesia*, 6th edition. Wolters Kluwer, 2019: pp. 370, 558, 560.

Kaplan, J.A. et al. *Kaplan's Cardiac Anesthesia*, 7th edition. Elsevier, 2017: pp. 315, 649, 745, 760–761.

Pieske, B. et al. How to diagnose heart failure with preserved ejection fraction: the HFA–PEFF diagnostic algorithm: a consensus recommendation from the Heart Failure Association (HFA) of the European Society of Cardiology (ESC). *Eur Heart J*, 2019;40:3297–3317.

Question 26: Answer

A. True.
B. True.
C. False.
D. True.
E. True.

Coeliac plexus block is a sympathetic block used to relieve pain related to upper gastrointestinal cancers and pain caused by pancreatitis. Diarrhoea and hypotension are common side effects of this particular sympathetic block. Pneumothorax might be a complication due to the close proximity of the needle to the pleura. Paraplegia can occur rarely due to damage to the artery of Adamkiewicz.

Stein, C. and Kopf, A. Anesthesia and treatment of chronic pain. In: R.D. Miller (ed.). *Miller's Anesthesia*, 7th edition. Churchill Livingstone, 2010: Chapter 58: pp. 1797–1818.

Waldman, S.D. *Atlas of Interventional Pain Management*, 4th edition. Elsevier Saunders, 2015: Chapter 77, Celiac plexus block: two needle retrocrural technique: pp. 374–380.

Question 27: Answer

A. False.
B. True.
C. True.
D. True.
E. True.

The active metabolite (normeperidine) of meperidine has potential CNS toxicity especially in patients with renal failure.

Stein, C. and Kopf, A. Anesthesia and treatment of chronic pain. In: R.D. Miller (ed.). *Miller's Anesthesia*, 7th edition. Churchill Livingstone, 2010: Chapter 58: pp. 1797–1818.

Question 28: Answer

A. True.
B. True.
C. False.
D. False.
E. True.

Characteristics of neuropathic pain are included in the Leeds Assessment of Neuropathic Symptoms and Signs, McGill Pain Short Form 2, Neuropathic Pain Scale and DN4. Available at: https://academic.oup.com/bjaed/article/8/6/210/405993

Question 29: Answer

   A. True.
   B. True.
   C. True.
   D. False.
   E. True.

Anti-inflammatory therapy and bed rest are the first-line treatment strategies for radicular pain caused by neural compression or oedema. As paracetamol is a centrally acting drug, it does not have a role in decreasing oedema.

Malik, K. and Benzon, H.T. Low back pain. In: H.T. Benzon et al. (eds.) *Raj's Practical Management of Pain*, 4th edition. Mosby Elsevier, 2008: pp. 367–387.

Question 30: Answer

   A. True.
   B. False.
   C. False.
   D. False.
   E. True.

A diabetic patient with burning foot pain is likely to have a painful diabetic neuropathy. Pregabalin and duloxetine are the first line treatment options. Nonsteroidal anti-inflammatory drugs are inefficient to relieve neuropathic pain.

Attal, N. et al. EFNS guidelines on the pharmacological treatment of neuropathic pain: 2010 revision. *Eur J Neurol*, 2010;17:1113–1123.

Khadilkar, S.V. et al. Neuropathic pain: approach, pathophysiology and management. In: D.K. Baheti et al. (eds.). *Symptom Oriented Pain Management*, 2nd edition. Jaypee Brothers Medical Publishers, 2017: pp. 297–306.

Stein, C. and Kopf, A. Anesthesia and treatment of chronic pain. In: R.D. Miller (ed.). *Miller's Anesthesia*, 7th edition. Churchill Livingstone, 2010: Chapter 58: pp. 1797–1818.

1. **Among postoperative complications**
   - **A.** the most common cause of respiratory insufficiency in the immediate postoperative period is airway obstruction due to loss of pharyngeal muscle tone
   - **B.** pharyngeal muscle dysfunction is not restored to normal until the adductor pollicis train-of-four ratio is at least 0.7
   - **C.** respiratory insufficiency can result from hypoxaemia due to hypoventilation even in a healthy patient with normal lungs
   - **D.** acute renal insufficiency can be the result of Grade III intra-abdominal hypertension
   - **E.** the development of postoperative delirium is associated with intraoperative hypotension

2. **Regarding cardiopulmonary resuscitation**
   - **A.** the recommended chest compression rate is 100–120 compressions/min
   - **B.** once an endotracheal tube is inserted, the recommended ventilation strategy is two breaths for every 15 chest compressions
   - **C.** an end-tidal carbon dioxide ($ETCO_2$) level of 10–20 mmHg immediately after the return of spontaneous circulation (ROSC) predicts failure to survive
   - **D.** cardiac output is a reliable variable to identify an adequate response to resuscitation of the cardiovascular system
   - **E.** monophasic or biphasic defibrillator waveforms are equally effective in achieving ROSC from cardiac arrest due to ventricular fibrillation

3. **Regarding non-surgical management of hypovolaemic shock due to perioperative bleeding**
   - **A.** data from structured patient interviews are a primary tool for preoperative assessment of bleeding risk
   - **B.** central venous pressure (CVP) is the primary tool to guide optimization of preload during severe bleeding
   - **C.** CVP is directly dependent on lung function
   - **D.** a target haemoglobin (Hb) concentration of 101 g/dl is recommended during active bleeding
   - **E.** if the plasma fibrinogen concentration is less than 1.5 g/l treatment with a fibrinogen concentrate at a dose of 50 mg/kg is appropriate

4. **In acute cardiogenic shock**
   A. mitral valve regurgitation is characterized by 'v' waves of greater than 10 mmHg in the pulmonary artery occlusion pressure (PAOP) tracing
   B. papillary muscle rupture can occur three to seven days after an infarct in the territory of the left circumflex artery
   C. caused by myocardial infarction resulting in ventricular septal defect, a 5% step-up in haemoglobin oxygen saturation occurs between the right atrium and the pulmonary artery
   D. airway end-tidal CO_2 levels are indicative of native cardiac output when using venoarterial extracorporeal membrane oxygenation support
   E. levosimendan and phosphodiesterase III inhibitors are not recommended for treatment

5. **In a patient with obstructive shock**
   A. stroke volume decreases due to decreased CVP
   B. due to pulmonary embolism (PE), monitoring CVP trend is more informative of severity than pulmonary arterial pressure
   C. computed tomographic pulmonary angiography demonstrating pulmonary embolization with a systolic blood pressure drop of more than 40 mmHg that lasts longer than 15 min identifies acute high-risk PE
   D. the Pulmonary Embolism Severity Index (PESI) should be calculated in confirmed pulmonary embolism to determine the early mortality risk
   E. due to PE, no benefit from systemic thrombolysis is expected if symptoms are older than 7 days

6. **A 34-year-old male is admitted to the intensive care unit (ICU) 21 days following haematopoietic stem cell transplantation (HSCT) with cough, chest pain, dyspnoea, and haemoptysis. Initial findings on admission show PaO$_2$ 60 mmHg (8 kPa) on 4 l/min O$_2$, blood pressure 88/40 mmHg, capillary refill time 3 sec, Glasgow Coma Scale score 15. Laboratory parameters highlight granulocytopenia, a five-times higher than normal C-reactive protein (CRP) with normal procalcitonin (PCT).**
   Suitable management includes
   A. a trial of non-invasive ventilation
   B. hydroxyethyl starch for initial volume resuscitation
   C. galactomannan antigen test
   D. administration of voriconazole
   E. if a computed tomography scan of the lung shows a thick-walled, cavity lesion with an air crescent sign and an intra-cavity mass, surgical resection is required

7. **The following interventions are adequate for the treatment of a hypertensive emergency resulting in thoracic aorta dissection**
   A. gradually decreasing mean arterial pressure to 70–80 mmHg
   B. heart rate should be maintained at around 60 bpm
   C. nifedipine 10 mg sublingual
   D. boluses of labetalol 10 mg intravenously
   E. the right radial artery is preferred over the left for invasive arterial blood pressure measurement

8. **When treating a patient with heart failure**
   A. the New York Heart Association (NYHA) Functional Classification Class III means that the patient is unable to carry out any physical activity without discomfort and symptoms of heart failure are present at rest
   B. acute heart failure is unlikely if N-terminal pro b-type Natriuretic Peptide (NT-proBNP) is less than 300 pg/ml
   C. tricuspid annular plane systolic excursion (TAPSE) less than 17 mm indicates right ventricular (RV) systolic dysfunction
   D. with preserved ejection fraction (HfpEF), no treatment has yet been shown convincingly to reduce morbidity or mortality
   E. routine use of an intra-aortic balloon pump cannot be recommended in acute heart failure

9. **In a patient with a cardiovascular implantable electronic device**
   A. distinguishing a conventional pacemaker (PM) from a transvenous cardioverter-defibrillator (T-ICD) can be accomplished by examining the chest radiograph
   B. nerve stimulators may cause asystole or ventricular fibrillation in patients with a PM or ICD
   C. PM asynchronous modes (VOO or DOO) can induce a lethal ventricular tachyarrhythmia
   D. should cardioversion or defibrillation be needed in a patient with a disabled T-ICD, the removal of the disabling magnet is sufficient
   E. prophylactic placement of an implantable cardioverter-defibrillator (ICD) is superior to drug therapy in patients with an ejection fraction < 0.3 and without evidence of arrhythmic inducibility

10. **In a patient with pulmonary hypertension (PH)**
   A. severity assessment of pulmonary arterial hypertension (PAH) is made by transthoracic echocardiogram
   B. vasoreactivity testing is considered positive in PAH if there is a reduction of mean pulmonary artery pressure (mPAP) more than 10 mmHg to reach an absolute value of mPAP less than 40 mmHg without decreasing cardiac output
   C. treatment of WHO group 2 PH should focus on treating the underlying lung disease
   D. specific therapy for PAH targets smooth muscle proliferation.
   E. oxygen saturation should be kept at more than 90–92%

11. **When using lung ultrasound for a systematic diagnostic approach to acute respiratory failure**
   A. low-frequency transducers visualize deep thoracic structures
   B. presence of lung point is diagnostic of pneumothorax
   C. lung ultrasound has higher sensitivity and similar specificity to chest X-ray in diagnosing pneumothorax
   D. B-pattern is characteristic of acute exacerbation of asthma
   E. it is reliable for titrating positive end-expiratory pressure and recruitment

12. **Regarding the intensive care of chronic obstructive pulmonary disease (COPD)**
    A. a patient with Global Initiative for Obstructive Lung Disease (GOLD) grade 3 severity COPD has a forced expiratory volume in 1 second/forced vital capacity less than 70% ($FEV_1/FVC < 70\%$) and FEV_1 50–80%
    B. in serious community-acquired infection, a third-generation cephalosporin is a suitable first-line agent
    C. anticholinergic agents should be used routinely to treat an acute exacerbation of COPD (AECOPD)
    D. the use of non-invasive ventilation (NIV) is preferred over invasive ventilation in the initial treatment of AECOPD
    E. pneumococcal vaccination is recommended as part of a post-intensive care bundle to prevent AECOPD

13. **When weaning from mechanical ventilation**
    A. clinicians initiate screening tests for successful weaning at an appropriate point in patient care
    B. a ratio of respiratory frequency to tidal volume (f/VT) of 105 or higher during a spontaneous breathing weaning trial predicts unsuccessful weaning
    C. ICU-acquired critical illness neuromyopathy may develop in patients receiving aminoglycosides for several days, and impair weaning
    D. in patients at risk of developing extubation failure because of ineffective clearing of secretions, extubation to NIV reduces mortality
    E. a single week of controlled mechanical ventilation is enough to induce severe diaphragm atrophy

14. **Thrombolysis is indicated for the treatment of acute pulmonary embolism (APE) in a patient with no comorbidities if**
    A. mean arterial pressure is less than 49 mmHg
    B. plasma D-dimer levels are elevated more than three times the normal range
    C. computed tomographic pulmonary angiography detects an embolism in the left main pulmonary artery with normal heart size
    D. the APE is eight days old with deteriorating RV dysfunction and elevated troponin levels
    E. a high-risk, life-threatening APE occurs during pregnancy

15. **A urea: creatinine ratio of 100:1 µmol/l (20:1 mg/dl) measured in a critical state patient is compatible with**
    A. severe liver dysfunction
    B. rhabdomyolysis
    C. dehydration due to insufficient intake of fluids (exsiccosis)
    D. administration of corticosteroids
    E. gastrointestinal haemorrhage

16. **A 28-year-old woman is admitted to ICU with a 24-hour history of somnolence, fever, vomiting, lower abdominal pain, and progressive respiratory failure. Her past medical history includes type 2 diabetes and hypertension. Regular medications: insulin glargine, metformin, empagliflozin, lisinopril. Arterial blood gas parameters pH 7.0, pCO_2 18 mmHg, pO_2 94 mmHg, HCO_3^- 17 mmol/l, lactate 2 mmol/l, glucose 10.6 mmol/l (190 mg/dl), sodium 149 mmol/l, potassium 5.3 mmol/l, chloride 100 mmol/l**

   A. diabetic ketoacidosis is unlikely

   B. pregnancy can cause these findings

   C. urinary tract infection should be investigated

   D. metformin is the likely cause of her critical state

   E. 100 mmol sodium bicarbonate should be given to treat metabolic acidosis

17. **The following interventions may worsen severe acute pancreatitis**

   A. calcium supplementation

   B. initiating enteral feeding before the pain resolves

   C. early cholecystectomy if pancreatitis is related to gallstones

   D. administration of probiotics

   E. routine prophylactic use of antibiotics

18. **When planning clinical nutrition**

   A. a patient who has lost more than 10% of their body weight in the past 6 months due to acute disease is considered severely malnourished

   B. if enteral nutrition is contraindicated, parenteral nutrition should be implemented after 48 hours

   C. it is reasonable to withhold enteral nutrition in critically ill patients with uncontrolled shock and acidosis regardless of their nutritional state

   D. bolus rather than continuous enteral nutrition should be used

   E. in critically ill patients with gastric feeding intolerance, intravenous erythromycin should be used as a first-line prokinetic therapy

19. **Which of the following conditions would preclude a conclusive diagnosis of brain death**

   A. core temperature of 35.2°C

   B. serum sodium level of 155 mmol/l

   C. free thyroxine (FT4) of 0.2 µg/dl with a thyroid-stimulating hormone (TSH) of 20 mIU/l

   D. a blood pressure of 190/100 mmHg

   E. use of rocuronium

20. Regarding the management of delirium

   A. Confusion Assessment Method for the ICU (CAM-ICU) can only be evaluated in patients with a Richmond Agitation-Sedation Scale (RASS) above −3

   B. a RASS score of −2 means movement or eye-opening to voice but no eye contact

   C. pain medication should be administered at a Critical Care Pain Observation Tool score above 8

   D. the use of benzodiazepines should be avoided in delirium

   E. blood transfusion is a modifiable risk factor associated with delirium

21. Regarding oncological emergencies requiring intensive care

   A. the treatment of malignant hypercalcaemia includes saline infusion and thiazide diuretics

   B. when administering vaptans for the treatment of hyponatraemia in the syndrome of inappropriate antidiuretic hormone (SIADH) serum sodium should not increase more than 0.5 mmol/l/hour

   C. anaemia should not be tolerated, and a liberal transfusion strategy is recommended in patients with leukostasis

   D. when treating extravasation injury due to chemotherapy, application of ice to the affected area is recommended for extravasation of vinca alkaloids

   E. the emergency treatment of cancer-related hypoglycaemia includes administration of glucagon, dextrose infusion, and diazoxide

22. A 25-year-old woman in her 34th week of pregnancy is admitted to ICU with thrombocytopenia (15 × 10⁹/l), mechanical haemolytic anaemia (haemoglobin level 6.5 g/dl, lactate dehydrogenase (LDH) more than three times the upper limit of normal, undetectable serum haptoglobin, presence of schistocytes on blood smear), and loss of consciousness and seizures. Appropriate management consists of

   A. rapid delivery

   B. plasma exchange

   C. platelet transfusion prior to plasma exchange

   D. anti-C5 treatment

   E. complement and ADAMTS-13 (von Willebrand factor-cleaving protease) tests should be performed after plasma exchange

Question 1: Answer

A. True. The persistent effects of inhaled and intravenous anaesthetics, neuromuscular blocking drugs, and opioids all contribute to the loss of pharyngeal tone, which is the most frequent cause of airway obstruction in the immediate postoperative period.

B. False. Pharyngeal muscle function is not restored to normal until the adductor pollicis train-of-four (TOF) ratio is greater than 0.9. The pharyngeal muscles are the last to recover from neuromuscular blockade, thus routine monitoring by the TOF ratio does not accurately reflect the return of pharyngeal muscle tone.

C. True. Even a healthy patient with normal lungs can become hypoxic if hypoventilating significantly while breathing room air.

Example:

if $P_AO_2 = FiO_2 (PB - PH_2O) - PaCO_2/RQ$

and $PaCO_2$ increases up to 80 mmHg (10.7 kPa) due to hypoventilation, then $P_AO_2 = 0.21$ $(760 - 47) - 80/0.8 = 150 - 100 = 50$ mmHg or in kPa $P_AO_2 = 0.21(101.3 - 6.3) -10.7/ 0.8 = 19.95 - 13.4 = 6.55$ kPa!

Where PAO_2 partial pressure of oxygen in the alveoli, PB barometric pressure, PH_2O vapour pressure of water, FiO_2 fraction of inspired oxygen, $PaCO_2$ partial pressure of CO_2 in arterial blood, RQ respiratory quotient.

D. True. Intra-abdominal hypertension is classified into four grades: I: 12–15 mmHg; II: 16–20 mmHg; III: 21–25 mmHg; and IV: greater than 25 mmHg. Abdominal compartment syndrome is defined as an intra-abdominal pressure greater than 20 mmHg. Postoperative renal impairment is independently associated with four factors: hypotension, sepsis, older age, and increased abdominal pressure.

E. False. Intraoperative factors that are predictive of postoperative delirium are: surgical blood loss; haematocrit less than 30%; and the number of intraoperative blood transfusions. Intraoperative factors that have not been shown to increase the risk of postoperative delirium in adults are intraoperative haemodynamic derangement, the administration of nitrous oxide, and anaesthetic technique (general versus regional).

Nicholau, T.K. The postanaesthesia care unit. In: R.D. Miller et al. (eds.). *Miller's Anesthesia*, 8th edition. Elsevier, 2015: Chapter 96.

Question 2: Answer

A. True. 100–120 compressions/min is the current recommended chest compression rate.

B. False. Once a definitive airway is placed the recommended ventilation strategy is ten breaths per minute.

C. False. An end-tidal carbon dioxide ($ETCO_2$) less than 10 mmHg following 20 minutes of high-quality chest compressions can predict failure to survive. However, $ETCO_2$ level should not be used as a criterion alone to decide to terminate resuscitation efforts.

D. False. The normal value for cardiac output for a particular patient is unknown and thus other markers need to be used to assess adequacy of resuscitation.

E. True. No specific defibrillator waveform (either monophasic or biphasic) is consistently associated with a greater incidence of ROSC or increased hospital discharge rates from cardiac arrest due to ventricular fibrillation. Nevertheless, recommendations for energy levels to be used for defibrillation vary according to the type of waveform.

Roberts, B.W. et al. Cardiac arrest and cardiopulmonary resuscitation. In: J.E. Parillo and R.P. Dellinger (eds.). *Critical Care Medicine Principles of Diagnosis and Management in the Adult*, 5th edition. Elsevier, 2019: Chapter 1.

Soar, J. et al. European Resuscitation Council Guidelines 2021: adult advanced life support. *Resuscitation*, 2021;*161*:115–151.

Question 3: Answer

A. True. The use of standardized questionnaires on bleeding and drug history is preferable to the routine use of conventional coagulation screening tests such as aPTT, INR, and platelet count in elective surgery patients according to 2017 guidelines from the European Society of Anaesthesiology and Intensive Care (ESAIC).

B. False. CVP is a static variable, insufficient to guide fluid therapy and optimization of pre-load during hypovolaemia, e.g., due to severe bleeding. CVP is the clinical measurement of right atrial pressure, an important haemodynamic indicator, but it is a dependent parameter so is not appropriate for assessing the volume state. Measurement of dynamic parameters of fluid responsiveness like stroke volume variation or pulse pressure variation should be considered instead. Fluid challenges and the leg-raising test are valid alternatives.

C. False. CVP depends on venous return, cardiac function, and external pressure on the heart.

D. False. 2017 ESAIC guidelines recommend a target haemoglobin concentration of 7–9 g/dl during active bleeding. Data from patients undergoing surgery or in intensive care indicate that a restrictive transfusion regimen (haemoglobin concentration maintained at 7–8 g/dl) is as effective and well-tolerated as a liberal transfusion regimen (target haemoglobin concentration from 9 to 11 g/dl). There is a lack of evidence indicating benefits from higher haemoglobin concentrations, and considering the potential side effects of transfusing allogeneic blood, blood transfusions to increase haemoglobin concentrations above 9 g/dl cannot be supported.

E. True. A fibrinogen concentration of less than 1.5–2 g/l indicates hypofibrinogenaemia in acquired coagulopathy and is associated with increased bleeding risk, and thus should be treated. The recommended starting dose of fibrinogen concentrate is 25–50 mg/kg.

Berlin, D.A. and Bakker, J. Starling curves and central venous pressure. *Crit Care*, 2015;*19*(1):55.

Kozek-Langenecker, S.A., et al. Management of severe perioperative bleeding: guidelines from the European Society of Anaesthesiology. *Eur J Anaesthesiol*, 2017;*34*:332–395.

Question 4: Answer

A. True. Mitral valve failure (e.g., due to rupture or dysfunction of chordae or papillary muscles) is characterized by 'v' waves of greater than 10 mmHg on a PAOP tracing.

B. False. Papillary muscle rupture frequently occurs 3 to 7 days after an infarct in the left anterior descending coronary artery territory.

C. True. Ventricular septal defects caused by acute ischaemia may also result in the abrupt onset of cardiogenic shock and can be diagnosed by a 5% step-up in haemoglobin oxygen saturation between the right atrium and the pulmonary artery (owing to the left to right shunting of blood through the septum).

D. True. Cardiac function can vary from absent to near-complete during different phases of venoarterial extracorporeal membrane oxygenation (VA ECMO) support. As CO_2 is only delivered to the lungs by the native cardiac output through the pulmonary circulation, airway end-tidal CO_2 excretion is indicative of native cardiac output.

E. False. According to the 2016 European Society of Cardiology (ESC) Guidelines, treatment includes short term intravenous infusion of inotropic agents—dobutamine, dopamine, levosimendan, phosphodiesterase III (PDE III) inhibitors—in patients with hypotension (systolic blood pressure (BP) < 90 mmHg) and/or signs/symptoms of hypoperfusion despite adequate filling status, to increase cardiac output, increase blood pressure, improve peripheral perfusion, and maintain end-organ function.

Kumar, A. et al. Shock: classification, pathophysiology, and approach to management. In: J.E. Parillo and R.P. Dellinger (eds.). *Critical Care Medicine Principles of Diagnosis and Management in the Adult*, 5th edition. Elsevier, 2019: Chapter 22.

Pellegrino, V. et al. Extracorporeal membrane oxygenation. In: A.D. Bersten et al. (eds.). *Oh's Intensive Care Manual*, 8th edition. Elsevier, 2019: Chapter 41.

Question 5: Answer

A. False. In obstructive shock, cardiac tamponade compromises cardiac function, and PE leads to right heart failure due to increased pulmonary vascular resistance (PVR) and increased RV afterload, and tension pneumothorax increases juxta-cardiac pressure and decreases preload of the right ventricle. CVP depends on venous return, cardiac function, and external pressure on the heart. All three changes described above will therefore result in compromised cardiac output accompanied by increased CVP. A marked increase in CVP (in the absence of juxta-cardiac pressure elevation or tricuspid valve insufficiency) is also a sign of right heart failure due to increased PVR in PE.

B. True. In PE monitoring CVP trend is more informative of the severity of the disease than following pulmonary arterial pressure (PAP). In the beginning PAP increases, but the increase in CVP will depend on how well cardiac function can compensate for the increasing afterload. As PVR exceeds the RV compensation threshold, the cardiac output (CO) and PAP decrease, however the CVP continues to rise.

C. True. According to the 2019 ESC Guidelines for the diagnosis and management of APE, high-risk PE is defined by haemodynamic instability, with one of the following clinical manifestations at presentation:

• Cardiac arrest: Need for cardiopulmonary resuscitation;
• Obstructive shock: Systolic BP less than 90 mmHg or vasopressors required to achieve a BP more than 90 mmHg despite adequate filling status.

And

• End-organ hypoperfusion (altered mental status; cold, clammy skin; oliguria/anuria; increased serum lactate);
• Persistent hypotension: Systolic BP less than 90 mmHg or systolic BP drop more than 40 mmHg, lasting longer than 15 min and not caused by new-onset arrhythmia, hypovolaemia, or sepsis.

    D. False. Confirmed PE (confirmation on computed tomography pulmonary angiography (CTPA) and/or evidence of RV dysfunction on transthoracic echocardiography (TTE)) in combination with haemodynamic instability is sufficient to place the patient in the high-risk PE category. In these cases, calculation of the PESI, or measurement of troponins or other cardiac biomarkers is unnecessary.

    E. False. The greatest benefit of systemic thrombolysis is observed when treatment is initiated within 48 h of symptom onset, nevertheless systemic thrombolysis can still be effective in patients who have had symptoms for 6–14 days.

Guyton, A.C., et al. The limits of right ventricular compensation following acute increase in pulmonary circulatory resistance. *Circ Res*, 1954;2(4):326–332.

Konstantinides, S.V., et al. 2019 ESC Guidelines for the diagnosis and management of acute pulmonary embolism developed in collaboration with the European Respiratory Society (ERS): The Task Force for the diagnosis and management of acute pulmonary embolism of the European Society of Cardiology (ESC). *Eur Respir J*, 2019;54(3):1901647.

Question 6: Answer

    A. True. Past medical history and recent parameters support the diagnosis of septic shock, a life-threatening organ dysfunction caused by a dysregulated host response to infection with circulatory and cellular/metabolic dysfunction associated with a higher risk of mortality. Regarding respiratory support, there is no evidence that sepsis and septic shock in patients with neutropenia need to be treated differently from non-neutropenic patients. Nevertheless, several studies that included selected immunosuppressed patients with pneumonitis and acute respiratory failure, showed that early initiation of NIV was associated with significant reductions in the rates of endotracheal intubation and serious complications together with an improved likelihood of survival to hospital discharge. Therefore, a trial of NIV in immunosuppressed (haemato-oncological) patients can be beneficial and avoid intubation. The trial should be closely monitored for signs of failure as an unnecessary delay in intubation is associated with increased mortality and should be avoided.

    B. False. According to recent guidelines, crystalloids are the fluid of choice for initial resuscitation and subsequent intravascular volume replacement in patients with sepsis and septic shock. Hydroxyethyl starches (HESs) are colloids for which there are safety concerns in patients with sepsis. The use of HESs resulted in a higher risk of death and the need for renal replacement therapy compared with crystalloids and albumin. There is a strong recommendation with high-quality evidence against the use of HES in the resuscitation of patients with sepsis or septic shock.

    C. True. High CRP accompanied by a negative PCT in sepsis in a HSCT patient with respiratory tract signs suggests a high probability of invasive fungal infection, especially invasive aspergillosis which remains a major cause of morbidity and mortality in immunosuppressed hosts. Definitive diagnosis requires tissue biopsy with direct visualization of the microorganism on microscopic examination. Given the challenges of obtaining tissue in thrombocytopenia or in hosts with coagulation disorders, non-culture-based diagnostics such as antigen detection of galactomannan (GM), a component of the Aspergillus cell wall, are the most frequently used methodology.

    D. True. Voriconazole, a second-generation triazole, is a mainstay of antifungal prophylaxis protocols in HSCT patients and remains the treatment of choice for invasive aspergillosis.

    E. True. Surgical intervention is required for proven anatomical sepsis source control. Aspergilloma can be seen on CT scan as a cavity lesion, most commonly in the upper lobes. Wall thickening is a sign of secondary infection and an intra-cavitary mass, with an air crescent sign is also characteristic. Clinical manifestations range from asymptomatic and incidentally discovered radiographic findings to life-threatening haemoptysis requiring emergency intervention. Symptomatic aspergilloma can be managed with surgical resection; however, in many patients, underlying structural lung disease, and low pulmonary reserve preclude operative intervention. In such a case a combination of embolization and antifungal therapy may achieve disease stabilization.

Cadena, J. et al. Invasive aspergillosis: current strategies for diagnosis and management. *Infect Dis Clin N Am*, 2016;*30*:125–142.

Kochanek, M., et al. Management of sepsis in neutropenic cancer patients: 2018 guidelines from the Infectious Diseases Working Party (AGIHO) and Intensive Care Working Party (iCHOP) of the German Society of Hematology and Medical Oncology (DGHO). *Ann Hematol*, 2019;*98*(5):1051–1069.

Rhodes, A., et al. Surviving Sepsis Campaign: international guidelines for management of sepsis and septic shock: 2016. *Intensive Care Med*, 2017;*43*(3):304–377.

Question 7: Answer

A. False. Aortic dissection is a dramatic and rapidly fatal complication of severe hypertension. The aim of therapy is to control BP and left ventricular ejection velocity to minimize propagation of the dissection. BP should be decreased as rapidly as possible to a normal or slightly hypotensive range, to achieve systolic BPs of 100–120 mmHg or mean arterial pressure of 55–65 mmHg with a heart rate of 60 bpm.

B. True. See answer A.

C. False. Intravenous administration of antihypertensive drugs is recommended during a hypertensive emergency as the absorption of drugs is guaranteed, and the patient is stabilized. The oral, intramuscular, or sublingual route may be used once an adequate BP level is maintained.

D. True. The preferred antihypertensives for the treatment of hypertensive emergencies resulting in aortic dissection are labetalol, beta-blockers, nitroprusside sodium. In particular, labetalol is preferred in patients with acute dissection. Boluses of 10–20 mg may be administered intravenously, or the drug may be infused at 1 mg/min rate until the target BP range is reached.

E. True. A right radial arterial catheter is used for aneurysms involving the proximal descending thoracic aorta because occasionally the cross-clamp is placed proximal to the left subclavian artery, thus occluding flow to the left upper extremity.

Norris, E.J. Anesthesia for vascular surgery. In: RD. Miller et al. (eds.). *Miller's Anesthesia*, 8th edition. Elsevier, 2015: Chapter 69.

Whelton, P.K. et al. 2017 ACC/AHA/AAPA/ABC/ACPM/AGS/AphA/ASH/ASPC/NMA/PCNA Guideline for the prevention, detection, evaluation, and management of high blood pressure in adults: executive summary: a report of the American College of Cardiology/American Heart Association Task Force on clinical practice guidelines. *Circulation*, 2018;*138*(17):e426–e483.

Question 8: Answer

A. False. NYHA Functional Classification Class III means: 'Marked limitation of physical activity. Comfortable at rest. Less than ordinary activity causes fatigue, palpitation, or dyspnoea.'

B. True. The upper limit of the normal range of natriuretic peptides varies according to the acuity of heart failure. In the non-acute setting for B-type natriuretic peptide (BNP) the upper limit is 35 pg/ml and for N-terminal pro-BNP (NT-proBNP) it is 125 pg/ml; in the acute setting, higher limits should be used (BNP < 100 pg/ml, NT-proBNP < 300 pg/ml).

C. True. RV systolic dysfunction is reflected by TAPSE < 17 mm and tissue Doppler-derived tricuspid lateral annular systolic velocity (s′) < 9.5 cm/s.

D. True. No treatment has yet been shown, convincingly, to reduce morbidity or mortality in heart failure with preserved ejection fraction, treatment so far is mainly symptomatic. Diuretics improve congestion and symptoms. Data are lacking or inconsistent regarding whether beta-blockers, mineralocorticoid receptor antagonists, angiotensin receptor blockers, or angiotensin-converting enzyme inhibitors can improve symptoms.

E. True. The SHOCK II trial demonstrated that the use of an intra-aortic balloon pump (IABP) did not improve outcomes in patients suffering from acute myocardial infarction and cardiogenic shock. Therefore, routine use of an IABP currently is not recommended.

Ponikowski, P. et al. 2016 ESC Guidelines for the diagnosis and treatment of acute and chronic heart failure: The Task Force for the diagnosis and treatment of acute and chronic heart failure of the European Society of Cardiology (ESC). Developed with the special contribution of the Heart Failure Association (HFA) of the ESC. *Eur J Heart Fail*, 2016;*18*(8):891–975.

Thiele, H. et al. Intraaortic balloon pump in cardiogenic shock complicating acute myocardial infarction: long-term 6-year outcome of the randomized IABP-SHOCK II trial. *Circulation*, 2019;*139*(3):395–403.

Question 9: Answer

A. True. Distinguishing a conventional pacemaker (PM) from a transvenous cardioverter-defibrillator (T-ICD) can be accomplished by examining the RV lead system on a chest radiograph. Chest radiography can also help identify the device manufacturer if there is a lack of documentation.

B. True. Nerve stimulators use a monopolar electrosurgical unit (ESU). A monopolar ESU is more likely to cause problems with cardiovascular implantable electronic devices (CIED) than a bipolar ESU. Nerve stimulators can cause PM oversensing, with resultant PM inhibition and cardiac arrest. In patients with an ICD, inappropriate detection of neuromuscular stimulators may result in ventricular tachycardia (VT) or ventricular fibrillation (VF).

C. True. During asynchronous modes (VOO or DOO) the pulse generator delivers a pacing stimulus at a fixed rate, without any sensing capabilities. As the pacemaker delivers a pacing stimulus, regardless of what the native conduction is doing, there is a small possibility that pacing could induce a pacing stimulus in the vulnerable period (on the T wave), which could potentially induce a lethal ventricular tachyarrhythmia. Therefore, these modes are rarely used for extended periods of time. The main indication for VOO or DOO is when electrocautery is used in a pacemaker dependent patient that could be sensed by the PM as native electrical conduction, which would inhibit PM output and be followed by profound bradycardia or even asystole.

D. False. Continuous electrocardiogram monitoring and the ability to deliver external cardioversion or defibrillation must be present during the time of ICD disablement. When a magnet is used to prevent ICD discharge, simple removal of the magnet may not be sufficient for immediate antiarrhythmic therapy. Lengthy treatment delays may be caused by the actual rate of tachycardia relative to the lowest treatment zone rate or by programmed therapy delays of the device.

E. True. Indeed, the Sudden Cardiac Death–Heart Failure Trial and Multicenter Unsustained Tachycardia Trial proved that prophylactic placement of an ICD is superior to drug therapy in any patient with an ejection fraction < 0.3 even without evidence of arrhythmic inducibility.

This evidence led to a significant increase in the number of patients for whom ICD therapy is indicated.

Moss, A. et al. Prophylactic implantation of a defibrillator in patients with myocardial infarction and reduced ejection fraction. *N Engl J Med*, 2002;346 (12):877–883.

Poole, L.J. et al. Long-term outcomes of implantable cardioverter-defibrillator therapy in the SCD-HeFT. *J Am Coll Cardiol*, 2020;76(4):405–415.

Buxton, A. E. et al. Prevention of sudden death in patients with coronary artery disease. Multicenter Unsustained Tachycardia Trial Investigators. *N Engl J Med*, 1999; 341(25):1882-1890. Accessed at: https://pubmed.ncbi.nlm.nih.gov/10601507/

Rozner, M.A. Implantable cardiac pulse generators. In: R.D. Miller et al. (eds.). *Miller's Anesthesia*, 8th edition. Elsevier, 2015: Chapter 48.

Question 10: Answer

A. False. Right heart catheterization (RHC) is the gold standard for diagnosis and assessing the severity of PAH.

B. True. Pulmonary vasoreactivity testing is recommended in three forms of PAH: idiopathic PAH, hereditary PAH, and drug-induced PAH. The test is considered positive if there is a reduction of mPAP $\geq$ 10 mmHg to reach an absolute value of mPAP $\leq$ 40 mmHg without decreasing CO.

C. False. PH has been classified by the WHO into five major groups: WHO group 1: PAH; WHO group 2: PH due to left heart disease; WHO group 3: PH due to pulmonary disease; WHO group 4: PH due to chronic thromboembolism pulmonary hypertension (CTEPH); and WHO group 5: PH due to unclear and multifactorial mechanisms. Thus, treatment of WHO group 2 PH should focus on treating the underlying cardiac aetiology causing left heart disease (e.g., therapy according to guidelines for heart failure with reduced or preserved function).

D. True. Specific therapy for PAH targets smooth muscle cell proliferation through three main pathways: endothelin receptor antagonists, prostacyclin analogues, and cyclic guanosine monophosphate (cGMP) pathway enhancers.

E. True. Alveolar and arterial hypoxia, acidosis, and hypercapnia can all cause pulmonary vasoconstriction, which may further worsen PH and can lead to RV failure. Measures should be taken to keep oxygen saturation above 90–92%. High-flow oxygen administered through nasal cannulae is a useful option.

Gupta, T. et al. A simplified diagnostic and therapeutic approach to pulmonary hypertension. *Curr Probl Cardiol*, 2022;47(4);100857.

Question 11: Answer

A. True. Low-frequency transducers visualize deep thoracic structures (e.g., between ribs), while high-frequency transducers are preferred to evaluate the surface of the pleura and lung.

B. True. The lung point is characterized by the alternation between normal and abolished lung sliding with respiration. This marker, representing the contact point between the aerated lung and the air collection of the pneumothorax, is 100% specific for pneumothorax.

C. True. Lung ultrasound is reported to have superior pooled sensitivity (78–90%) compared with chest X-ray (39–52%). The specificity of the two diagnostic modalities is similar (> 98%).

D. False. B-pattern, also known as alveolar-interstitial syndrome, is the phenomenon when three or more B-lines are seen per BLUE point. B-lines result from widening of the pulmonary interlobular septa due to fluid accumulation (cardiogenic pulmonary oedema), inflammation (pneumonia, acute respiratory distress syndrome (ARDS)), or fibrosis.

E. True. The transition of lung image from consolidation to B-lines and then to A-lines with increasing positive end-expiratory pressure (PEEP) by titration is reflective of successful alveolar recruitment. Ultrasound-guided alveolar recruitment improves respiratory compliance and helps to lower driving pressures, which has been associated with survival benefits in ARDS.

Islam, M. et al. Lung ultrasound for the diagnosis and management of acute respiratory failure. *Lung*, 2020;*198*(1):1–11.

Question 12: Answer

A. False. The management strategy for COPD is based on the assessment of airflow limitation, symptoms, and future risk of exacerbations. The severity of airflow limitation is determined by post-bronchodilator spirometry and classified according to GOLD.

B. True. If acute exacerbation of chronic obstructive pulmonary disease (AECOPD) is of infective origin the most common bacterial isolates are *Streptococcus pneumoniae* and *Haemophilus influenzae*. A third-generation cephalosporin (e.g., ceftriaxone) is a suitable empirical choice until the results of microbiological cultures can facilitate targeted antibiotic choice.

C. True. Anticholinergic agents, such as ipratropium bromide, have been shown to have a similar or greater bronchodilator action and fewer side effects than β-agonists (e.g., tachycardia, tremor, reduction in serum potassium) in COPD, and thus should be used routinely to treat AECOPD.

D. True. The use of NIV is preferred over invasive ventilation as the initial mode to treat AECOPD. NIV has shown a success rate of 80–85% in this patient population.

E. True. The GOLD guidelines indicate that the 23-valent pneumococcal vaccine has demonstrated a reduction in community-acquired pneumonia in patients with COPD who are younger than 65 years. In patients with COPD who are 65 years or older, the 13-valent pneumococcal vaccine has been effective in reducing bacteraemia and serious invasive pneumococcal disease. To prevent *Streptococcus pneumoniae* infection, pneumococcal vaccination is recommended in COPD patients and is part of the post-intensive care bundle.

Global Initiative for Chronic Obstructive Lung Disease. Global strategy for the diagnosis, management, and prevention of chronic obstructive pulmonary disease: 2022 report. Available at: https://goldcopd. org/2022-gold-reports-2/

Mandell, L.A. et al. Infectious Diseases Society of America/American Thoracic Society consensus guidelines on the management of community-acquired pneumonia in adults. *Clin Infect Dis*, 2007;*44*(S2):S27–S72.

Question 13: Answer

A. False. Considerable evidence suggests that most patients weaned successfully could have tolerated the weaning attempts had they been initiated a day or more earlier. Such data emphasize the need for the early use of screening tests as these have the greatest potential for enhancing clinical management if performed at a time when the clinician still has considerable doubt as to whether a patient is ready for extubation.

B. True. Rapid shallow breathing developing right after being disconnected from the ventilator, quantified as the ratio of respiratory frequency to tidal volume (f/VT) is a physiologic indicator of weaning failure. An f/VT measured during spontaneous breathing, through an endotracheal tube for a relatively short period of time, commonly 30–120 minutes (spontaneous breathing trial) is a screening test that can discriminate between successful and unsuccessful attempts of weaning with high sensitivity. Depending on studies, an f/VT > 80–105 has been associated with weaning failure.

C. True. Prolonged use of the following drugs is related to ICU-acquired critical illness neuromyopathy: neuromuscular blocking agents, steroids, and aminoglycosides.

D. False. Ineffective clearing of secretions leads to extubation failure and is also a relative contraindication for NIV.

E. True. Histobiochemical examination found signs of diaphragmatic injury and atrophy present after 5–6 days of controlled mechanical ventilation with the force-generating capacity of the diaphragm reduced by two-thirds.

Baptistella, A.R. et al. Predictive factors of weaning from mechanical ventilation and extubation outcome: a systematic review. *J Crit Care*, 2018;48:56–62.

Carlucci, A. and Navalesi, P. Weaning failure in critical illness. In: A. Webb et al. (eds.). *Oxford Textbook of Critical Care*, 2nd edition. Oxford University Press, 2016: Chapter 103.

Question 14: Answer

A. True. The critical factor determining outcome following APE is the presence or absence of RV dysfunction. Patients with signs of haemodynamic instability (shock or systemic hypotension), RV dysfunction, or myocardial injury due to APE are candidates for thrombolysis treatment.

B. False. Plasma D-dimer levels (a degradation product of cross-linked fibrin) rise with excessive degrees of coagulation and fibrinolysis. This phenomenon can be observed with diverse aetiologies: trauma, sepsis, cancer, in pregnancy, in the elderly, or hospitalized patients. Plasma D-dimer has a poor positive predictive value but remarkably high negative predictive value, thus is frequently used to rule-out PE. An elevated value *per se* is neither diagnostic for APE nor relevant in assessing its mortality risk.

C. False. CTPA is the current gold standard diagnostic tool for APE, however it is not diagnostic for RV dysfunction. In acute shock states, the RV may not have time to dilate so its size may appear relatively normal while its functionality may already be severely compromised. An embolism in the main pulmonary arteries does not necessarily result in RV dysfunction.

D. True. In normotensive patients with intermediate-risk APE, defined as the presence of RV dysfunction and elevated troponin levels, thrombolytic treatment was associated with a significant reduction in the risk of haemodynamic decompensation or collapse (Pulmonary Embolism Thrombolysis trial) and overall mortality of as much as 50–60% versus heparin treatment. Rescue thrombolytic therapy is recommended for patients who deteriorate haemodynamically. The greatest benefit of thrombolytic therapy is usually observed when treatment is initiated within 48 h of the onset of symptoms, but thrombolysis can still be useful in patients who have had symptoms for 6–14 days.

E. True. Thrombolysis or surgical embolectomy should be considered for pregnant women with high-risk APE.

Konstantinides, S.V. et al. 2019 ESC Guidelines for the diagnosis and management of acute pulmonary embolism developed in collaboration with the European Respiratory Society (ERS). *Eur Heart J*, 2020;41:543603.

Singer, M. Pathophysiology and causes of pulmonary embolism. In: A. Webb et al. (eds.). *Oxford Textbook of Critical Care*, 2nd edition. Oxford University Press, 2016: Chapter 170.

Question 15: Answer

A. False. The reference range for normal urea/creatinine serum ratio is 40:1–100:1 µmol/l in SI Units and 10:1–20:1 mg/dl in Imperial Units. Urea is synthetized in the process of deamination of amino acids during the urea (Krebs) cycle mainly in the liver. The urea cycle plays an essential role in the detoxification of excess ammonia produced during the protein metabolism of the body and in allowing the formation of new amino acids through the degradation of proteins and alterations of amino acids. Severe liver dysfunction is compatible with a decreased urea/creatinine ratio.

B. True. Plasma urea concentration is influenced by the concentration of its amino acid precursors. Excessive amino acid supply may be a consequence of muscle breakdown and can lead to increased urea/creatinine serum ratio.

C. True. Urea also contributes to the renal medullary osmotic gradient. It is reabsorbed in the inner medullary collecting ducts of the nephrons and increases the osmolarity in the medullary interstitium surrounding the descending limb of the loop of Henle, thus facilitating water reabsorption. Increased urea reabsorption and a disproportionately elevated serum level relative to creatinine in serum is compatible with hypoperfusion of the kidneys due to dehydration.

D. True. Some medications, e.g., corticosteroids inducing relative insulin resistance may also be responsible for excess protein catabolism and reduced amino acid uptake, resulting in an excessive supply of amino acid precursors and an increased urea/creatinine serum ratio.

E. True. Gastrointestinal bleeding is compatible with an increased urea/creatinine serum ratio due to increased urea production consequent on digestion of blood and increased absorption of derived amino acids. Hypoperfusion of the kidneys associated with volume loss may also contribute to increased urea reabsorption.

Haines, R.W. et al. Diagnostic implications of creatinine and urea metabolism in critical illness. In: J.-L. Vincent (ed.). *Annual Update in Intensive Care and Emergency Medicine*. Springer, 2019: Chapter 25, pp. 327–338.

Question 16: Answer

A. False. Patients with diabetic ketoacidosis (DKA) present with classic symptoms of volume depletion: weakness, fatigue, somnolence, headache, and ketosis-related symptoms (nausea, vomiting, and abdominal pain). DKA develops quickly, frequently within 24 hours. The diagnosis of DKA according to the American Diabetes Association is made in the presence of a pH less than 7.3, bicarbonate less than 18 mEq/l, anion gap greater than 10 mEq/l, glucose level greater than 250 mg/dl (13.9 mmol/l), and ketonaemia. While DKA is usually associated with elevated blood glucose levels, in people taking sodium glucose co-transporter-2 (SGLT-2) inhibitors (e.g., empagliflozin) DKA may be diagnosed with normal blood glucose levels, a phenomenon called euglycemic ketoacidosis. Patients at greatest risk are those with type 2 diabetes mellitus on insulin along with a SGLT-2 inhibitor who omit their insulin, patients with decreased oral intake or an acute illness, or infection.

B. True. Euglycemic ketoacidosis may occur in pregnant patients (due to the presence of increased counterregulatory hormones). Bicarbonate can also be normal in DKA, in patients with gastric loss of hydrogen ions (H^+) (e.g., hyperemesis gravidarum).

C. True. Blocking SGLT-2—which is found almost exclusively in the proximal tubules in the kidneys—reduces blood glucose by blocking glucose reabsorption in the kidney and thereby excreting glucose via the urine. The most common precipitating factors for DKA are infection (most commonly pneumonia and urinary tract infection-UTI) and omission of antidiabetic therapy. In this case, lower abdominal pain, fever, and SGLT-2 therapy are highly suggestive of UTI.

D. False. Biguanides such as metformin may cause type B lactic acidosis presenting with nausea, abdominal pain, tachycardia, hypotension, and tachypnoea. This occurs through inhibition of gluconeogenesis by blocking pyruvate carboxylase, the first step of gluconeogenesis, mainly in the gut, and also by decreasing the hepatic metabolism of lactate. In this case, metformin is unlikely to be the cause as the patient's lactate level is normal, and her anion gap metabolic acidosis is not related to lactic acidosis.

E. False. The patient has a high anion gap metabolic acidosis due to euglycemic ketoacidosis. In the management of ketoacidosis replacement of bicarbonate (e.g., 100 mmol in 400 ml of water at a rate of 200 ml/h, repeated every 2 hours until the pH is above 7) is only suggested at a pH of 6.9 or lower as bicarbonate may increase the risk of cerebral oedema and can worsen hypokalaemia. So far there is no evidence that administration of bicarbonate improves outcome or recovery in patients with a pH of 7.0 or above.

Krowl, L., Al-Khalisy, H., and Kaul, P. Metformin-induced lactic acidosis (MILA): review of current diagnostic paradigm *Am J Emerg Med*, 2018;36(5):908.e3–908.e5.

Morgan, F. et al. Acute diabetic emergencies, glycemic control, and hypoglycemia. In: J.E. Parillo and R.P. Dellinger (eds.). *Critical Care Medicine Principles of Diagnosis and Management in the Adult*, 5th edition. Elsevier, 2019: Chapter 55.

Rosenstock, J. and Ferrannini, E. Euglycemic diabetic ketoacidosis: a predictable, detectable, and preventable safety concern with SGLT2 inhibitors. *Diabetes Care*, 2015;38(9):1638–1642.

Question 17: Answer

A. True. Primary acinar injury may be caused by supplementation with calcium, which regulates trypsin activation. Enhanced entry of extracellular calcium may lead to a sustained increase in cytosolic calcium in the acini. This increase leads to premature activation of trypsinogen to trypsin, resulting in further acinar injury.

B. False. Several recent guidelines recommend initiating enteral feeding within 24 to 72 hours. The evidence clearly supports enteral over total parenteral nutrition. Early enteral nutrition presumably exerts its beneficial effect through the maintenance of gut microbiota integrity, subsequently preventing mucosal damage, increased intestinal permeability, translocation of bacteria to the portal circulation, and mesenteric lymphatics leading to multiple organ dysfunction syndrome.

C. True. Early cholecystectomy should not be performed in patients who have peripancreatic collections or severe acute pancreatitis related to gallstones because of the risk of superinfection of the peripancreatic fluid collections. The operation should be delayed until the fluid collections resolve or after 6 weeks following the episode of acute pancreatitis so that cholecystectomy can be combined with internal drainage. Endoscopic retrograde cholangio-pancreatography with sphincterotomy can be considered to minimize pancreatic duct obstruction from migrating gallstones in such a case. Nevertheless, this intervention is not a definitive solution and may not prevent subsequent cholecystitis.

D. True. Probiotics are not recommended in severe acute pancreatitis. An increase in gut ischaemia (5.9% vs. 0, p-value 0.004) and mortality in the probiotic arm compared with placebo (16% vs. 6%, RR, 2.53; 95% CI, 1.22–5.25) was observed in the PROPATRIA study. A possible explanation is that the elevated level of lactic acid produced by excess bacterial fermentation of carbohydrates was a key contributing factor to the increase in gut ischaemia.

E. True. The routine use of prophylactic antibiotics in patients with acute pancreatitis is not associated with a significant decrease in secondary pancreatic infection and mortality and thus it is discouraged. Overuse of antibiotics leads to antibiotic resistance and dysbiosis which has a clear correlation with worse outcomes. Antibiotics should be used in patients who develop pancreatic and/or extrapancreatic infection or sepsis.

Al-Omran, M. et al. Enteral versus parenteral nutrition for acute pancreatitis. *Cochrane Database Syst Rev*, 2010;*2010*(1):CD002837.

Besselink, M.G. et al. Probiotic prophylaxis in predicted severe acute pancreatitis: a randomised, double-blind, placebo-controlled trial. *Lancet*, 2008;*371*(9613):651–659.

Mederos, M.A. et al. Acute pancreatitis: a review. *JAMA*, 2021;*325*(4):382–390.

Question 18: Answer

A. True. According to current European Society for Clinical Nutrition and Metabolism (ESPEN) guidelines, malnutrition is defined by the association of a phenotype criteria (weight loss %, decrease in body mass index (kg/m^2 or muscle mass)), and an aetiology criterion (decrease in food intake, malabsorption or gastrointestinal symptoms, disease burden, or inflammation). A patient who has lost > 10% of their bodyweight within the past 6 months due to acute disease should be considered severely malnourished.

B. False. If oral and enteral nutrition are contraindicated, parenteral nutrition should be implemented within three to seven days.

C. True. The European Society of Intensive Care Medicine (ESICM) and the ESPEN guidelines suggest withholding enteral nutrition in critically ill patients with uncontrolled shock, uncontrolled hypoxemia and acidosis, uncontrolled upper gastrointestinal (GI) bleeding, gastric aspirate > 500 ml/6 h, bowel ischaemia, bowel obstruction, abdominal compartment syndrome, and high-output fistula without distal feeding access.

D. False. Continuous rather than bolus enteral nutrition should be used. Several studies and meta-analyses have found a significant reduction in diarrhoea with continuous versus bolus administration without any differences identified in other outcomes.

E. True. According to recent studies and meta-analyses, prokinetic use is associated with a trend towards better enteral feeding tolerance. This difference becomes significant when intravenous erythromycin is used but cannot be observed for other prokinetics like metoclopramide. The effectiveness of erythromycin or other prokinetics is significantly decreased after 72 h, thus should be discontinued after three days.

Singer, P. et al. ESPEN guideline on clinical nutrition in the intensive care unit. *Clin Nutr*, 2019;*38*(1):48–79.

Question 19: Answer

To diagnose brain death, the following factors should be absent so that the results of brain death testing are not jeopardized: hypothermia, electrolyte abnormalities, acid-base abnormalities, endocrine crises, neuromuscular blockade, sedative medications, and intoxication.

A. True. Hypothermia precludes a conclusive brain death diagnosis. A core temperature higher than 36°C is mandatory to attempt to determine brain death.

B. True. Hypernatraemia (serum sodium concentration exceeding 145 mmol/l) precludes a conclusive brain death diagnosis.

C. True. A low free thyroxine (FT4; normal range: 0.9–1.7 ng/dl) level and a high TSH; normal range: 0.40–4.50 mIU/ml) level is suggestive of primary hypothyroidism which precludes a conclusive brain death diagnosis.

D. False. Hypertension does not preclude a conclusive brain death diagnosis.

E. True. The use of rocuronium and other neuromuscular blocking agents precludes a conclusive brain death diagnosis.

Rincon, F. Neurologic criteria for death in adults. In: J.E. Parillo and R.P. Dellinger (eds.). *Critical Care Medicine Principles of Diagnosis and Management in the Adult*, 5th edition. Elsevier, 2019: Chapter 59.

Question 20: Answer

Delirium that is a severe complication of critical illness and critical care is associated with short- and long-term adverse outcomes. According to recent evidence, monitored, goal-directed sedation and analgesia improve outcome.

A. True. At deeper levels of consciousness (RASS −4 or −5) the patient is not responsive. These levels are referred to as stupor or coma, and in these situations CAM-ICU cannot be assessed. Patients can display at least the beginnings of meaningful responsiveness (e.g., response to voice) at the lighter levels of consciousness (RASS −3 to +4), thus the RASS score should be > −3 to be able to assess for clarity of thought, specifically delirium.

B. False. A RASS score of −2 means light sedation: patient briefly awakens with eye contact to voice (< 10 seconds). Movement or eye-opening to voice, but no eye contact indicates a RASS score of −3, moderate sedation.

C. False. The Critical Care Pain Observation Tool score range is 0–8. Significant pain needing prompt intervention and administration of pain medication is present at a score ≥ 3. The Prevention and Management of Pain, Agitation/Sedation, Delirium, Immobility, and Sleep Disruption in Adult Patients in the ICU (PADIS) guidelines make several strong recommendations for treating pain in ICU, also for the effective prevention of delirium.

D. True. Randomized controlled trials demonstrated that the prevalence of delirium was lower in patients who were sedated with dexmedetomidine versus benzodiazepines. Based on these studies, the PADIS guidelines recommend the avoidance of benzodiazepines in patients with delirium.

E. True. Strong evidence indicates that certain modifiable (e.g., blood transfusion and benzodiazepine use) and non-modifiable (e.g., age, dementia, pre-ICU emergency surgery or trauma, high Acute Physiology and Chronic Health Evaluation (APACHE) score) risk factors are associated with delirium.

Devlin, J.W. et al. Clinical practice guidelines for the prevention and management of pain, agitation/sedation, delirium, immobility, and sleep disruption in adult patients in the ICU. *Crit Care Med*, 2018;46(9):e825–e873.

Question 21: Answer

A. False. The treatment of malignant hypercalcaemia includes saline infusion, furosemide, calcitonin, and bisphosphonates. Thiazide diuretics should be avoided as they increase calcium reabsorption from the urine.

B. True. The vaptans bind competitively to V2 receptors in the collecting duct of the kidney where they induce almost pure aquaresis. Vaptan-induced excessive correction of hyponatraemia may lead to central pontine myelinolysis, and thus should be closely monitored. The serum sodium should not increase at a higher rate than 0.5 mmol/l/hour.

C. False. In leukostasis, whole blood viscosity is usually not dramatically increased because the rise in the white blood cell count is often counterbalanced by a decrease in the erythrocyte count. This is the reason why packed red blood cell transfusions in patients with asymptomatic hyperleukocytosis can easily provoke leukostasis; thus packed red blood cells should only be given when tissue oxygenation is inadequate due to significant anaemia or after leukapheresis.

D. False. Extravasation of chemotherapy may lead to serious soft tissue damage or infection requiring surgical intervention. Infusion should be discontinued, and the affected limb elevated. Treatment is drug-specific. While certain irritants react positively to cooling (application of ice to the affected area) which causes vasoconstriction and reduces the extent of local injury and pain, in the case of others (like vinca alkaloids), heat is recommended to increase perfusion and drug removal. For vinca alkaloids cooling is contraindicated as it worsens ulceration.

E. True. The emergency treatment of cancer-related hypoglycaemia includes glucagon (1 mg iv/im), dextrose infusion, and diazoxide (3 mg/kg/day). Non-selective beta-blockers that may blunt adrenergic response to low blood sugar should be reconsidered. Exogenous glucocorticoids and regimented carbohydrate intake may be beneficial. The definitive treatment is surgical removal of the underlying tumour.

Lewis, M.A. et al. Oncologic emergencies: pathophysiology, presentation, diagnosis, and treatment. *CA Cancer J Clin*, 2011;*61*(5):287–314.

Question 22: Answer

A. True. Pregnancy has long been recognized as a high-risk period for different forms of thrombotic microangiopathy (TMA). TMA in pregnancy is diagnosed based on the presence of a platelet count < 100 × 10⁹/l, a haemoglobin level < 10 g/dl, lactate dehydrogenase (LDH) > 1.5 times the upper limit of normal, undetectable serum haptoglobin, negative direct erythrocyte antiglobulin test, and the presence of schistocytes on blood smear, or TMA features in kidney biopsy. Rapid delivery should be considered, as it may be sufficient to control some forms of pregnancy-associated TMA (pre-eclampsia/eclampsia, haemolysis elevated liver enzymes, and low platelet count (HELLP) syndrome) or allow for more rapid remission of other types of pregnancy-associated TMA such as thrombotic thrombocytopenic purpura (TTP) and atypical haemolytic uremic syndrome, (aHUS).

B. True. After initial blood testing (especially sFlt-1/PlGF, complement, and ADAMTS13 tests), plasma exchange should be initiated if TMA diagnosis is suspected in a patient with atypical presentation of eclampsia or HELLP syndrome, life-threatening neurological (seizures, altered consciousness, coma) signs and potentially profound thrombocytopenia (< 30 × 10⁹/l). Plasma exchange should be performed as for acute TTP until ADAMTS13 test results are available. TTP is the consequence of a severe deficiency in ADAMTS13, the specific metalloproteinase that cleaves ultra large multimers of von Willebrand factor. Pregnancy-associated TTP is defined by a severe deficiency in ADAMTS13 activity (< 20%).

C. False. Platelet transfusions, which may be required for procedures (e.g., caesarean section, central catheter insertion), should be avoided in patients with TTP due to a high risk of thrombosis and worsening of neurological symptoms. If platelet transfusion is urgently needed, it should be administered along with plasma exchange (PEX).

D. False. Anti-C5 treatment is the specific treatment of aHUS, which is caused by a dysregulation of the complement alternative pathway and characterized dominantly by renal involvement.

E. False. The treatment of immune TTP during pregnancy is plasma exchange performed by administration of fresh-frozen plasma (1.0–1.5 plasma volume, 40–60 ml/kg fresh-frozen plasma), which may jeopardize the correct assessment of sFlt-1/PlGF, complement, and ADAMTS-13 levels needed for differential diagnosis. Diagnostic blood sampling thus must be performed before starting PEX.

Fakhouri, F. et al. Management of thrombotic microangiopathy in pregnancy and postpartum: report from an international working group. *Blood*, 2020;*136*(19):2103–2117.

1. **In patients with a recent history of myocardial infarction**
   A. warfarin is indicated for one year after the ischaemic event
   B. beta-blockers should be introduced in the absence of any contraindication
   C. non-urgent, scheduled surgery may take place two months after insertion of a coronary artery drug-eluting stent
   D. if urgent surgery is necessary 15 days after the insertion of a stent, then dual antiplatelet therapy with aspirin and clopidogrel should be withheld during the perioperative period
   E. angiotensin-converting enzyme (ACE) inhibitors are contraindicated in the presence of heart failure

2. **ECG changes associated with hyperkalaemia include**
   A. flat T waves
   B. a prolonged PR interval
   C. an enlarged QRS complex
   D. emergence of a U wave
   E. right bundle branch block

3. **Untreated severe hypertension**
   A. is associated with an increased incidence of perioperative myocardial infarction
   B. is associated with a right-shift of the cerebral blood flow autoregulation curve
   C. is a contraindication to the use of sevoflurane
   D. predisposes to deep venous thrombosis
   E. is a contraindication to the intraoperative use of sodium nitroprusside

4. **In a patient with recent-onset atrial fibrillation (AF)**
   A. hypothyroidism is a possible cause
   B. if the duration of AF is over 48 hours, anticoagulation is not recommended before cardioversion
   C. digoxin is contraindicated if the patient has Wolff-Parkinson-White (WPW) syndrome
   D. mitral stenosis is a possible cause
   E. intravenous beta-blockers are indicated to control a rapid ventricular rate that is poorly tolerated

5. **The following signs are associated with COVID-19 infection**
    A. hypothermia
    B. a decrease in the plasma level of D-dimers
    C. diarrhoea
    D. thrombocythaemia
    E. cough

6. **The following diseases are associated with a decrease in the ratio of forced expiratory volume in one second to forced vital capacity (FEV$_1$/FVC)**
    A. chronic obstructive pulmonary disease
    B. asthma
    C. pneumonectomy
    D. kyphoscoliosis
    E. bronchiectasis

7. **When analysing a preoperative chest X-ray**
    A. an enlargement of the superior mediastinum is compatible with pericarditis
    B. a normal chest X-ray shows a higher right than left diaphragmatic dome
    C. the association of parenchymal opacities and bilateral hilar enlargement is compatible with a diagnosis of sarcoidosis
    D. an opacity of the lower pulmonary field associated with an ipsilateral mediastinal deviation is typical of a pleural effusion
    E. vessels should normally be visible at the lung periphery

8. **Concerning cystic fibrosis**
    A. changes in coagulation respond to vitamin K treatment
    B. elevated Cl⁻ values in sweat are always found
    C. chronic infection, with *Staphylococcus aureus* and *Pseudomonas aeruginosa*, is the most common cause of death
    D. cholecystitis and cholelithiasis are common complications
    E. during anaesthesia, anticholinergic drugs are recommended

9. **In a patient with diabetes mellitus**
    A. a glycosylated haemoglobin (HbA1c) level of 8% is associated with adequate short-term glycaemic control
    B. treatment with metformin should be interrupted 5 to 7 days prior to major surgery
    C. the risk of perioperative infection is increased
    D. frequent silent ischaemic events are common
    E. the risk of bronchial aspiration is increased

10. **In a patient with morbid obesity**
    A. during general anaesthesia, ventilation/perfusion mismatch is worse in the supine position
    B. polycythaemia improves oxygenation
    C. the risk of colorectal cancer is increased
    D. the dose of neuromuscular blocking agent should be based on ideal body weight
    E. pain-related respiratory complications are avoided by opioid administration

11. **Acute intermittent porphyria**
    A. after an acute attack resolves, paresis disappears within hours
    B. seizures should be treated immediately with phenytoin
    C. is an inherited autosomal dominant disorder
    D. patients requiring surgery, should have a preoperative fasting period longer than 6 hours
    E. nitrous oxide is a safe inhaled anaesthetic in patients with porphyria

12. **In a patient with Addison's disease**
    A. atypical abdominal pain is common
    B. haemodynamic instability is observed in uncompensated cases
    C. etomidate should not be used
    D. routine urea and electrolyte levels show changes from an early stage of the disease
    E. hypermagnesaemia can be found

13. **Complications of chronic kidney disease include**
    A. platelet dysfunction
    B. hypercalcaemia
    C. autonomic neuropathy
    D. neutropenia
    E. hepatitis

14. **In Guillain–Barré syndrome**
    A. succinylcholine should not be administered for tracheal intubation
    B. fever is frequently present when neurological clinical symptoms start
    C. a segmental sensory neuropathy is typically observed
    D. autonomic dysfunction is uncommon
    E. sphincter disturbance is an associated symptom

15. **The following are compatible with a diagnosis of sickle cell disease**
    A. anaemia with a haematocrit of 20% and a low reticulocyte count
    B. atypical abdominal pain following fever
    C. pneumococcal infection
    D. onset of organ damage in adulthood
    E. onset of haemolytic anaemia in the perioperative period

Question 1: Answer

A. False. Warfarin is not indicated for coronary artery thrombosis prevention after acute myocardial infarction (AMI), even after stenting.

B. True. Beta-blocker therapy introduced in the early period after AMI reduces infarct size. There is also a reduction in both early mortality and long-term mortality when beta-blockade is continued after the acute phase.

C. False. Elective surgery should not be scheduled until six months to one year after insertion of a drug-eluting stent and three months after bare-metal stenting.

D. False. Dual anti-platelet therapy should be maintained at least one month after the insertion of a bare metal stent and six months after a drug-eluting stent. Whenever possible, surgery should be delayed until the full dual platelet therapy course is finished. In an emergency, if at all possible, surgery should be performed without discontinuation of aspirin.

E. False. ACE inhibitors and aldosterone receptor antagonists are indicated following AMI, when they should not be discontinued in the perioperative period. Particular attention should be paid to intraoperative blood pressure control, due to the risk of hypotension, especially if patients are also treated with beta-blockers.

De Hert, S. et al. Pre-operative evaluation of adults undergoing elective noncardiac surgery: updated guideline from the European Society of Anaesthesiology. *Eur J Anaesthesiol*, 2018;35:407–465.

Reed, G.W., Rossi, J.E., and Cannon, C.P. Acute myocardial infarction. *Lancet*, 2017;389:197–210.

Question 2: Answer

A. False. Hyperkalaemia is responsible for repolarization abnormalities, with peaked T waves.

B. True. Atrial conduction is depressed, and the PR interval may become prolonged.

C. True. Hyperkalaemia leads to conduction abnormalities with an enlarged QRS complex, and bradycardia.

D. False. U waves are typically observed in hypokalaemia.

E. True. Hyperkalaemia is associated with conduction abnormalities and can lead to any kind of conduction block.

Lin, T., Smith, T., and Pinnock, C. *Fundamentals of Anaesthesia*, 4th edition. Cambridge University Press, 2017: Section 1, Chapter 1, Electrolyte disturbances: pp. 6–8.

Morgan, G.E., Mikhail, M.S., and Murray, M.J. *Clinical Anesthesiology*. Lange Medical Books/McGraw Hill Medical Pub Division, 2018: Section III, Anesthetic management: Chapter 49, Management of patients with fluid and electrolyte disturbances.

Question 3: Answer

A. True. Uncontrolled severe hypertension significantly increases the risk of major cardiovascular events such as coronary events, strokes, or dissecting aneurysm in the perioperative period.

B. True. Cerebral blood flow is autoregulated over a mean arterial pressure range of 50–150 mmHg in healthy patients. This range is shifted to the right in patients with chronic severe hypertension.

C. False. Sevoflurane is the halogenated agent with the least cardiovascular effect, and little effect on blood pressure. It is not contraindicated in patients with severe hypertension.

D. True. Hypertension is a risk factor for deep venous thrombosis in patients with lung cancer and those undergoing orthopaedic surgery, especially in the case of severe hypertension.

E. False. Sodium nitroprusside is a potent vasodilator, acting through nitric oxide release. It is used for the control of acute hypertension. Its rapid onset and short duration of action make it a good option for acute severe hypertension control. Marked hypertension in patients with limited cardiac reserve requires direct intra-arterial pressure monitoring; additional treatments include an intravenous infusion of nitroglycerin, nicardipine, or clevidipine.

Gilbert-Kawai, E. and Montgomery, H. Cardiovascular assessment for non-cardiac surgery: European guidelines. *Br J Hosp Med (Lond)*, 2017;78:327–332.

Lin, T., Smith, T., and Pinnock, C. *Fundamentals of Anaesthesia*, 4th edition. Cambridge University Press, 2017: Section 1, Chapter 36, Cardiovascular pharmacology: pp. 695–707.

Morgan, G.E., Mikhail, M.S., and Murray, M.J. *Clinical Anesthesiology*. Lange Medical Books/McGraw Hill Medical Pub Division, 2018: Section III, Anesthetic management: Chapter 56, Postanesthesia care.

Question 4: Answer

A. True. Possible causes of AF include hypertension, myocardial infarction, hypothyroidism, hyperthyroidism, or other metabolic disorders, valvular disorders, exposure to stimulants, sick sinus syndrome, virus infections, and pulmonary diseases.

B. False. For AF of 48 hours duration or longer, anticoagulation is recommended for a period of three weeks before, and four weeks after cardioversion. If the patient requires urgent cardioversion, anticoagulation must be initiated as soon as possible and continued for four weeks.

C. True. Adenosine, verapamil, and digoxin are contraindicated during AF in patients with WPW syndrome because they can dangerously accelerate the ventricular response, and amiodarone is not recommended. The most useful pharmacological agents are class Ia drugs (such as procainamide).

D. True. Valvular disorders that provoke atrial dilation, such as mitral stenosis, increase the risk of AF.

E. True. Beta-blockers are indicated to reduce heart rate and improve tolerance to AF. Alternative drugs are calcium antagonists and digoxin. Pharmacological cardioversion is possible using class Ic (flecainide, propafenone) or class III (amiodarone) antiarrhythmic drugs.

January, C.T. et al. 2019 AHA/ACC/HRS focused update of the 2014 AHA/ACC/HRS guideline for the management of patients with atrial fibrillation: a report of the American College of Cardiology/ American Heart Association task force on clinical practice guidelines and the Heart Rhythm Society in collaboration with the Society of Thoracic Surgeons. *Circulation*, 2019;140:e125–e51.

Question 5: Answer

A. False. Fever is the most common sign of COVID-19 (88% of cases).

B. False. COVID-19 is responsible for disseminated intravascular coagulopathy (DIC), associated with an elevation of the plasma level of D-dimers. Patients with a plasma level greater than 1 mcg/ml have a high risk of mortality (OR: 18.42, 95% CI 2.64–128.55).

C. True. Gastrointestinal symptoms like nausea and vomiting or diarrhoea are regularly encountered during COVID-19 infection.

D. False. COVID-19 is associated with thrombocytopenia.

E. True. Respiratory symptoms are the second most frequent clinical signs during COVID-19, both non-productive cough (68%) and dyspnoea (19%) are common.

Guan, W.J. et al. Clinical characteristics of coronavirus disease 2019 in China. *N Engl J Med*, 2020;*382*:1708–1720.

Zhou, F. et al. Clinical course and risk factors for mortality of adult inpatients with COVID-19 in Wuhan, China: a retrospective cohort study. *Lancet*, 2020;*395*:1054–1062.

Question 6: Answer

The ratio of the forced expiratory volume in the first second of exhalation (FEV_1) to the total forced vital capacity (FVC) is proportional to the degree of airway obstruction. Normally, FEV_1/FVC is 80% or greater.

A. True. All patients affected by an obstructive pulmonary disease will have spirometry showing a decreased FEV_1/FVC ratio. Chronic obstructive pulmonary disease (COPD) is an example of obstructive pulmonary disease.

B. True. Asthma is an obstructive pulmonary disease.

C. False. Pneumonectomy by itself decreases the total pulmonary capacity, but not the FEV_1/FVC ratio. It presents as a restrictive pulmonary pattern, but in the absence of co-existing disease, not an obstructive pulmonary pattern.

D. False. Kyphoscoliosis produces a restrictive pulmonary pattern, so FEV_1/FVC is not affected.

E. True. Bronchiectasis is another cause of obstructive pulmonary disease.

Haynes, J.M. Basic spirometry testing and interpretation for the primary care provider. *Can J Respir Ther*, 2018;*54*(4):10.29390/cjrt-2018-017.

Moore, V.C. Spirometry: step by step. *Breathe*, 2012;*8*:232–240.

Question 7: Answer

A correct systematic analysis and interpretation are necessary to assess a chest X-ray adequately.

A. False. The cardiac silhouette is enlarged in pericarditis, but only in the lower part of the mediastinum. Causes of an enlarged cardiac silhouette also include cardiomegaly, anterior mediastinal mass, and an anterior-posterior (AP) projection (the technical set-up for taking a chest X-ray can influence interpretation of the cardiothoracic index).

B. True. The hemidiaphragms are not at the same level, and a height difference of one intercostal space is encountered on the normal chest X-ray.

C. True. Pulmonary signs are found in 90% of patients with sarcoidosis. The association of bilateral adenopathy and pulmonary infiltrates corresponds to stage 2 of the disease.

D. False. The association of a lower chest opacity with an ipsilateral mediastinal deviation is mostly due to pulmonary atelectasis; the mediastinum is drawn towards the affected lung.

Pleural effusion does not usually affect mediastinal position, even though it can be associated with atelectasis.

E. False. Vessels should be almost invisible at the lung periphery.

Hines, R.L. and Marschall, K.E. *Stoelting's Anesthesia and Co-existing Disease*, 7th edition. Elsevier, 2018: Chapter 322: pp. 2135–2142; Chapter 158: pp. 1006–1020.

Klein, J.S. and Rosado-de-Christenson M.L. A systematic approach to chest radiographic analysis. In: J. Hodler, R. Kubik-Huch, and G. von Schulthess (eds.). *Diseases of the Chest, Breast, Heart and Vessels 2019–2022*. IDKD Springer Series. Springer, 2019: pp. 1–16.

Question 8: Answer

Cystic fibrosis (CF) is an autosomal recessive disorder. Most patients with CF present with signs and symptoms of the disease in childhood.

A. True. CF can impair coagulation due to hepatic dysfunction or if absorption of fat-soluble vitamins from the gastrointestinal tract is impaired. Vitamin K treatment may be necessary.

B. False. The presence of a sweat Cl⁻ concentration greater than 70 mEq/l plus clinical manifestations (cough, chronic purulent sputum production, dyspnoea) or a family history of the disease confirms the diagnosis of CF. Nevertheless between 1 and 2% of patients with clinical signs of CF have normal sweat Cl⁻ values.

C. True. The primary cause of morbidity and mortality in patients with CF is chronic pulmonary infection. Chronic infection with *Staphylococcus aureus* and *Pseudomonas aeruginosa* is the most frequent.

D. True. Cholecystitis and cholelithiasis are common complications, as well as pancreatic and hepatic dysfunction.

E. False. Humidification of inspired gases, adequate hydration, and avoidance of anticholinergic drugs are very important during general anaesthesia because they ensure maintenance of fluid secretions.

Fauci, A. et al. (eds.). *Harrison's Internal Medicine*, 17th edition. McGraw Hill Education, 2008: Part 10: Chapter 253, Cystic fibrosis: pp. 1865–1868.

Hines, R L. and Marschall, K.E. *Stoelting's Anesthesia and Co-existing Disease*, 7th edition. Elsevier, 2018: Chapter 2, Obstructive respiratory diseases: pp. 30–32.

Question 9: Answer

A. False. In a controlled diabetic patient, glycosylated haemoglobin should not exceed 6.5%.

B. False. Metformin should be continued until 48 h before surgery and restarted if renal and hepatic functions are not altered.

C. True. Diabetes mellitus is associated with immunosuppression, which increases susceptibility to infection.

D. True. Electrocardiographic anomalies of ST segment, T-wave, or even silent myocardial ischaemia or infarct are typical in diabetic patients even in the absence of clinical signs. This silent ischaemia is due to diabetic autonomic neuropathy.

E. True. Autonomic dysfunction during diabetes mellitus is responsible for diabetic gastroparesis leading to delayed emptying of the stomach, which can be treated with antacids and prokinetics.

Morgan, G.E., Mikhail, M.S., and Murray, M.J. *Clinical Anesthesiology*. Lange Medical Books/McGraw Hill Medical Pub. Division, 2006: Chapter 35, Anesthesia for patients with endocrine diseases: pp. 753–772.

Question 10: Answer

Obesity is defined as a body mass index (BMI) of 30 or higher, and morbid obesity as a BMI of more than 40.

A. True. Patients with morbid obesity should be positioned on a 30° upward ramp as the functional residual capacity of obese patients deteriorates in the supine position. Reduction in lung volumes is accentuated by the supine and Trendelenburg positions. In particular, functional residual capacity may fall below closing capacity.

B. True. Obstructive sleep apnoea is a complication of obesity characterized by hypercapnia, cyanosis-induced polycythaemia, right-sided heart failure, and somnolence.

C. True. The WHO International Agency for Research on Cancer estimates that obesity and lack of physical activity are responsible for 25–33% of breast, colon, endometrial, renal, and oesophageal cancers. Prostate and uterine cancer are also seen in a higher percentage of overweight patients. Hiatus hernia, gastroesophageal reflux disease, delayed gastric emptying, and hyper-acidic gastric fluid all increase the risk of gastric cancer.

D. True. Water-soluble drugs (such as neuromuscular blocking agents) have small volumes of distribution, which are minimally increased by body fat. Therefore, the dosing of water-soluble drugs should be based on ideal body weight to avoid overdosage.

E. False. During the postoperative period, obese patients are more vulnerable to sedatives or opioids.

Hines, R.L. and Marschall, K.E. *Stoelting's Anesthesia and Co-existing Disease*, 7th edition. Elsevier, 2018: Chapter 20, Nutritional diseases: obesity and malnutrition: pp. 385–403.

Morgan, G.E., Mikhail, M.S., and Murray, M.J. *Clinical Anesthesiology*. Lange Medical Books/McGraw Hill Medical Pub. Division, 2006: Chapter 35, Anesthesia for patients with endocrine diseases: pp. 753–772.

Question 11: Answer

Porphyria is a metabolic disorder, resulting from the deficiency of a specific enzyme in the haem biosynthetic pathway. Of all the presentations of porphyria, acute intermittent porphyria is the most serious and can cause severe problems during anaesthesia.

A. False. When an acute attack resolves, abdominal pain disappears within hours, but paresis begins to improve within days and may continue up to several years.

B. False. Most anticonvulsant drugs can exacerbate symptoms. Clonazepam is safe.

C. True. Acute porphyria is an inherited autosomal dominant disorder with a variable expression.

D. False. Preoperative fasting should be minimized because caloric restriction has been linked to attacks of acute porphyria. The first line of treatment for an acute porphyria crisis is to remove any known triggering factor so adequate hydration and carbohydrate loading are recommended.

E. True. Nitrous oxide is a safe inhaled anaesthetic in patients with porphyria. Isoflurane, sevoflurane, and desflurane are also safe.

Fauci, A. et al. (eds.). *Harrison's Internal Medicine*, 17th edition. McGraw Hill Education, 2008: Part 15: Chapter 352, The porphyrias: pp. 2434–2444.

Hines, R.L. and Marschall, K.E. *Stoelting's Anesthesia and Co-existing Disease*, 7th edition. Elsevier, 2018: Chapter 19, Inborn errors of metabolism: pp. 377–384.

Question 12:   Answer

Addison's disease results from progressive destruction of the adrenals. It must involve more than 90% of the glands before clinical signs of adrenal insufficiency appear.

   A. True. Clinical signs are characterized by fatigue, weakness, anorexia, abdominal pain, nausea and vomiting, cutaneous and mucosal hyperpigmentation, hypovolaemia, hyponatraemia, and hyperkalaemia.

   B. True. Arterial hypotension with postural accentuation is common during uncompensated Addison's disease. The patient should be managed aggressively with invasive monitoring, IV corticosteroids, and fluid and electrolyte resuscitation.

   C. True. Etomidate transiently inhibits cortisol synthesis and should be avoided in this population.

   D. False. In the early phase of gradual adrenal destruction, there may be no demonstrable abnormalities in routine laboratory tests. At an advanced stage of adrenal destruction, serum sodium, chloride, and bicarbonate levels are reduced, and serum potassium is elevated.

   E. True. Causes of hypermagnesaemia include hypothyroidism, hyperparathyroidism, Addison's disease, and lithium therapy.

Fauci, A. et al. (eds.). *Harrison's Internal Medicine*, 17th edition. McGraw Hill Education, 2008: Part 15: Chapter 336, Disorders of the adrenal cortex: pp. 2247–2269.

Hines, R.L. and Marschall, K.E. *Stoelting's Anesthesia and Co-existing Disease*, 7th edition. Elsevier, 2018: Chapter 23, Endocrine disease: pp. 468–470.

Question 13:   Answer

   A. True. Platelet function is impaired in patients with kidney failure. Clinically this is manifest as a prolonged bleeding time. Most patients have decreased platelet factor III activity as well as decreased platelet adhesiveness and aggregation.

   B. False. Chronic kidney disease provokes multiple metabolic abnormalities including hyperkalaemia, hyperphosphatemia, hypocalcaemia, hypermagnesaemia, hyperuricaemia, and hypoalbuminaemia. Changes in calcium and phosphate metabolism are due to alterations in the synthesis of 1,25-dihydroxycholecalciferol in the kidney, which causes hypocalcaemia. Hypocalcaemia triggers secondary hyperparathyroidism with hyperphosphataemia.

   C. True. Autonomic and peripheral neuropathies are common in patients with chronic kidney disease, being more frequent and severe if patients also suffer from diabetes mellitus.

   D. True. Chronic kidney disease is responsible for complications directly or indirectly related to renal replacement therapy. These include hypotension, neutropenia, hypoxaemia, and dialysis disequilibrium syndrome.

   E. True. Patients with chronic kidney disease are prone to transfusion-related hepatitis.

Butterworth, J.F., Mackey, D.C., and Wasnick, J.D. *Morgan and Mikhail's Clinical Anesthesiology*, 6th edition. McGraw Hill, 2018: Chapter 31, Anesthesia for patients with kidney disease.

Hines, R.L. and Marschall, K.E. *Stoelting's Anesthesia and Co-existing Disease*, 7th edition. Elsevier, 2018: Chapter 22, Renal disease: pp. 432–441.

Question 14: Answer

The stem of this question refers to Guillain–Barré syndrome (GBS), an acute, severe, ascending polyradiculoneuropathy of autoimmune nature.

A. True. Succinylcholine should not be administered: there is a risk of excessive potassium release from denervated skeletal muscle.

B. False. 70% of cases of GBS occur 1–3 weeks after a respiratory or gastrointestinal infection, so patients do not present with fever at the onset of neurological symptoms.

C. False. There are mild sensory symptoms or signs, but no segmental sensory level is observed.

D. False. Autonomic involvement is common and may occur even in patients with mild neurological symptoms of GBS. The autonomic disturbances usually observed are loss of vasomotor control with wide fluctuation in blood pressure, postural hypotension, and cardiac dysrhythmias.

E. False. GBS does not affect sphincters. If patients present with sphincter disorder, a different diagnosis should be sought, especially acute myelopathies associated with prolonged back pain.

Fauci, A. et al. (eds.). *Harrison's Internal Medicine*, 17th edition. McGraw Hill Education, 2008: Part 16, Neurological disorders: Chapter 380, Guillain–Barré syndrome and other immune-mediated neuropathies: pp. 2667–2670.

Hines, R.L. and Marschall, K.E. *Stoelting's Anesthesia and Co-existing Disease*, 7th edition. Elsevier, 2018: Diseases of the autonomic and peripheral nervous systems: pp. 315–326.

Question 15: Answer

Hb-S (the abnormal haemoglobin (Hb) in sickle cell disease) has an error in Hb with a single amino acid substitution that results in reduced solubility and precipitation of the abnormal Hb.

A. False. Most patients with sickle syndromes suffer from haemolytic anaemia, with a haematocrit between 15–30%, but there is significant reticulocytosis.

B. True. Factors that precipitate a crisis include infection, excessive exercise, anxiety, abrupt changes in temperature, hypoxia, and hypertonic dyes.

C. True. Splenic failure is frequently observed within the first 18–36 months of life, causing susceptibility to infection, particularly with pneumococcus.

D. False. Organ damage can start early in childhood.

E. True. In the perioperative period patients are at risk of haemolytic crisis, which can be precipitated by perioperative hypothermia, hypoxia, dehydration, acidosis, and the use of an occlusive orthopaedic tourniquet.

Fauci, A. et al. (eds.). *Harrison's Internal Medicine*, 17th edition. McGraw Hill Education, 2008: Part 6: Education: Chapter 99, Disorders of hemoglobin, pp. 635–643.

Hines, R.L. and Marschall, K.E. *Stoelting's Anesthesia and Co-existing Disease*, 7th edition. Elsevier, 2018: Chapter 24, Hematological disorders: pp. 477–506.

1. **With regards to pneumothorax**
   A. it is a recognized cause of acute chest pain
   B. spontaneous pneumothorax is associated with physical exertion
   C. the size of a pneumothorax is generally overestimated on a posteroanterior (PA) chest X-ray
   D. arterial blood gas values are commonly abnormal
   E. treatment of a spontaneous pneumothorax with high flow oxygen therapy improves hypoxaemia but does not affect the rate of resolution of the pneumothorax

2. **In an adult patient with central chest pain**
   A. if there is new-onset left bundle branch block (LBBB) the patient should be assessed urgently for coronary reperfusion therapy
   B. relief of the pain with sublingual glyceryl trinitrate is diagnostic of cardiac chest pain
   C. who remains unconscious after cardiopulmonary arrest secondary to acute ST-elevation myocardial infarction (STEMI), Percutaneous Coronary Intervention (PCI) is contraindicated
   D. the differential diagnosis should include unstable angina which is an acute coronary syndrome
   E. if the pain is due to an acute myocardial infarction, blood cardiac troponin levels may remain elevated for up to two weeks

3. **Elevated blood cardiac troponin levels may occur in**
   A. subarachnoid haemorrhage
   B. thermal injury
   C. sepsis
   D. pheochromocytoma
   E. the presence of chest pain despite a normal coronary angiogram

4. In acute paracetamol (acetaminophen) poisoning

A. hepatic damage can be detected on routine liver function tests within 12 hours of ingestion

B. a high plasma alanine aminotransferase (ALT) level 72 hours following ingestion is of prognostic value

C. acute renal failure may occur in the absence of hepatic failure

D. following ingestion of a single overdose, it is critical to determine the actual dose of paracetamol ingested to predict the likelihood of liver damage

E. in a staggered overdose (multiple doses taken over a period of time) it is essential to refer to the treatment nomogram to determine whether treatment with acetylcysteine is required

5. In an adult patient with an isolated traumatic head injury

A. bleeding in the oral cavity is associated with a base of skull fracture

B. the target blood pressure in the resuscitation phase is a systolic blood pressure ≥ 90 mmHg

C. in patients with a Glasgow Coma Scale score (GCS) < 9, prehospital intubation of the trachea has been shown to protect against secondary brain injury

D. hyperventilation may result in secondary brain injury

E. 10% of patients presenting with a GCS of 12 will not survive

6. Concerning anaphylaxis

A. anaphylaxis in response to radiocontrast medium is most often IgE mediated

B. hypotension following administration of a drug may herald the onset of anaphylaxis

C. ischaemic changes may be seen on the electrocardiogram (ECG) following successful resuscitation in a patient with normal coronary arteries

D. treatment with intravenous adrenaline (epinephrine) is the first priority

E. patients may complain of abdominal pain

7. In the management of major trauma

A. a correctly fitted cervical collar must not be undone while securing a definitive airway

B. administration of tranexamic acid is associated with improved outcome if administered in the first three hours following major trauma

C. airway compromise is the leading cause of preventable death following trauma

D. talking to the patient should be avoided while conducting the primary survey so that the team remains focused on identifying life-threatening injuries

E. in a multiple casualty scenario, the number of injured and the severity of their injuries exceeds the capability of the facility and personnel

8. Concerning trauma in older people

A. motor vehicle accidents are the commonest cause of major trauma

B. there is a marked seasonal variation in the incidence of major trauma

C. head injury is the most prevalent mechanism of major trauma

D. current trauma triage methods have been shown to be highly effective in identifying older patients who have sustained major injuries

E. mechanisms of injury involving low energy transfer are the commonest cause of major trauma

9. Concerning button batteries

   A. ingestion may result in pneumothorax
   B. when lodged in the oesophagus, erosion is more likely to occur at the positive pole of the battery
   C. may be differentiated from a coin by the presence of a 'halo sign' on a radiograph
   D. tissue erosion may continue for weeks following removal of a battery lodged in the oesophagus
   E. ingestion of honey is beneficial in children aged over one year in the prehospital management of battery ingestion

10. Concerning diabetic ketoacidosis (DKA)

   A. a diagnosis of DKA is highly unlikely if the patient does not have a history of diabetes mellitus
   B. in adults the commonest cause is discontinuation of insulin therapy
   C. DKA may be triggered by cocaine ingestion
   D. DKA is frequently associated with abdominal pain of ischaemic origin
   E. initial resuscitation should be with either colloid or crystalloid fluids

11. A suspected internal drug trafficker is brought to the emergency department for assessment

   A. proctoscopy or examination with a vaginal speculum may be useful for confirming the presence of concealed drugs
   B. most often drugs are concealed in handmade packages using condoms or other materials
   C. any packages recovered from the patient should be safely destroyed as soon as possible
   D. acute abdominal pain is an indication for emergency surgical intervention
   E. an abdominal X-ray is a reliable test for detecting ingested drug packages

12. Toxicology

   A. serotonin syndrome may ensue following ingestion of cocaine
   B. cyanosis is commonly observed in cyanide poisoning
   C. in amitriptyline overdose a QRS interval > 100 msec is predictive of complications
   D. methylthioninium chloride (methylene blue) may be used in the treatment of serotonin syndrome
   E. salicylate poisoning may result in cerebral oedema

13. In the emergency treatment of hyperkalaemia

   A. intravenous sodium bicarbonate is recommended
   B. the ECG may be completely normal in severe hyperkalaemia
   C. a patient with a serum potassium level of 5.5 mmol/l with peaked T waves on the ECG should be considered to have severe hyperkalaemia.
   D. 10 ml of 10% calcium gluconate contains the same amount of calcium as 10 ml of 10% calcium chloride.
   E. sodium zirconium cyclosilicate is used in conjunction with insulin-glucose and salbutamol in the treatment of severe hyperkalaemia

14. In paediatric resuscitation

A. the parents should be allowed to stay during resuscitation if they wish to do so

B. it is important to be cautious when performing chest compressions in a child due to the risk of causing rib fractures

C. an adult automated external defibrillator (AED) is not suitable for use in a child

D. amiodarone should not be given via the intraosseous route

E. hyperoxia should be avoided following the return of spontaneous circulation (ROSC)

15. Concerning sepsis

A. at least half of all hospital inpatients will satisfy the criteria for systemic inflammatory response syndrome (SIRS) during their hospital stay

B. patients with septic shock are likely to be hypovolaemic

C. an advantage of the Sequential Organ Failure Assessment (SOFA) scoring tool is that it does not rely on laboratory testing

D. if there is no response to initial crystalloid resuscitation, hydroxyethyl starch solution should be added

E. patients with septic shock may have warm peripheries and rapid capillary refill

16. In the assessment and management of acute severe asthma

A. medical air should be used as the driving gas for nebulized drugs

B. a modest dose of a benzodiazepine may be useful for relieving the anxiety of a severe asthma attack

C. nebulized magnesium sulfate may be useful

D. a $PaCO_2$ of 6.5 kPa (49 mmHg) should trigger an immediate referral to critical care

E. a gas mixture containing 21% oxygen and 79% helium (heliox) is of benefit in acute severe asthma

17. In adults who have a cardiac arrest

A. there is a reduction in the health-related quality of life in neurologically intact long-term survivors

B. there is a higher likelihood of survival for inpatient cardiac arrest if the first recorded ECG rhythm is ventricular fibrillation (VF) and the cardiac arrest occurs during working hours

C. for shockable rhythms, chest compressions should be continued during defibrillator charging, and the process of defibrillation should not interrupt chest compressions for more than 5 seconds

D. if pulmonary embolism (PE) is suspected as the cause it may be necessary to continue CPR for up to 90 minutes after administration of thrombolysis

E. an attempt at intravenous access should be made before attempting intraosseous access

18. **Concerning trauma in pregnancy**
    A. trauma is a rare cause of maternal mortality
    B. increased joint laxity predisposes to falls in pregnancy
    C. left lateral tilt is the preferred method for relief of aortocaval compression during cardiopulmonary resuscitation
    D. in the event of cardiopulmonary arrest, the patient should be transferred immediately to an operating theatre for resuscitative hysterotomy
    E. if an intercostal catheter (chest drain, thoracostomy tube) is indicated it should be placed in the fifth intercostal space in the midaxillary line

19. **In trauma resuscitation**
    A. the use of crystalloids is associated with an increased risk of multiple organ failure
    B. permissive hypotension is associated with improved mortality
    C. crystalloid, platelets, and red blood cells should be transfused in a ratio of 1:1:1
    D. human albumin infusion is associated with reduced mortality in haemorrhagic shock
    E. needle cricothyroidotomy is the fastest and most reliable technique to oxygenate a patient when a 'can't intubate can't oxygenate' (CICO) emergency has been declared

20. **Concerning bradycardia**
    A. sinus bradycardia is often associated with haemodynamic instability
    B. the presence of a biphasic P wave in lead V1 is abnormal
    C. bradycardia resulting from an acute myocardial infarction (MI) is associated with increased mortality
    D. may present with acute confusion
    E. temporary transvenous pacing increases the risk of subsequent infection following permanent pacemaker insertion

Question 1: Answer

A. True. Spontaneous pneumothorax classically presents with dyspnoea and chest pain. However, there is wide variation in the presentation between individuals. Some may remain asymptomatic for several days, while others may have severe dyspnoea. The degree of dyspnoea does not necessarily reflect the size of the pneumothorax. If breathlessness is present active intervention is indicated.

B. False. There is no association between spontaneous pneumothorax and physical exertion. Following resolution of the pneumothorax, patients can be reassured that they can resume normal physical activity once they are asymptomatic. However, the pneumothorax should be fully resolved before patients undertake intense physical activity.

C. False. The size of the pneumothorax tends to be *under*estimated when a standard erect inspiratory posteroanterior chest radiograph is used. The addition of an expiratory chest X-ray is not considered to be of additional diagnostic value.

D. True. However, it is not necessary to measure arterial blood gases in a stable patient who is maintaining blood oxygen saturation ≥ 92% while breathing room air.

E. False. In addition to correcting hypoxaemia, treatment with high flow oxygen increases the rate of resolution of a spontaneous pneumothorax.

MacDuff, A., Arnold, A., and Harvey J. Management of spontaneous pneumothorax: British Thoracic Society pleural disease guideline *Thorax*, 2010;*65*(Suppl 2): ii18–ii31.

Question 2: Answer

A. True. In STEMI the electrocardiograph (ECG) shows > 1 mm ST elevation in two consecutive limb leads, 2 mm ST elevation in two consecutive chest (V) leads, or the presence of new-onset LBBB. According to the National Institute for Health and Care Excellence (NICE) guidelines, patients with acute STEMI should immediately be assessed for eligibility for reperfusion therapy.

B. False. Relief of chest pain with nitrates is not reliable for the diagnosis of cardiac chest pain.

C. False. Unconsciousness is not a contraindication to PCI following cardiopulmonary arrest due to STEMI.

D. True. The term acute coronary syndrome (ACS) encompasses several conditions resulting in myocardial ischaemia. These include STEMI, non-ST-elevation myocardial infarction (NSTEMI), and unstable angina. The key difference between these is that in STEMI there is necrosis of cardiac muscle due to the sudden complete occlusion of a coronary artery, whereas in NSTEMI and unstable angina there is a sudden reduction in blood flow to a region of myocardium.

E. True.

National Institute for Health and Care Excellence. Myocardial infarction with ST-segment elevation: acute management (NICE Guideline CG167). 2013. Available at: https://www.nice.org.uk/Guidance/CG167.

Reed-Poysden, C. and Gupta, K.J. Acute coronary syndromes. *BJA Education*, 2015;*15*(6):286–293.

Question 3: Answer

A. True.

B. True.

C. True.

D. True.

E. True.

Blood cardiac troponin levels generally indicate myocardial necrosis. However, there are many non-ACS causes of elevated cardiac troponins. Therefore, the history, examination findings, and results of all investigations must be considered when making a diagnosis. Other conditions where elevated cardiac troponin levels may occur include severe cardiac failure, myocarditis, cardiac arrhythmias (including atrial fibrillation), rhabdomyolysis, PE, chronic obstructive pulmonary disease, and strenuous exercise.

Lee, T.W., et al. Pheochromocytoma mimicking both acute coronary syndrome and sepsis: a case report. *Med Princ Pract*, 2013;22(4):405–407.

Menke-van der Houven van Oordt C.W., et al. Pheochromocytoma mimicking an acute myocardial infarction. *Neth Heart J*, 2007;15:248–251.

Reed-Poysden, C. and Gupta, K.J. Acute coronary syndromes. *BJA Education*, 2015;15:286–293.

Question 4: Answer

Paracetamol toxicity is the commonest cause of acute hepatic failure and is the commonest drug taken in deliberate overdose in many countries. Paracetamol toxicity may also occur when therapeutic doses of the drug are taken in susceptible individuals, or an incorrect dose is calculated.

A. False. Routine liver function tests usually remain unaffected until at least 18 hours after ingestion of an overdose of paracetamol. Hepatic damage can be assessed by plasma levels of the liver enzymes alanine aminotransferase (ALT) and aspartate transaminase (AST), or by measurement of the International Normalized Ratio (INR) 72–96 hours following ingestion.

B. False. The rate of rise of ALT rather than the magnitude of increase in ALT correlates with the severity of hepatic injury following paracetamol ingestion. Thus, the actual ALT level is of little prognostic value.

C. True. In the presence of clinically significant hepatic injury, acute renal failure is regarded as a key prognostic indicator. However, acute renal failure can occur in the absence of hepatic injury following paracetamol ingestion due to the direct toxic effects of paracetamol on the renal tubules.

D. False. The severity of paracetamol poisoning is related to the dose ingested. However, a single measurement of the plasma paracetamol concentration > 4 hours following ingestion is a more reliable predictor of hepatic damage than the actual dose of paracetamol ingested. It becomes complicated when the patient has ingested the drug over a longer period of time (i.e., multiple doses). Patients who present late (> 24 hours after ingestion) are at greater risk of hepatic and renal failure.

E. False. Treatment nomograms are used to determine whether acetylcysteine treatment is indicated in patients who have ingested a single acute overdose of paracetamol. If the patient has taken a staggered overdose or has ingested modified-release paracetamol preparations the nomogram cannot be relied upon. Acetylcysteine should be administered to all patients where the dose ingested over the preceding 24 hours is believed to be ≥150 mg/kg.

Dear, J.W. and Bateman, N. Paracetamol poisoning. *Medicine*, 2020;48:208–210.

Question 5: Answer

A. True. Profuse bleeding from the mouth or nose may be due to a base of skull fracture, although this is not the only cause of bleeding in the mouth following head trauma. Other possible signs of a base of skull fracture include cerebrospinal fluid leak from the nose or ear, haemotympanum, bruising around the eyes ('Panda' or 'Racoon' eyes) and bruising over the mastoid process (Battle's sign). A computerized tomography (CT) scan of the head is indicated in the presence of any of these signs.

B. True. In isolated head trauma systolic blood pressure should be maintained at ≥ 90 mmHg, ideally in the normal physiological range, to minimize the risk of secondary brain injury.

C. False. Prevention of secondary brain injury is the cornerstone of effective management at all stages of traumatic brain injury including prehospital care. Hypotension and hypoxia should be avoided. Although securing a definitive airway is essential, evidence suggests an increase in mortality in patients where tracheal intubation is performed in suboptimal conditions. The reasons for this are likely to be multifactorial and include transient hypoxia during intubation, hypotension, impaired cerebral blood flow due to over ventilation, and delayed transfer to definitive care.

D. True. Although hyperventilation can bring about a reduction in intracranial pressure through hypocarbic vasoconstriction, hyperventilation also results in reduced cerebral perfusion and may result in cerebral ischaemia.

E. True. Traumatic brain injury (TBI) is the commonest cause of death in people aged under 25 and is also the commonest form of traumatic injury in older people (age ≥ 65). The GCS is inversely related to the severity of TBI and has a prognostic value (Table 15.1).

Table 15.1 Severity of TBI and prognostic value

GCS	Classification of TBI	Mortality
13–15 *	Mild	0.1%
9–12	Moderate	10%
< 9	Severe	40%

* In some countries the classification of Mild TBI is restricted to GCS 14–15 because of the poor outcome in many patients with GCS 13.

Dinsmore, J. Traumatic brain injury: an evidence-based review of management. *Continuing Education in Anaesthesia Critical Care & Pain*, 2013;13:189–195.

Haydel, M.J. Assessment of traumatic brain injury. *BMJ Best Practice*, 2018. Available at: https://bestpractice.bmj.com/topics/en-gb/515.

Vella, M.A., Crandall, M.L., and Patel, M.B. Acute management of traumatic brain injury. *Surg Clin N Am*, 2017;97:1015–1030.

Question 6: Answer

Anaphylaxis is an acute severe potentially fatal generalized systemic reaction due to the sudden release of mast cell and basophil derived inflammatory mediators into the circulation. It may have an immunological (IgE mediated) basis (most common) or a non-immunological cause. Regardless of the mechanism, the clinical syndrome is the same.

A. False. Anaphylaxis to radiocontrast agents is usually a consequence of non-immunological anaphylaxis. Other triggers of non-immunological anaphylaxis include non-steroidal anti-inflammatory agents (NSAIDs) and opioids. The commonest causes of IgE mediated anaphylaxis include foodstuffs (peanuts, seafood, dairy products), insect stings and drugs, notably antibiotics, especially penicillins.

B. True. The clinical presentation of anaphylaxis varies widely. It is often not recognized quickly enough, and undertreated. The diagnosis is made based on clinical signs and symptoms. A high index of clinical suspicion is required, and prompt intervention is of critical importance.

C. True. ECG changes suggestive of myocardial ischaemia can occur following treatment with adrenaline (epinephrine) in patients with normal coronary arteries.

D. False. When there is suspicion of anaphylaxis the immediate management is to assess the airway, breathing, circulation, disability, and to expose the patient as required (ABCDE approach), call for help, and raise (elevate) the patient's legs. If anaphylaxis is suspected, treatment with intramuscular (IM) adrenaline is then recommended without delay—0.01 mg/kg to a maximum of 500 µg IM (0.5 ml of 1/1000 adrenaline) in adults, repeated every 5 minutes if necessary. Intravenous (IV) adrenaline should only be used by experienced specialists (such as anaesthesiologists and intensivists) with careful heart rate and blood pressure monitoring. The IV dose of adrenaline is 50 µg in adults and 1 µg/kg in children.

E. True. In addition to the more usual clinical manifestations of anaphylaxis such as respiratory and cardiovascular symptoms and signs, patients may report a wide variety of symptoms including gastrointestinal symptoms of nausea, vomiting, abdominal pain, and diarrhoea.

Fischer, D. et al. Anaphylaxis. *Allergy Asthma Clin Immunol*, 2018;14:54.

Lott, C. et al. ERC Special Circumstances Writing Group Collaborators. European Resuscitation Council Guidelines 2021: cardiac arrest in special circumstances. *Resuscitation*, 2021;161:152–219.

Question 7: Answer

A. False. All trauma patients should be triaged and assessed according to European Trauma Course (ETC) guidelines. Maintenance of the airway with restriction of cervical spine motion is the cornerstone of all trauma management. Assessment and management of the airway is the first priority. During this process, it is essential that the cervical spine is protected from excessive movement. However, it is not possible to perform tracheal intubation in a patient with a properly fitting hard cervical collar. Therefore, the collar is undone while a trained member of the trauma team performs manual in-line stabilization (MILS) of the head and neck.

B. True. Tranexamic acid (TXA) is a synthetic analogue of the amino acid lysine. It acts by competitively inhibiting the activation of plasminogen into the enzyme plasmin which is involved in the dissolution of fibrin blood clots. TXA has been shown to improve survival in major trauma patients when administered within three hours of injury.

C. False. Haemorrhage is the commonest cause of preventable death following trauma. Trauma patients should undergo structured assessment according to the mnemonic ABCDE (**A**irway maintenance with restriction of cervical spine movement; **B**reathing and ventilation; **C**irculation with haemorrhage control; **D**isability (assessment of neurological status); **E**xposure—undress; and **E**nvironment—temperature control). This initial assessment where life-threatening conditions are identified, and treatment is initiated is termed the primary survey. The secondary survey consists of a head-to-toe examination of the patient carried out once the primary survey has been completed.

D. False. If the patient can talk and give an appropriate verbal response to questions (e.g., what is your name?) it is unlikely that the airway is in danger of immediate compromise, they are demonstrating that they are able to breathe (as they can move enough air to generate speech), and their level of consciousness is not significantly decreased. Verbal response is a key part of assessing the GCS. It is also reassuring to a frightened patient to hear someone talking to them in a calm voice.

E. False. This is the definition of a mass casualty event. In a multiple casualty scenario, the facility and personnel have the necessary capability to deal with the number of injured patients.

Leibner, E. et al. Damage control resuscitation. *Clin Exp Emerg Med*, 2020;7:5–13.

The European Trauma Course. *The Team Approach*, course manual, 4th edition. The ETC Course Management Committee. 2018. Available at: https://www.europeantraumacourse.com.

Question 8: Answer

A. False. Motor vehicle collision is the commonest mechanism of injury in younger patients. The commonest mechanism of injury in older patients is a fall from a height of fewer than two metres (typically a fall from standing height).

B. False. There is little evidence of seasonal variation in the incidence of major trauma in older people. Most falls occur indoors so factors such as weather have little bearing on the incidence throughout the year.

C. True. TBI is the leading type of injury seen in older people. Thoracic injury is the second most common anatomical site for major injury in older people.

D. False. A key finding in a recent report from the Trauma Audit and Research Network (TARN) was that current triage methods often fail to identify older people who have major injuries. This is probably because triage in a trauma setting is focused on the identification of high-energy transfer trauma.

E. True. Older people can sustain major injuries from seemingly trivial mechanisms of injury characterized by low energy transfer. Other factors include comorbidities such as cognitive impairment which may mask the presentation.

The Trauma Audit and Research Network (TARN). Major trauma in older people. 2017. Available at: https://www.tarn.ac.uk/Content.aspx?c=3793.

Question 9: Answer

A. True. Button batteries can lead to perforation of the oesophagus resulting in pneumomediastinum and pneumothorax. Other complications associated with oesophageal perforation include tracheobronchial fistula, recurrent laryngeal nerve damage, and major haemorrhage and death from erosion into major blood vessels, including the aorta.

B. False. An electrical current can be generated if both sides of the battery are in contact with the fluid milieu of the oesophagus. Highly caustic hydroxide is generated at the negative pole of the battery, which in turn leads to tissue necrosis.

C. True. Button batteries are round and flat in construction, resembling two thin discs of different diameters stacked together. The negative terminal side of the battery is smaller in diameter than the positive side. The characteristic appearance of two superimposed concentric circles gives the appearance of a ring or 'halo' around the outer edge of the disc when seen face-on in a radiograph. The construction of the battery also gives rise to a 'step off' sign when viewed edge-on, due to the change in diameter between the two poles of the battery (Fig 15.1). The presence of these radiological signs is highly suggestive, but not pathognomonic of the presence of an ingested button battery.

D. True. Once a battery has been removed from the oesophagus, erosion may occur for days or weeks in some cases. Death due to complications of late erosion have been reported. It is essential that an appropriate period of observation and follow-up is undertaken. The precise nature of follow up will vary according to the clinical scenario.

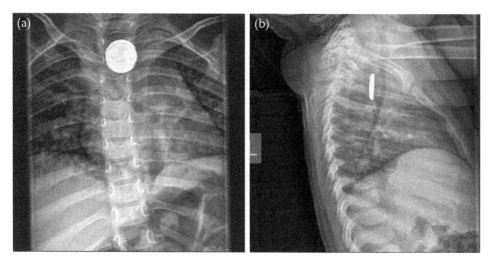

Fig 15.1 Typical radiographic appearances of a button battery lodged in the oesophagus of a child. (a) AP chest X-ray showing the characteristic 'halo sign'. (b) Lateral chest X-ray: The smaller diameter negative pole stacked immediately adjacent to the larger positive pole gives rise to the 'step off' sign.

Reprinted from Sahn B, Mamula P, Ford CA. (2014) Review of foreign body ingestion and esophageal food impaction management in adolescents. *J Adolesc Health*. 52: 260–6, with permission from Elsevier.

    E. True. Removal of a battery lodged in the oesophagus within two hours of ingestion is ideal but rarely achievable. Ingestion of small amounts of acidic liquid (lemon or orange juice) has been shown to help neutralize the alkaline environment in the oesophagus. Honey (and sucralfate) have a higher viscosity and are believed to coat the battery. Giving 10 ml of honey every 10 minutes until the presence of a battery in the oesophagus has been excluded is recommended but procuring honey should not delay going to the emergency department. Other than treatment with honey (or in hospital sucralfate) the patient should be kept nil by mouth. Any exothermic reaction associated with pH neutralization is believed to be minimal.

Eck, J.B. and Ames, W.A. Anesthetic implications of button battery ingestion in children. *Anesthesiology*, 2020;*132*:917–924.

Sahn, B., Mamula, P., and Ford, C.A. Review of foreign body ingestion and esophageal food impaction management in adolescents. *J Adolesc Health*, 2014;*52*:260–266.

Question 10: Answer

DKA is a common preventable life-threatening complication of diabetes. Three criteria need to be met to make the diagnosis: 1. A blood glucose concentration of > 11 mmol/l or the patient is known to be diabetic. 2. A capillary blood ketone concentration of > 3.0 mmol/l or the presence of significant ketonuria (2 + or more on standard urine test sticks). 3. A serum bicarbonate concentration of < 15.0 mmol/l and/or venous blood pH < 7.3.

    A. False. Up to a quarter of cases of DKA are the first presentation of diabetes. Thus, the absence of a history of diabetes does not exclude the diagnosis of DKA.

    B. False. Voluntary discontinuation of insulin therapy is frequently the cause of DKA in adolescents. Most adults with recurrent episodes of DKA have an underlying cause, the most frequent being infection.

C. True. Sympathomimetic drugs such as cocaine may trigger DKA. Other drugs that can trigger DKA include thiazide diuretics, corticosteroids, and some antipsychotic agents.

D. False. Abdominal pain is common in DKA, but it is usually of idiopathic origin.

E. False. There is an increased risk of morbidity and mortality associated with the use of colloids for resuscitation. Crystalloid fluid resuscitation is recommended.

Joint British Diabetes Societies for Inpatient Care and the UK Chemotherapy Board. The management of diabetic ketoacidosis in adults. 2021. Available at: https://abcd.care/sites/abcd.care/files/site_uploads/JBDS_Guidelines_Current/JBDS_02%20_DKA_Guideline_amended_v2_June_2021.pdf.

Question 11: Answer

A. False. Internal examination either with a finger or using a proctoscope or speculum carries a risk of rupturing drug packages. It is also unlikely to detect most concealed packages. Low dose computerized tomography (LDCT) scan is the most useful investigation for detecting (or excluding the presence of) ingested drug packages. Informed consent is required from the patient.

B. False. In the past handmade packaging from items such as condoms was commonplace, but it is now more common for them to be machine manufactured.

C. False. Any packages or other items recovered from the patient should be given to the police as soon as possible in order to preserve the chain of evidence in their criminal investigation.

D. True. Acute abdominal pain may be due to obstruction or ileus and is an indication for the urgent removal of any internal packages. Other indications for urgent surgical intervention include evidence of worsening drug toxicity, and radiological evidence of the presence of packages that are too large to pass through the gastrointestinal tract.

E. False. Although some concealed packages may show up on an abdominal X-ray and ultrasound, CT imaging has greater sensitivity and specificity and is the recommended imaging modality. A low-dose CT protocol should be used. The ingested packages are often prepared using methods which can give radiological appearances similar to faeces. Imaging can only be carried out with the informed consent of the patient.

Heymann-Maier, L. et al. Emergency department management of body packers and body stuffers. *Swiss Med Wkly*, 2017;147:w14499.

The Royal College of Emergency Medicine Best Practice Guideline. Management of suspected internal drug trafficker (SDIT). 2020. Available at: https://rcem.ac.uk/wp-content/uploads/2021/10/Management_of_Suspected_Internal_Drug_Trafficker_December_2020.pdf.

Tsang, H.K.P. et al. Radiological features of body packers: an experience from a regional accident and emergency department in close proximity to the Hong Kong International Airport. *Hong Kong Journal of Emergency Medicine*, 2018;25(4):202–210.

Question 12: Answer

A. True. Serotonin syndrome (SS) is a potentially fatal condition due to excessive serotonergic activity in the central nervous system. Any substance that affects the synthesis, release, metabolism, or reuptake of serotonin (5-hydroxytryptamine) has the potential to cause serotonin syndrome.

B. False. Cyanide compounds reversibly inhibit cytochrome oxidase which in turn halts cellular respiration, the process by which oxygen is utilized to generate adenosine triphosphate (ATP). The resulting cellular hypoxia and ATP depletion leads to metabolic acidosis.

However, there is an excess of oxygen in the circulation as oxygen uptake by the tissues is inhibited, so cyanosis is not a feature of cyanide poisoning.

C. True. A QRS interval > 100 ms is reliably predictive of complications including seizures and ventricular arrhythmias following tricyclic antidepressant (TCAD) overdose. TCADs cause reduced cardiac contractility, hypotension, and arrhythmias via sodium channel antagonism. Other ECG indices predictive of complications include a QTc > 430 ms and an R:S ratio > 0.7 in lead aVR.

D. False. Methylthioninium chloride is a phenothiazine derivative which inhibits monoamine oxidase. It can therefore *cause* serotonin syndrome in patients taking selective serotonin reuptake inhibitors (SSRIs) such as fluoxetine. Methylthioninium chloride is used in the treatment of methaemoglobinemia.

E. True. Salicylates are salts or esters of salicylic acid and include aspirin (acetylsalicylic acid) and diflunisal. In overdose, patients may develop hearing loss, tinnitus, epigastric pain, vomiting, diaphoresis, dehydration, hyperventilation, respiratory alkalosis, metabolic acidosis, tachycardia, and hyperthermia. Agitation and altered mental state may herald the onset of cerebral oedema, which may be fatal.

Bartakke, A., Corredor, C., and van Rensburg, A. Serotonin syndrome in the perioperative period. *BJA Education*, 2020;*20*:10–17. Corrigendum. *BJA Education*, 2020;20:139.

Body, R. et al. Guidelines in Emergency Medicine Network (GEMNet): guideline for the management of tricyclic antidepressant overdose. *Emerg Med J*, 2011;28:347–368.

Ward, C. and Sair, M. Oral poisoning update. *Contin Educ Anaesth Crit Care Pain*, 2010;10:6–11.

Question 13: Answer

A. False. Although widely used in the past, evidence shows that sodium bicarbonate does not lower serum potassium within 60 minutes of administration and is of no use in the emergency treatment of hyperkalaemia. In addition, sodium bicarbonate may result in sodium and volume overload, and tetany in individuals with chronic renal failure if there is hypocalcaemia.

B. True. Abnormal ECG changes in hyperkalaemia may include peaked T waves, prolonged PR interval, decreased P wave amplitude, or absent P waves, atrioventricular block, and sine wave QRST pattern. However, the ECG may also be completely normal even in severe hyperkalaemia.

C. True. Hyperkalaemia is classified as follows (all values are serum potassium values in mmol/l): Mild: 5.5–5.9; Moderate: 6.0–6.5; Severe: ≥ 6.5. However, hyperkalaemia should be considered severe at any serum K^+ ≥ 5.5 mmol/l in any patient with ECG changes and/or symptoms of palpitations, paraesthesia, flaccid paralysis, or muscle weakness.

D. False. 10 ml of 10% calcium gluconate contains 2.3 mmol Ca^{2+} compared with 6.8 mmol in 10 ml of 10% calcium chloride.

E. True. Sodium zirconium cyclosilicate and Patiromer are orally administered potassium binders used in the treatment of life-threatening hyperkalaemia (serum K^+ ≥ 6.5 mmol/l) in addition to insulin-glucose and salbutamol therapy.

Alfonzo, A. et al. Clinical practice guidelines treatment of acute hyperkalaemia in adults. Renal Association, 2020. Available at: https://renal.org/sites/renal.org/files/RENAL%20ASSOCIAT ION%20HYPERKALAEMIA%20GUIDELINE%202020.pdf.

Lindner, G. et al. Acute hyperkalemia in the emergency department: a summary from a Kidney Disease: Improving Global Outcomes conference. *Eur J Emerg Med*, 2020;27:329–337.

Question 14: Answer

A. True. The parents should be allowed to remain with their child during resuscitation and a member of staff should be designated to support them. They should be allowed to maintain physical contact with their child wherever possible. If the parents are impeding resuscitation, they should be asked to leave in a sensitive way.

B. False. The chest should be compressed by at least one-third of its depth. Rib fractures are very rarely caused during paediatric resuscitation. Good quality chest compressions are an essential part of cardiopulmonary resuscitation.

C. False. AEDs can be used in children. Over the age of 8 years, adult pads can be applied in the anterolateral position, as for an adult, but in children less than 8 years it may not be possible to apply them in the 'normal' anterolateral position without the pads being in contact with one another. Therefore, in smaller children one pad is applied to the front of the chest and one to the back.

D. False. For the treatment of pulseless ventricular tachycardia or VF ('shockable rhythms') defibrillation should be attempted. If three shocks have been delivered without successful cardioversion, amiodarone 5 mg.kg^{-1} (up to a maximum of 300 mg) should be given, and it can safely be given via the intraosseous route.

E. True. Following ROSC, oxygen delivery should be titrated to maintain an oxygen saturation of 94–98%. Hyperoxia is believed to induce the production of reactive oxygen species (free radicals) which can lead to reperfusion injury.

Ali, U. and Bingham, R. Current recommendations for paediatric resuscitation. *BJA Education*, 2018;18:116–121.

Resuscitation Council UK. 2021 Resuscitation guidelines. 2021. Available at: https://www.resus.org.uk/library/2021-resuscitation-guidelines.

Question 15: Answer

A. True. The criteria for SIRS are non-specific. They consist of two or more of: 1. Temperature > 38.0°C or < 36.0°C; 2. Heart rate > 90 beats/min; 3. Respiratory rate > 20 breaths/min, or PaCO$_2$ < 4.3 kPa (32 mmHg); 4. White blood cell count > 12000 or < 4000 per µl.

B. False. In a patient with sepsis, septic shock is defined as low systemic arterial blood pressure requiring vasopressors to maintain a mean arterial pressure≥ 65 mmHg, or a serum lactate level > 2 mmol/l after adequate fluid resuscitation. Sepsis is defined as life-threatening organ dysfunction due to a dysregulated host response to infection.

C. False. The SOFA score predicts mortality based on a combination of clinical data and laboratory results. However, the quick SOFA (qSOFA) score is a simple tool used to identify high-risk patients that does not require laboratory testing. It outperforms the SOFA score in non-critical care patient populations. The criteria for qSOFA are: 1. Respiratory rate ≥ 22 breaths/min; 2. Altered mental status; 3. Systolic blood pressure ≤ 100 mmHg.

D. False. The ideal approach to fluid resuscitation in sepsis-related hypotension is still the subject of ongoing research. There is widespread agreement that initial fluid resuscitation should be with crystalloid solution. There is also widespread consensus that hydroxyethyl starch should not be used. Hydroxyethyl starch increases the risk of acute kidney injury and death.

E. True. Patients with high output vasodilated shock may have these physical signs.

Nunnally, M.E. Sepsis for the anaesthetist. *Br J Anaesth*, 2016;117:iii44–iii51.

Thompson, K., Venkatesh, B., and Finfer, S. Sepsis and septic shock: current approaches to management. *Intern Med J*, 2019;49:160–170.

Question 16:   Answer

A. False. Oxygen should be used as the driving gas for nebulized drugs in the treatment of acute severe asthma.

B. False. Sedatives should not be administered in the treatment of acute severe asthma. They are likely to cause a deterioration due to respiratory depression.

C. False. Nebulized magnesium sulfate is not effective in acute severe asthma. A single dose of intravenous magnesium sulfate (1.2–2 g) given as an intravenous infusion over 20 min may be beneficial in severe, or life-threatening asthma. Repeated dosing may result in respiratory failure secondary to muscle weakness caused by hypermagnesaemia.

D. True. In acute asthma, there is increased respiratory drive. This leads to hypocapnia and respiratory alkalosis. The presence of a normal $PaCO_2$ is a sign of life-threatening asthma, and a $PaCO_2$ level of 6.5 kPa (49 mmHg) indicates near-fatal asthma. Beware of the asthmatic patient with a normal or elevated $PaCO_2$.

E. False. There is no evidence that heliox is of use in the treatment of acute severe asthma.

Carlsson, J.A. and Bayes, H.K. Acute severe asthma in adults. *Medicine*, 2020;48:297–302.

Question 17:   Answer

A. True. Long-term outcome following cardiac arrest varies between countries. Cardiac arrest survivors with a good neurological outcome experience fatigue, cognitive impairment, and emotional problems, leading to a reduction in health-related quality of life. In addition, their family members may develop post-traumatic stress disorder.

B. True. Factors determining the likelihood of survival for inpatient cardiac arrest fall into two categories: non-modifiable (e.g., age, sex, comorbidities) and modifiable (e.g., the site within the hospital the cardiac arrest occurs, whether the ECG is being monitored at the time of the cardiac arrest, time of day, time to delivery of treatment).

C. True. There should be minimal disruption of chest compressions during defibrillation, but care must be taken to ensure the safety of the rescuers. Cardiopulmonary resuscitation (CPR) should continue while a defibrillator is sourced, and the pads are applied. Chest compressions should be continued during defibrillator charging and resumed immediately upon delivery of the shock.

D. True. However, the evidence in support of thrombolysis for suspected PE is very low-level evidence.

E. True. This is the current recommendation of the International Liaison Committee on Resuscitation (ILCOR) 2020 and the European Resuscitation Council (ERC) guidelines 2021.

Gräsner, J.T. et al. European Resuscitation Council Guidelines 2021: epidemiology of cardiac arrest. 2021. Available at: https://doi.org/10.1016/j.resuscitation.2021.02.007.

Soar, J. et al. European Resuscitation Council Guidelines 2021: adult advanced life support. 2021. Available at: https://doi.org/10.1016/j.resuscitation.2021.02.010.

Question 18:   Answer

A. False. Trauma is a leading cause of maternal and foetal mortality.

B. True. Increased joint laxity, weight gain, and an altered centre of gravity in pregnancy can affect mobility and predispose to falls, especially in the third trimester. Approximately 25% of pregnant women report at least one fall during pregnancy.

C. False. Aortocaval compression becomes an issue beyond 20 weeks' gestation. It can be relieved by left lateral tilt or manual sidewards displacement of the uterus. Manual displacement of the uterus is preferable in cardiopulmonary arrest as left lateral tilt makes resuscitation difficult.

D. False. Resuscitative hysterotomy should be performed immediately when there is the expectation of imminent maternal death, or within four minutes of cardiopulmonary arrest (although this standard is rarely achieved). It should be carried out where the patient is and may be lifesaving for both the mother and foetus.

E. False. In pregnancy, intercostal catheters should be placed one or two intercostal spaces above (cranial) to the classical fifth intercostal space in the midaxillary line to avoid abdominal contents. The second intercostal space in the midclavicular line may also be used.

Irving, T., Menon, R., and Ciantar, E. Trauma during pregnancy. *BJA Education*, 2021;*21*:10–19.

Mendez-Figueroa, H. et al. Trauma in pregnancy: an updated systematic review. *Am J Obstet Gynecol*, 2013;*209*:1–10.

Question 19: Answer

A. True. The use of crystalloids has been shown to increase mortality in trauma resuscitation. Studies have shown crystalloids cause dilutional coagulopathy, worsen metabolic acidosis, and are associated with an increased incidence of acute respiratory distress syndrome (ARDS), abdominal compartment syndrome, and multiple organ failure.

B. True. Although the optimum target blood pressure is yet to be determined, current evidence supports the use of hypotensive resuscitation as part of a damage control resuscitation strategy.

C. False. Fluid management in massive haemorrhage has long been controversial. The focus has changed from large volume fluid resuscitation to damage control resuscitation. There is evidence that the transfusion of plasma, platelets, and red blood cells in a ratio of 1:1:1 reduces mortality from blood loss in the first 24 hours. In addition to the added risk of multiple organ failure, resuscitation with crystalloid is associated with an increased risk of ARDS and abdominal compartment syndrome.

D. False. Human albumin solution does not reduce mortality in patients with trauma and in those patients with severe TBI, resuscitation with 4% albumin has been shown to increase mortality significantly.

E. False. Although successful cricothyroidotomy can be performed using either a scalpel or cannula technique, the fastest and most reliable front of neck access technique is scalpel cricothyroidotomy.

Frerk, C. et al. Difficult Airway Society intubation guidelines working group, Difficult Airway Society 2015 guidelines for management of unanticipated difficult intubation in adults. *Br J Anaesth*, 2015;*115*:827–848.

Leibner E, et al. Damage control resuscitation. *Clin Exp Emerg Med*, 2020;*7*:5–13.

SAFE Study Investigators. Saline or albumin for fluid resuscitation in patients with traumatic brain injury. *N Engl J Med*, 2007;*357*:874–884.

Sen, J.P.B. and Wiles, M.D. Fluids in traumatic haemorrhage. *BJA Educ*, 2021;*21*(10):366–368.

Question 20: Answer

A. False. Sinus bradycardia (a heart rate < 60 beats/min) is rarely associated with haemodynamic instability. It is frequently seen in athletes and in older people.

B. False. The sinus P wave is generated by the sinoatrial node close to the junction of the superior vena cava with the right atrium. On a normal 12-lead electrocardiogram (ECG) the P wave is typically positive in leads II, II, and aVF, and biphasic in lead V1.

C. True. Post MI bradycardia is usually due to atrioventricular block.

D. True. Due to cerebral hypoperfusion.

E. True. The risk of infection is doubled following temporary transvenous pacing.

Burri, H. and Dayal, N. Acute management of bradycardia in the emergency setting. *Cardiovasc Med*, 2018;21:98–104.

Sidhu, S. and Marine, J.E. Evaluating and managing bradycardia. *Trends Cardiovasc Med*, 2020;30:265–272.

EDAIC PART II: ORAL GUIDED QUESTIONS

APPLIED PHYSIOLOGY

QUESTIONS

SOE 1 Oxygen transport in the blood

1.1 Tell me how oxygen is carried in blood.

1.2 What is the structure of haemoglobin (Hb)?

1.3 How does foetal Hb differ from adult Hb?

1.4 What is 2,3-DPG?

1.5 How does the saturation of Hb occur?

1.6 What is the oxygen dissociation curve (ODC)?

1.7 Can you draw the oxyhaemoglobin dissociation curve and explain what shifts it to the right or to the left?

1.8 What is the Bohr effect?

1.9 What is the Haldane effect?

SOE 2 Cerebral physiology

2.1 Please discuss the production, circulation, and contents of cerebrospinal fluid (CSF).

2.2 What functions does the CSF fulfil?

2.3 Please explain the mechanism behind the CSF's ability to protect the brain from ischaemia (The Monro–Kellie doctrine).

2.4 What is cerebral perfusion pressure?

2.5 What is the blood-brain barrier?

2.6 Why does the anaesthetist have to consider the blood-brain barrier when choosing anaesthetic drugs?

2.7 What are the circumventricular organs and what is their function?

2.8 What are the main functions of the hypothalamus?

SOE 3 Respiratory physiology

3.1 Please describe the relationship between ventilation and perfusion in different parts of the lungs.

3.2 What is a pulmonary shunt and under which clinical conditions does shunt occur?

3.3 What is dead space and what types of dead space are there?

3.4 Tell me about the factors influencing the diffusion of gases between pulmonary capillaries and alveoli.

3.5 Why does carbon dioxide equilibrate faster than oxygen between the alveoli and the pulmonary capillaries?

3.6 How can the body compensate for the increased ventilation and perfusion during physical activity?

3.7 What is hypoxic pulmonary vasoconstriction?

SOE 4 Renal physiology

4.1 Please describe the physiological functions of the kidneys.

4.2 Please describe the three mechanisms involved in urine production.

4.3 What is glomerular filtration rate?

4.4 What is renal clearance? How can it be measured?

4.5 What is autoregulation of renal blood flow? What are the mechanisms?

4.6 How does the kidney contribute to the regulation of the water balance in the body?

4.7 Please describe the renin-angiotensin-aldosterone system (RAAS).

SOE 5 Calcium metabolism and regulation

5.1 How is calcium stored in the body?

5.2 Is calcium mainly an intra- or an extracellular ion?

5.3 What is the normal plasma level of calcium?

5.4 How is calcium represented in plasma?

5.5 What are the functions of calcium in the body?

5.6 How is the metabolism of calcium regulated in the body?

5.7 Tell me about the role of parathyroid hormone in calcium homeostasis.

5.8 What is the role of calcitonin in calcium regulation?

5.9 How is Vitamin D involved in calcium regulation?

Answers to SOE 1

1.1 Tell me how oxygen is carried in blood.

Most of the oxygen (97%) in blood is transported bound to haemoglobin (Hb). Once the Hb is saturated, oxygen content can only marginally be increased by dissolved oxygen (at atmospheric pressure). Dissolved oxygen is a linear function of P_AO_2 and is 0.023 ml/kPa/100 ml (0.003 ml/mm Hg/100 ml) of plasma.

1.2 What is the structure of haemoglobin?

Hb is a conjugated protein with a molecular weight of 66,700 Daltons and is composed of four haem subunits. Each subunit has a central ferrous (Fe^{2+}) atom and is conjugated to a polypeptide chain. The four polypeptide chains collectively form the globin moiety. Different forms of Hb exist, identified by their polypeptide chains. Normal adult Hb consists of HbA1 (98%) containing two α and two β polypeptide chains, and HbA2 (2%) containing two α and two δ chains.

1.3 How does foetal Hb differ from adult Hb?

Foetal erythrocytes contain HbF with two α and two γ chains. HbF has an increased affinity for oxygen, which adapts its transport and delivery characteristics to the lower oxygen tensions in the placento-foetal circulation. HbA replaces HbF during the first year of life. HbF is also modified by having a lower affinity for binding 2,3-diphosphoglycerate (2,3-DPG) than adult forms of Hb.

1.4 What is 2,3-DPG?

2,3-Diphosphoglycerate (2,3-DPG) is a highly anionic intermediate (organic phosphate) of glycolysis. It binds to the deoxygenated form of Hb, significantly reducing the affinity of Hb for oxygen. This facilitates the 'unloading' of oxygen in tissues with low oxygen tensions.

1.5 How does the saturation of haemoglobin occur?

The iron (Fe^{2+}) ion is a site for oxygen binding in Hb. One molecule of Hb can bind four molecules of oxygen—one per each haem subunit. This is not a chemical reaction as in oxidation but is a readily reversible bond. Oxygen binding produces an allosteric change in the structure of Hb from a 'Taut' (deoxygenated) form to a 'Relaxed' form. The T form predominates in tissues where the pH is lower and PCO_2 is higher. The R form predominates in the areas of higher pH, lower PCO_2 and higher PO_2 (alveoli). This switching between R and T forms underlies the oxygenation and delivery mechanisms. This binding process is 'cooperative', meaning that the binding of O_2 at each site promotes binding at the remaining sites due to allosteric changes in Hb. This increases the amount of O_2 delivered under physiological conditions, compared with a carrier having independent binding sites.

1.6 What is the oxygen dissociation curve (ODC)?

The ODC defines the relationship between the partial pressure of oxygen and the percentage saturation of oxygen. In solutions of blood substitutes, such as perfluorocarbons, this curve is linear, with saturation being directly proportional to partial pressure. With haemoglobin containing solutions, however, the curve is sigmoid shaped. This is because as Hb binds each of its four molecules of oxygen, its affinity for the next increases.

1.7 Can you draw the oxyhaemoglobin dissociation curve and explain what shifts it to the right or to the left?

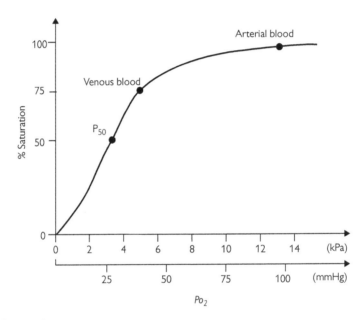

Fig 16.1 Oxygen dissociation curve.

Reprinted from Chambers D, Huang C, and Matthews G (2015) 'Basic Physiology for Anaesthetists'. Cambridge University Press: Cambridge, with permission from Cambridge University Press.

The curve can be displaced in either direction along the X-axis. This movement is usually described using the P_{50}, which is the partial pressure of oxygen at which haemoglobin is 50% saturated. This is normally 3.5 kPa (26 mmHg). The P_{50} is decreased (leftward shift) by alkalosis, by reduced PCO_2, by hypothermia, and by reduced concentrations of 2,3-DPG. A shift to the right is caused by acidosis, by increased PCO_2, by pyrexia, by anaemia, and by increases in 2,3-DPG. In most instances, a shift to the right is accompanied by increased tissue oxygenation.

1.8 What is the Bohr effect?

This is a process that occurs in the tissues. The Bohr effect is the shift in position of the ODC caused by CO_2 entering or leaving blood. This describes the change in the affinity of oxygen for Hb, which is associated with changes in pH. It enhances the 'unloading' of oxygen in the tissues, where PCO_2 levels are high compared with the pulmonary capillaries. In the tissues CO_2 enters the red cells, combining with water and dissociating into H^+ and HCO_3^-:

$$CO_2 + H_2O \leftrightarrow H_2CO_3 \leftrightarrow H^+ + HCO_3^-$$

The increased $[H^+]$ shifts the ODC to the right facilitating the release of oxygen from Hb.

1.9 What is the Haldane effect?

This process occurs in the lungs. The Haldane effect describes the ability of the deoxygenated Hb to carry more carbon dioxide. The decrease in P_{50} causes a leftward shift of the ODC allowing more oxygen to bind to Hb. The attachment of oxygen to Hb reduces its ability to bind to carbon dioxide facilitating removal of the latter by the lungs. Thus, the binding of oxygen will facilitate the release of carbon dioxide in the lungs. In the periphery, deoxygenation will increase the ability of uptake and transport of carbon dioxide back to the lungs.

References

Dunn, J.-O.C., Mythen, M.G., and Grocot, M.P. Physiology of oxygen transport. *BJA Education*, 2016;16(10):341–348.

Kam, P. and Power, I. *Principles of Physiology for the Anaesthetist*, 3rd edition. CRC Press, 2015.

Answers to SOE 2

2.1 Please discuss the production, circulation, and contents of cerebrospinal fluid (CSF).

CSF is produced in the plexuses in the lateral ventricles of the brain. It circulates from the lateral ventricles, through the third and fourth ventricles to the outside of the brain and spinal cord. It fills the subarachnoid space and is absorbed by arachnoid granulations on the outside of the brain. The daily production of CSF is about 500–600 ml, but at any time, there are about 125 ml of CSF surrounding the brain. The normal CSF contains no red blood cells and a negligible number of white blood cells (fewer than 5/ml). CSF is derived from blood plasma and has electrolyte levels similar to it, except for a slightly higher chloride level than blood plasma. Normal CSF has markedly lower protein levels than blood plasma, normally about 0.35 g/l (plasma: 70 g/l). The level of glucose in CSF is normally about two-thirds the value of plasma glucose.

2.2 What functions does the CSF fulfil?

The CSF gives the brain buoyancy. A normal brain weighs around 1500 g, however, when the brain is immersed in CSF, the net weight is equivalent to a mass of 25–50 g. This allows the brain to maintain its density without being impaired by its weight.

The CSF works as a fluid buffer and protects the brain from movement when the head is moved abruptly or hit by a hard object.

The CSF transports electrolytes and nutrients and also contributes to waste clearance.

The CSF protects the brain from ischaemia by being able to compensate for small changes in intracerebral volumes.

2.3 Please explain the mechanism behind the CSF's ability to protect the brain from ischaemia (The Monro–Kellie doctrine).

The Monro–Kellie doctrine describes the relationship between the contents of the cranium and the intracranial pressure. The original theory was that the sum of the volume of the brain (blood, CSF, and brain tissue) was constant and that a change in one of the factors would lead to alteration in one or both of the others. The skull is a rigid box, and a net increase in the contents must lead to an increase in intracranial pressure. With an increase in solid content, such as intracranial haemorrhage or tumour formation, by regulating either the blood volume or the CSF volume, the intracranial net volume and pressure can be maintained. This is true only within certain limits. When those limits are exhausted, the intracranial pressure will rise steeply with a small increase in volume.

2.4 What is cerebral perfusion pressure?

Cerebral perfusion pressure (CPP) is the net pressure that is driving blood through the brain and is a determinant of oxygenation of the brain. The CPP is calculated as the mean arterial pressure (MAP) minus the intracranial pressure (ICP). CPP should always be measured at the level of the ear.

2.5 What is the blood-brain barrier (BBB)?

The BBB is a physiological barrier that prevents harmful substances, such as toxins, macromolecules, and pathogens, from entering the brain from the blood. It is a highly selective semipermeable border of endothelial cells and functions as a filter. Some molecules are allowed to pass the BBB without delay, for example, oxygen and carbon dioxide. Small, fat-soluble molecules such as caffeine and alcohol can pass easily. For some larger molecules, like glucose, there are transport proteins that facilitate movement from plasma into the brain tissue.

2.6 Why does the anaesthetist have to consider the blood-brain barrier when choosing anaesthetic drugs?

Different drugs will have different permeability through the blood-brain barrier. Small, fat-soluble molecules will pass quickly and easily, while other drugs will have a time delay in passing or cannot pass at all. The volatile anaesthetics desflurane and sevoflurane will pass quickly, while isoflurane will pass more slowly. Fat-soluble opioids such as sufentanil will pass quickly, while more water-soluble drugs, such as morphine, will have a delayed onset. If the blood-brain barrier is damaged, for example, by infection or trauma, the barrier will be weaker and substances that do not normally pass the barrier may pass more easily.

2.7 What are the circumventricular organs and what is their function?

The circumventricular organs of the brain are small structures in the brain characterized by extensive and highly permeable capillaries; areas where the blood-brain barrier is weaker than in the rest of the brain. They are organized along the surface of the brain ventricles and have an important role in the measurement of homeostatic parameters. They are involved in the maintenance of body fluid balance, blood pressure, temperature, respiration, energy balance, mediation of immune and host-defence responses, pain modulation, protection against toxic substances (e.g., emesis and conditioned taste aversion), biological rhythms, reproduction, parental behaviour, lactation, growth, sleep, arousal, and attention.

2.8 What are the main functions of the hypothalamus?

The hypothalamus is the main centre for the connection between the endocrine and the central nervous system. The hypothalamus regulates hormone production in many endocrine systems through the production of stimulatory or inhibitory neurohormones acting on the pituitary gland. The hypothalamus also produces anti-diuretic hormone (ADH) and oxytocin, which are neuronally transported to the posterior pituitary gland from where they are released. The hypothalamus has a central role in regulating and controlling the autonomic nervous system. It regulates the activity of the autonomic reflex centres in the pons and medulla, and connects the autonomic nervous system with the limbic system which links autonomic responses to emotional reactions. The hypothalamus also has an important role in temperature regulation.

Answers to SOE 3

3.1 Please describe the relationship between ventilation and perfusion in different parts of the lungs.

Optimal gas exchange in the lungs requires an optimal relationship between ventilation and perfusion. At rest, the normal ventilation/perfusion ratio is 0.8. The V/Q ratio is lower towards the lung base (dependent parts) and higher in the upper parts of the lungs. For normal, healthy adults, the differences in V/Q ratio between the different parts of the lungs have no real consequence for gas exchange since areas with a lower V/Q ratio will be compensated by other areas with a higher V/Q ratio.

3.2 What is a pulmonary shunt and under which clinical conditions does shunt occur?

A pulmonary shunt is defined by a V/Q ratio below 0.8. This happens when a proportion of the blood passes through the pulmonary circulation without being oxygenated. This condition leads to non-oxygenated blood mixing with oxygenated blood leading to a lower oxygen partial pressure of arterial blood. The extent of the reduction in oxygen partial pressure will be dependent on the size of the shunt. Typical clinical conditions that lead to shunting of blood are atelectasis, pneumonia, and pulmonary oedema.

3.3 What is dead space and what types of dead space are there?

Dead space arises from lung regions that have a V/Q ratio above 0.8. They are areas that are ventilated but not perfused. There are two types of dead space: **anatomical dead space** (the upper airways that conduct air down to the alveoli but do not take part in gas exchange—nose, pharynx, trachea, and bronchi) and alveolar dead space. The **alveolar dead space** is the sum of all alveoli which have little or no blood flow through the adjacent capillaries. One pathologic condition that increases the alveolar dead space is pulmonary embolism. The normal anatomical dead space of a healthy adult is approximately 150 ml. The sum of the anatomical and alveolar dead space is known as the **physiological dead space**.

3.4 Tell me about the factors influencing the diffusion of gases between pulmonary capillaries and alveoli.

All gases will try to equilibrate their partial pressure between the pulmonary capillaries and the alveoli. Factors influencing the rate of equilibration include: the concentration difference; the solubility of the gas in blood; the distance between capillary and alveolus; and the velocity of the blood through the capillaries. Conditions that increase the diffusion distance, for example, interstitial pulmonary oedema, will delay diffusion.

3.5 Why does carbon dioxide equilibrate faster than oxygen between the alveoli and the pulmonary capillaries?

The solubility of carbon dioxide in blood is 20 times that of oxygen. If the difference in their partial pressures is exactly the same, then carbon dioxide equilibrates much more quickly than oxygen. However, there is a greater concentration gradient for oxygen, which compensates for its slower passage through the alveolar membrane.

3.6 How does the body compensate for increased ventilation and perfusion during physical activity?

During physical activity, the body may need as much as 20 times more oxygen than at rest. The heart can increase cardiac output only by a factor of 5–6. During hard physical exercise, lung capillaries that are normally closed at rest will open, which reduces pulmonary resistance and blood flow velocity. This will give the blood more time to equilibrate on its way through the capillaries. Under resting conditions, all gases will be equilibrated about halfway along the capillary, but during physical exercise, the whole distance may be utilized. In addition, peripheral oxygen extraction will increase together with increased production of CO_2, so the differences in their partial pressures in the lung will be greater and lead to faster diffusion.

3.7 What is hypoxic pulmonary vasoconstriction (HPV)?

HPV (also called the Euler-Liljestrand mechanism) is a mechanism where small pulmonary vessels react to hypoxia with local vasoconstriction. This leads to perfusion being diverted away from areas that are poorly ventilated. This vasoconstriction may lead to acute pulmonary hypertension when the hypoxic areas are large, such as during one-lung ventilation during pulmonary surgery, or climbing to high altitudes.

Answers to SOE 4

4.1 Please describe the physiological role of the kidneys

The kidneys play an important role in the homeostasis of the extracellular fluid volume. They regulate the concentration of ions in the extracellular space, remove unwanted molecules and toxins from the blood and play an important role in acid-base balance. Another important function is the production of hormones: renin, erythropoietin, and the active form of vitamin D_3 (calcitriol). The kidneys can also produce glucose (gluconeogenesis) and play a (small) role in the regulation of the blood glucose level.

4.2 Please describe the three mechanisms involved in urine production.

Urine is produced by filtration, reabsorption, and excretion. Fluid is **filtered** from the glomerular capillaries into the tubular system. This ultrafiltrate contains approximately the same ion concentrations as blood plasma. Proteins are normally not filtered. The normal filtration fraction is about 20% of the renal plasma flow. In 24 hours, 180 litres of ultrafiltrate are produced.

The **reabsorption** process starts immediately. Most of the ultrafiltrate is reabsorbed from the tubules to the peritubular capillaries, following the osmotic gradient. In addition, some ions undergo active transport out of the tubule, and some are involved in an ion-exchange mechanism, for example, potassium can be exchanged with hydrogen ions to regulate acid-base-balance. While all small molecules are filtered, reabsorption is a much more selective process. The 'unwanted' molecules are not reabsorbed but are excreted in the urine. 99% of the ultrafiltrate is reabsorbed and only about 1500 ml is excreted every 24 h.

The third mechanism is **secretion.** Organic ions and many drugs are bound to proteins, so not filtered by the glomerulus. Their removal depends on secretion into the tubular fluid. There is a very non-specific organic anion transport system in the proximal tubule that is extremely efficient, removing all such anions from plasma. Para-aminohippuric acid (PAH) is one such organic anion and PAH clearance is a method of calculating renal blood flow.

4.3 What is glomerular filtration rate (GFR)?

The GFR is the total volume of fluid filtered by the glomeruli per unit time. In a healthy adult, this is normally about 125 ml/min. For comparing values between individuals of varying body mass, GFR is normally indexed in relation to a standard body surface of 1.73 m^2. The values for males are a little higher than for females. The filtration rate depends on hydrostatic and oncotic pressure gradients across the glomerular membrane. Variations in GFR are normally the result of either a change in hydrostatic or oncotic pressure. The GFR falls with increasing age.

4.4 What is renal clearance? How can it be measured?

Renal clearance is the volume of plasma from which a substance is totally removed in a given time. For substances that are 100% filtered, plasma clearance of that substance will be the same as the renal plasma flow. Creatinine clearance is the plasma volume that is cleared of creatinine per time unit and is a useful measure for approximating the GFR. Since creatinine is also excreted, the clearance exceeds GFR. For substances that are secreted in addition to being filtrated, the clearance will be higher than renal plasma flow.

4.5 What is autoregulation of renal blood flow? What are the mechanisms?

Autoregulation is the kidney's ability to maintain a constant blood flow within a wide range of blood pressures. This will ensure a stable GFR, even with comparatively large variations in blood pressure (including in a denervated kidney). It is mediated through several mechanisms. First: a rapid myogenic response will lead to contraction of the afferent arteriole and thus reduce blood flow to the nephrons. The second mechanism is tubuloglomerular feedback. This is specifically designed to maintain a constant sodium chloride concentration in the distal tubule. If the sodium concentration or blood pressure in the juxtaglomerular complex decrease, this will be sensed in the macula densa. As a result, renin will be released, which in turn leads to an increased concentration of angiotensin II. The efferent arterioles will then contract, and the afferent arterioles will dilate thus leading to increased hydrostatic pressure in the afferent arterioles.

4.6 How does the kidney contribute to the regulation of the water balance in the body?

The kidneys play an important role in the water balance of the human body. When osmoreceptors in the hypothalamus sense an increased osmolality of the extracellular fluid, ADH (antidiuretic hormone, produced in the hypothalamus and transported to the pituitary) will be released from the posterior lobe of the pituitary gland. An increased ADH level will lead to increased reabsorption of water in the distal convoluted tubules and collecting ducts thus resulting in more concentrated urine and decreased plasma osmolality.

4.7 Please describe the renin-angiotensin-aldosterone system (RAAS)?

A decrease in arterial blood pressure is sensed in the macula densa in the juxtaglomerular complex and in the baroreceptor areas in the aortic arch and carotid area. This triggers the release of renin, either directly or through sympathetic nervous innervation. Renin will convert angiotensinogen to angiotensin I. Angiotensin I will be converted by ACE (angiotensin-converting enzyme, mainly found in lung tissue) to angiotensin II. Angiotensin II causes potent vasoconstriction of small arterioles and leads to increased systemic vascular resistance (SVR) and blood pressure. In addition, angiotensin II triggers increased reabsorption of sodium, chloride, and water in the kidney and the release of aldosterone, which in turn enhances sodium reabsorption and potassium excretion. Water and sodium will be retained, potassium will be excreted, and normal blood pressure will be restored.

Answers to SOE 5

5.1 How is calcium stored in the body?

Calcium is the most abundant mineral in the human body with a total weight of about 1 kg (25,000 mmol) and 99 % of it is stored within the skeletal system as calcium phosphate, carbonate, and hydroxyapatite. The remaining calcium is in the extracellular fluid, including plasma (about 9 mmol in total). The daily turnover of calcium is 15,000 mmol, mainly from bone remodelling.

5.2 Is calcium mainly an intra- or an extracellular ion?

The concentration of calcium ions inside cells (in the intracellular fluid) is more than 7000 times lower than in the blood plasma, hence calcium, like sodium and chloride, is mainly an extracellular ion.

5.3 What is the normal plasma level of calcium?

The total plasma concentration of calcium is 2.2–2.6 mmol/l

5.4 How is calcium represented in plasma?

Plasma calcium is divided into ionized (free) calcium (about 45%), protein bound to albumin and globulin (45%), and in a complex with citrate, carbonate, or hydrogen phosphate. However, it is free ionized calcium that is biologically active. Ionized calcium concentration in the plasma is 1.3–1.5 mmol/l.

5.5 What are the functions of calcium in the body?

Calcium has many functions in the body:

1. Excitable membranes of muscles and nerves contain specific calcium channels; calcium ions control the excitability of these membranes.

2. Calcium is required for the activation of clotting factors in the plasma. Clotting factor IV is ionized calcium, which plays an important role in all three (intrinsic, extrinsic, and common) clotting pathways.

3. Calcium is essential in excitation-contraction coupling of muscles ensuring muscle contraction.

4. Calcium provides structural support in cell surfaces ensuring membrane stability and is also an important component of bones and teeth.

5.6 How is the metabolism of calcium regulated in the body?

There are three substances that tightly regulate the plasma concentration of calcium within a very narrow range. They are parathyroid hormone (PTH), calcitonin, and vitamin D. These three substances act on bone, kidney, and intestine. In the gastrointestinal tract (GIT) calcium is absorbed by both passive (in a plasma-level-dependent manner) and active processes, the latter being stimulated by 1,25-dihydroxycholecalciferol. In the kidney, 98% of calcium is reabsorbed and only 2% is excreted (5 mmol/day). More calcium is excreted via faeces (15 mmol/day).

5.7 Tell me about the role of parathyroid hormone in calcium homeostasis.

PTH is produced by the chief cells of the four parathyroid glands located within the superior and inferior poles of both lobes of the thyroid gland. PTH is involved in a negative feedback mechanism regulating plasma calcium levels. If the plasma concentration of ionized calcium drops, PTH is released in response to a Ca^{2+} sensing receptor on the plasma membrane of the chief cells. PTH acts on bones, kidneys, and indirectly, on GIT. In the kidney, PTH increases active calcium reabsorption in distal tubules and collecting ducts in exchange for phosphate excretion. As a result, plasma ionized calcium concentration increases and phosphate falls. In bones, PTH increases the rate of bone resorption by stimulating the activity of osteoclasts to raise the serum calcium concentration.

5.8 What is the role of calcitonin in calcium regulation?

Calcitonin is secreted by the parafollicular cells in the thyroid gland. If the plasma concentration of calcium rises over 2.4 mmol/l, calcitonin is released due to the binding of calcium to the calcium-sensing receptors located on the parafollicular cells. Calcitonin decreases both calcium and phosphate concentration by direct inhibition of osteoblasts. It also increases renal excretion of calcium and phosphate by decreasing their reabsorption.

5.9 How is vitamin D involved in calcium regulation?

Vitamin D is a steroid compound derived from cholecalciferol (D_3). The active form is 1,25- dihydroxycholecalciferol (calcitriol). D_3 is produced in the skin by ultraviolet light. In the liver, D_3 is converted to 25-hydroxycholecalciferol and then, in the proximal nephron of the kidney, converted to 1,25- dihydroxycholecalciferol by the enzyme 1-hydroxylase which is in turn stimulated by PTH. The main action of vitamin D is to raise plasma calcium concentration by promoting the absorption of both calcium and phosphate from the GIT. 1,25-dihydroxycholecalciferol increases the synthesis of calcium-binding protein in the GIT and this, in turn, increases calcium absorption in the small intestine. It also mobilizes calcium and phosphate from bone to raise their plasma concentration.

Reference

Kam, P. and Power, I. *Principles of Physiology for the Anaesthetist*, 3rd edition. CRC Press, 2015: Chapter 11: pp. 342–345.

chapter 17

APPLIED PHARMACOLOGY

QUESTIONS

SOE 1 Local anaesthetic agents

1.1 What different groups of local anaesthetics do you know?
1.2 Can you tell me how local anaesthetics work?
1.3 Can you tell me how some of the local anaesthetics vary in their pharmacological and clinical properties and explain why?
1.4 What does protein binding determine?
1.5 What is the significance of the pKa?
1.6 Tell me more about lipid solubility.
1.7 What do you know about local anaesthetic metabolism?
1.8 What can you tell me about additives to local anaesthetics that influence their action?
1.9 Tell me about the different routes of administration of local anaesthetics.
1.10 What do you understand by the term 'differential block'?

SOE 2 Agonists and antagonists

2.1 What do you understand by the term 'agonist'?
2.2 What is an 'antagonist'?
2.3 You have mentioned two terms: 'affinity' and 'intrinsic activity'. Tell me more about them.
2.4 What is the difference between an agonist and an antagonist if they both bind to the same receptor?
2.5 What types of agonists are you aware of?
2.6 Give me some clinical examples of full and partial agonists?
2.7 What is the difference between full and partial agonists?
2.8 What is an inverse agonist?
2.9 How can we graphically compare the efficacy of different agonists?
2.10 What kind of plot is this?
2.11 What is so useful about this plot that could be used to compare two different agonists?
2.12 Tell me what the dose/response curve looks like for a partial agonist.
2.13 What kind of antagonists are there?
2.14 What do you understand by the term competitive antagonist?
2.15 Can the action of competitive antagonists be reversed?
2.16 What about non-competitive antagonists? How do they produce their effects?
2.17 What are the irreversible antagonists?
2.18 What is the difference between an inverse agonist and a competitive antagonist?

SOE 3 Inhalational anaesthetic agents

3.1   How can general anaesthesia be administered?
3.2   When would you prefer an inhalational versus an intravenous induction?
3.3   What are the features of an ideal inhalational anaesthetic agent?
3.4   What is 'saturated vapour pressure' and how is it clinically relevant?
3.5   How do you define the 'blood:gas partition coefficient' and how is it clinically relevant?
3.6   What is the 'oil:gas partition coefficient' and how is it clinically relevant?
3.7   What do you understand by 'MAC' and how is it clinically relevant?
3.8   What factors can increase or decrease MAC?
3.9   Which inhalational anaesthetic agents are currently in clinical use?
3.10 Which two inhalational anaesthetic agents do you use most frequently?
3.11 Compare and contrast the properties of these two agents.
3.12 What is nitrous oxide?
3.13 What are the advantages and disadvantages of using nitrous oxide?

SOE 4 Intravenous induction agents

4.1   How can general anaesthesia be administered?
4.2   What are the properties of the ideal intravenous induction agent?
4.3   Which central receptors do the intravenous induction agents act on?
4.4   Which intravenous induction agent do you use most often?
4.5   Why is propofol your preferred option?
4.6   What are the disadvantages of using propofol as an induction agent?
4.7   Can you compare and contrast propofol and thiopental as induction agents?
4.8   What are the advantages and disadvantages of etomidate as an induction agent?
4.9   What are the advantages and disadvantages of ketamine as an induction agent?
4.10 What other intravenous agents can be used to induce general anaesthesia?

SOE 5 Muscle relaxants

5.1   What do you understand by the term 'muscle relaxant'?
5.2   What types of muscle relaxants are you aware of?
5.3   Tell me about depolarizing muscle relaxants first.
5.4   Describe the side effects of succinylcholine.
5.5   Classify the non-depolarizing muscle relaxants.
5.6   Describe the pharmacology of your preferred muscle relaxant.
5.7   Which drugs are used to reverse the action of muscle relaxants?
5.8   How can the effect of muscle relaxants be monitored?
5.9   What can potentiate or prolong the effects of muscle relaxants?
5.10 What are the indications for using muscle relaxants in anaesthetic practice?
5.11 What are the problems with using muscle relaxants in anaesthetic practice?

Answer to SOE 1

1.1 What different groups of local anaesthetics do you know?

Local anaesthetics (LA) are divided into esters and amides, depending on the linkage of the aromatic lipophilic and the hydrophilic group. Examples of esters are cocaine, procaine, and amethocaine. Esters are more unstable in solution than amides. Examples of amide anaesthetics are lidocaine, prilocaine, bupivacaine, and ropivacaine.

1.2 Can you tell me how local anaesthetics work?

LA work by blocking sodium channels along the axonal membrane, therefore preventing conduction of an action potential along that nerve. This causes loss of sensation and motor function in that area of the body. The effect is reversible. Unionized lipid-soluble drug passes through the phospholipid membrane. Inside the axoplasm the drug is protonated, i.e., becomes ionized and binds to the internal surface of a sodium channel. This prevents the channel from opening. Another possible mechanism involves the dissolution of the unionized drug into the phospholipid membrane causing expansion of the sodium channel/lipoprotein matrix resulting in its inactivation.

1.3 Can you tell me how some of the local anaesthetics vary in their pharmacological and clinical properties and also explain why?

All LAs differ according to their protein binding, pKa, and lipid solubility.

1.4 What does protein binding determine?

The extent of protein binding influences the **duration of action**. The more protein bound the drug, the more prolonged its action. Esters are minimally protein bound while amides are more extensively bound. Bupivacaine is the amide drug with the highest protein binding, followed by ropivacaine, lidocaine, and prilocaine. An increase in plasma proteins (i.e., during pregnancy, renal failure, and postoperatively) will decrease the free fraction of the drug.

1.5 What is the significance of the pKa?

The **onset of action** is closely related to the pKa of the drug. The pKa is the pH at which the ionized and unionized forms of that LA are in equilibrium, i.e., 50% is ionized and 50% is unionized. All LAs are weak bases and exist mainly in the ionized form at normal physiological pH. Those drugs with a higher pKa have a greater ionized fraction, which is unable to penetrate the phospholipid membrane. The onset of action is therefore slower. Conversely, a lower pKa means a more unionized drug and a faster onset. This also explains why LAs are less effective in infected and therefore more acidic tissues.

1.6 Tell me more about lipid solubility.

Lipid solubility is also important and determines the anaesthetic **potency** of the drug. Bupivacaine, for instance, is highly lipid soluble and effective at low concentrations. Lidocaine, in contrast, is effective only at higher concentrations because of its lower lipid solubility.

1.7 What do you know about local anaesthetic metabolism?

Esters are rapidly hydrolysed by plasma esterases to inactive compounds. Cocaine, which undergoes hepatic hydrolysis, is the exception. Amides undergo hepatic metabolism by amidases. This is much slower than plasma hydrolysis, and amides are therefore prone to accumulation, especially when administered by continuous infusion. This becomes even more important when reduced hepatic blood flow or hepatic dysfunction decrease amidase activity.

1.8 What can you tell me about additives to local anaesthetics that influence their action?

Different additives are used to change their clinical effects. Bicarbonate, for instance, is sometimes added to lidocaine for epidural top-ups in urgent caesarean sections. The additive will raise the pH of the solution nearer to its pKa, thereby increasing the fraction of unionized lidocaine and therefore speed up onset of action of the drug. Different vasoconstrictors are also combined with LAs, the most popular being adrenaline (epinephrine). These slow the rate of systemic uptake of the drug and prolong its action.

1.9 Tell me about the different routes of administration of local anaesthetics.

LA can be given via topical, infiltration, nerve blocks, ganglion blocks, plexus blocks, paravertebral blocks, epidural, subarachnoid injections, and intravenous routes. Topically LA can be administered alone (tetracaine) or as a mixture (EMLA cream where lidocaine and prilocaine are mixed) to numb the skin before intravenous cannulation. Infiltration of LA is used wildly to numb an area of the body before or after an incision/procedure. LAs are used in a wide range of blocks (upper limb, lower limb, trunk blocks, eye blocks) to perform an operation with or without sedation or in combination with general anaesthetic (GA). Epidural administration of LA is used to perform a variety of procedures but this route is also suitable for continuous LA infusion for postoperative pain as well as analgesia in labour. Intravenous regional anaesthesia can be used for minor short procedures (Colles' fracture) where a special double cuff tourniquet is required.

1.10 What do you understand by the term 'differential block'?

Different nerve fibres are affected by local anaesthetics at different rates. This may be related to the size of the nerve. Small sensory nerves are usually blocked before large motor nerves. Frequency-dependence may play a role in this differential block. LA can enter the axoplasm while the sodium channel is in the open state, during depolarization. This happens at higher frequencies in smaller fibres, which get blocked more rapidly and easily. Larger motor fibres, by contrast, operate at lower frequencies so block occurs more slowly.

Reference

Peck, T.E. and Hill, S. *Pharmacology for Anaesthesia and Intensive Care*, 4th edition. Cambridge University Press, 2014.

Answer to SOE 2

2.1 What do you understand by the term 'agonist'?

An agonist is a substance that has a specific affinity for a receptor and full intrinsic activity.

2.2 What is an 'antagonist'?

An antagonist is a substance that also has an affinity for a receptor but has no intrinsic activity.

2.3 You have mentioned two terms: 'affinity' and 'intrinsic activity'. Tell me more about them.

Affinity is a measure of how avidly the drug binds to its receptor. Intrinsic activity, known more commonly as efficacy, is the size of the effect that it produces after binding to the receptor.

2.4 What is the difference between an agonist and an antagonist if they both bind to the same receptor?

An agonist binds to the receptor leading to a full effect: its intrinsic activity is one. An antagonist also binds to the receptor but elicits no effect at all: its intrinsic activity is zero. An antagonist simply blocks the receptor so that the agonist cannot exert its effect. In other words, it blocks the activity of an agonist.

2.5 What types of agonists are you aware of?

Full agonists and partial agonists.

2.6 Give me some clinical examples of full and partial agonists?

Morphine is a full agonist that acts on mu opioid receptors and buprenorphine is a partial agonist that also acts on those receptors.

2.7 What is the difference between full and partial agonists?

Although they both can bind to the receptors and fully occupy them, only the full agonist is able to elicit a maximal response. A partial agonist will also occupy all available receptors, but its efficacy will be less than 1, but above 0. Hence it will produce a lower maximum effect; for example, buprenorphine has a lower maximal analgesic action than morphine.

2.8 What is an inverse agonist?

It is a substance that binds to the same receptor as an agonist but produces the opposite effect to the endogenous agonist when activating the receptor, i.e., its intrinsic activity is less than zero. A necessary condition for inverse agonist action is that the receptors have a constitutive (intrinsic or basal) level of activity in the absence of any ligand. An agonist increases the activity of a receptor above its basal level (above 0), whereas an inverse agonist decreases its activity below the basal level (below 0). An inverse agonist preferentially binds to the inactive form of the receptor, so reducing any intrinsic activity. Inverse agonists can be strong or weak with an intrinsic activity of −1 (blocks all intrinsic activity), or between −1 and 0 (blocks only some intrinsic activity), respectively. The effects of an inverse agonist can be blocked by an antagonist. Many drugs previously classified as antagonists actually have inverse agonist properties, for example, certain antihistamines at H_1 receptors.

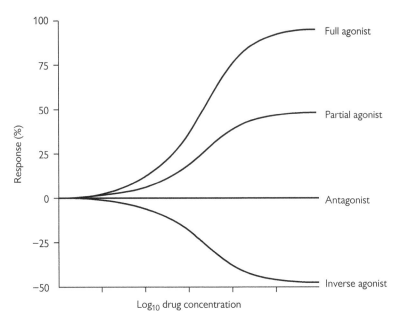

Fig 17.1 Semilog dose-response curve for different types of agonists.

2.9 How can we graphically compare the efficacy of different agonists?

We can create a plot where we have drug concentration on the X-axis, and the receptor occupancy, or the response, on the Y-axis (Fig 17.1)

2.10 What kind of graph is this?

It is a semi-logarithmic graph that has one axis on a logarithmic scale, and the other on a linear scale. It is useful for data with exponential relationships, or where one variable covers a large range of values.

2.11 What is so useful about this graph that could be used to compare two different agonists?

It's the shape of that curve (sigmoid shape) that is nearly straight in the middle that makes it so useful to compare different drugs.

2.12 Tell me what the dose/response curve will look like for the partial agonist.

For the partial agonist, the curve will resemble the curve for the full agonist but never reach the same maximum.

2.13 What kind of antagonists do you know?

Antagonists can be reversible or irreversible. Reversible antagonists can be competitive or non-competitive.

2.14 What do you understand by the term competitive antagonists?

A competitive antagonist is a substance that binds to receptors at the same binding site ('compete') as the agonist, but does not activate the receptor. Once bound, an antagonist will block agonist binding. The effect of this type of antagonist can be overcome by an increased dose of an agonist. Examples of competitive antagonists include naloxone and flumazenil.

2.15 Can the action of competitive antagonists be reversed?

Yes. If a sufficient concentration of an agonist is given, then this will displace the antagonist from the binding sites.

2.16 How do non-competitive antagonists produce their effects?

They work in one of two ways: by binding to an allosteric (non-active) site of the receptor or by irreversibly binding to the active site of the receptor. Their antagonism results from preventing receptor activation through conformational distortion of the receptor. Non-competitive antagonists decrease the maximum response that can be achieved by any amount of agonist. This is in contrast to competitive antagonists that will increase the amount of agonist required to elicit the response, but do not affect the maximum response. Increasing the concentration of an agonist cannot reverse non-competitive antagonists. An example includes ketamine, which antagonizes glutamate at the N-methyl-D-aspartate (NMDA) receptor in the central nervous system.

2.17 What are irreversible antagonists?

These are substances that effectively bind permanently to a receptor, preventing agonist binding and activity. Increasing the dose of an agonist does not overcome their effect. Examples are: phenoxybenzamine, which binds to alpha adrenoceptors and prevents the effect of noradrenaline/adrenaline; aspirin, which blocks COX-1 enzyme in platelets making them inactive for the duration of their life span (7-10 days). This is why both drugs need to be stopped for a long time before normal function of the receptors can return.

2.18 What is the difference between an inverse agonist and a competitive antagonist?

An inverse agonist binds preferentially to inactive receptors, which has the effect of reducing basal activity, an effect opposite to that of the agonist. A competitive antagonist binds equally to active and inactive receptors and prevents the agonist from binding. It has no effect of its own.

References

Berg, K.A. and Clarke, W.P. Making sense of pharmacology: inverse agonism and functional selectivity. *Int J Neuropsychopharmacol*, 2018;21(10):962–977.

Kenakin T. Principles: receptor theory in pharmacology. *Trends Pharmacol Sci*, 2004;25(4):186–192.

Peck, T.E. and Hill, S. *Pharmacology for Anaesthesia and Intensive Care*, 4th edition. Cambridge University Press, 2014.

Answer to SOE 3

3.1 How can general anaesthesia be administered?

General anaesthesia is usually administered via the intravenous or the inhalational route. Intravenous anaesthetics include propofol, thiopental, etomidate, and ketamine. Inhalational anaesthetics include isoflurane, sevoflurane, and desflurane. Anaesthesia can also be administered intramuscularly, for example using ketamine, or through intraosseous access.

3.2 When would you prefer an inhalational versus an intravenous induction?

I would usually perform an inhalational induction in paediatric anaesthetic practice. In adults, I would consider inhalational anaesthesia for patients with very difficult intravenous access, in cases where I would like the patient to keep breathing spontaneously such as in a difficult airway scenario, or in a patient with severe needle phobia.

3.3 What are the features of an ideal inhalational anaesthetic agent?

The ideal inhalational anaesthetic agent would have a number of features that can be grouped into physical, pharmacological, and logistical.

Ideal physical properties include: the agent should be a stable chemical, not affected by light or heat; it should not interact with materials that it is stored in or comes into contact with, such as glass or soda lime; it should be non-flammable and non-explosive and should ideally be odourless.

Pharmacologically, the ideal inhalational agent should have a high saturated vapour pressure, a low blood:gas partition coefficient, a high oil:gas partition coefficient, and a low minimum alveolar concentration (MAC). This agent should not have any potentially harmful side effects on any of the body systems. It should produce a smooth induction of and emergence from anaesthesia. Ideally, this agent should undergo minimal metabolism and should be eliminated unchanged through the lungs.

Logistical features include: the ideal inhalational anaesthetic agent should be inexpensive and easy to produce and administer; it should have a long shelf-life and should not require complicated transport or storage requirements; it should ideally have no preservatives and should not exert a greenhouse gas effect.

3.4 What is 'saturated vapour pressure' and how is it clinically relevant?

The saturated vapour pressure (SVP) is the pressure exerted by a vapour in equilibrium with its liquid, in a closed system. This occurs when the number of molecules escaping the liquid through evaporation equals the number of molecules returning to the liquid. Once this point is reached, the vapour can be described as 'saturated'. The SVP is often measured in mmHg and is dependent only on temperature. As the temperature rises, the SVP rises.

Clinically, the SVP is a measure of the volatility of the liquid inhalational anaesthetic and, therefore, the vaporizers are specifically designed for a particular inhalational agent. For example, the SVP of desflurane is close to one atmosphere so desflurane is close to boiling at room temperature. As a result, the desflurane vaporizer needs to be warmed to 39°C to make it a vapour/gas blender rather than a variable bypass type as seen with other agents. Because SVP changes with temperature, variable bypass vaporizers must be temperature-compensated to maintain a stable working temperature, giving a reliable and predictable inhalational anaesthetic agent output.

3.5 How do you define the 'blood:gas partition coefficient' and how is it clinically relevant?

The blood:gas partition coefficient is the ratio of the amount of inhalational agent in blood versus the amount of inhalational agent in gas. Both phases should be of equal volume and pressure and should be in equilibrium at 37°C.

The ideal inhalational agent should have a low blood:gas partition coefficient, meaning that the agent is relatively insoluble in blood. This means that equilibrium is reached more quickly between the gas and blood phases. Being relatively insoluble, the partial pressure of the gas in the blood increases faster, and it is this partial pressure of inhalational agent in the blood that produces the anaesthetic effect on the brain.

Therefore, a low blood:gas partition coefficient is related to the speed of onset of anaesthesia with inhalational agents. Desflurane has the lowest blood:gas partition coefficient of the inhalational agents in common use (0.42), while halothane has the highest (2.3).

3.6 What is the 'oil:gas partition coefficient' and how is it clinically relevant?

The oil:gas partition coefficient is the ratio of the amount of inhalational agent in oil versus the amount of inhalational agent in gas. It is therefore a measure of the lipid solubility of the inhalational agent.

The ideal inhalational agent should have a high oil:gas partition coefficient, meaning that the agent should be highly lipid soluble. This is related to the potency of the inhalational agent and expressed by its MAC. The Meyer-Overton hypothesis relates these two concepts by stating that when a certain amount of agent is dissolved into the neuronal lipid membrane, then the agent causes anaesthesia. Therefore, a high oil:gas partition coefficient is related to the potency of anaesthesia of the inhalational agents. Halothane has the highest oil:gas partition coefficient of the inhalational agents in common use (224), with isoflurane second (97) and nitrous oxide last (1.4).

3.7 What do you understand by 'MAC' and how is it clinically relevant?

MAC is the minimal alveolar concentration of inhalational agent needed to prevent 50% of non-premedicated patients from responding to a standard surgical stimulus. It is measured at one atmosphere of pressure (sea level) in 100% oxygen. Therefore, the MAC is equivalent to an ED_{50}. Clinically, an ED_{95} would be more useful, i.e., the concentration required to prevent 95% of non-premedicated patients from responding to a standard stimulus. It is expressed as a percentage and is important when monitoring the depth of anaesthesia, to reduce the chance of awareness.

Clinically, the MAC shows an inverse relationship with potency. The higher the MAC, the lower the potency of the inhalational anaesthetic agent. For example, desflurane—with a MAC of 6–7%—is less potent than sevoflurane (MAC 1.7–2.0%) or isoflurane (MAC 1.2%).

3.8 What factors can increase or decrease MAC?

MAC is increased in paediatric patients; in those with an activated sympathetic response such as very anxious patients; in patients with hypermetabolic states such as thyrotoxicosis; and in hyperthermic and hypercapnic patients. MAC is decreased by increasing age; pregnancy; hypoxia; hypovolaemia; and when other centrally acting drugs are used such as nitrous oxide, benzodiazepines, or opioids.

3.9 Which inhalational anaesthetic agents are currently in clinical use?

Currently, isoflurane, sevoflurane, desflurane, and enflurane are available for use. Nitrous oxide is also considered an inhalational anaesthetic agent. Halothane is still used in some developing countries and xenon is available in some resource-rich countries.

3.10 Which two inhalational anaesthetic agents do you use most frequently?

Here you can choose which of the inhalational anaesthetic agents you want to speak about. We will use sevoflurane and isoflurane as an example.

Of the inhalational anaesthetic agents, I use isoflurane and sevoflurane most frequently.

3.11 Compare and contrast the properties of these two agents.

Isoflurane and sevoflurane are both halogenated ether inhalational anaesthetics and are administered via plenum vaporizers. For induction of anaesthesia, sevoflurane is usually preferred due to its sweet smell and minimal pungency. In contrast, the use of isoflurane in the induction of anaesthesia is limited by its powerful smell and the risk of coughing and laryngospasm. Both agents are used for the maintenance of anaesthesia. Isoflurane, having a lower MAC and higher oil:gas partition coefficient, is more potent. Sevoflurane, having a lower blood:gas partition coefficient, is faster in onset and offset of anaesthesia. Both isoflurane and sevoflurane are potent bronchodilators, making them useful in clinical conditions such as severe status asthmaticus. Finally, isoflurane is less expensive than sevoflurane, but both are potent greenhouse gases.

3.12 What is nitrous oxide?

Nitrous oxide is a gas with the chemical formula N_2O. In anaesthetic practice, it is available as a piped gas through wall-mounted ports that are connected to a central cylinder bank, or as cylinders with French blue shoulders that are mounted to a yoke of the anaesthetic machine via the Pin Index system. It can also be provided as part of a 50:50 mixture by volume with oxygen, Entonox®, in cylinders with French blue and white shoulders, or through wall-mounted French blue and white ports.

It is a colourless gas, often described as having a sweet or metallic scent and taste. It is non-flammable but does support combustion. It has a MAC above 100%, which means that it cannot be used as the sole inhalational anaesthetic agent but can contribute towards one MAC in conjunction with another agent. It has a low blood:gas partition coefficient, giving a fast onset of action; and a relatively low oil:gas partition coefficient showing a low potency.

3.13 What are the advantages and disadvantages of using nitrous oxide?

The advantages of nitrous oxide are: it is easily available in routine anaesthetic practice; is relatively inexpensive; and, through the second-gas effect, it speeds up the induction of anaesthesia by increasing the alveolar concentration of the other inhalational anaesthetic agents. It also reduces the MAC of the co-administered volatile agent during the maintenance phase of general anaesthesia, and it has analgesic properties.

The disadvantages include: it increases pressure in non-compliant air-filled cavities such as the middle ear; it will increase the volume of compliant air-filled cavities such as bowel and pneumothoraxes; it has emetogenic effects; long term it has been shown to impair bone marrow function and exert neurotoxic effects; it is also a negative inotrope. Finally, nitrous oxide is a greenhouse gas and so contributes to climate change.

Reference

Peck, T.E. and Hill, S. *Pharmacology for Anaesthesia and Intensive Care*, 4th edition. Cambridge University Press, 2014.

Answer to SOE 4

4.1 How can general anaesthesia be administered?

General anaesthesia is usually administered via the intravenous or the inhalational route. Intravenous anaesthetics include propofol, thiopental, etomidate, and ketamine. Inhalational anaesthetics include isoflurane, sevoflurane, and desflurane. Anaesthesia can also be administered intramuscularly, for example using ketamine, or through intraosseous access.

4.2 What are the properties of the ideal intravenous induction agent?

The ideal intravenous anaesthetic agent would have a number of properties that can be grouped into physical, pharmacokinetic, pharmacodynamic, and logistical.

Ideal physical properties include compatibility with commonly used anaesthetic drugs and that it is chemically stable. It would be optimal if the drug preparation would contain no preservatives. It should also be water soluble and bacteriostatic.

Pharmacokinetically, the ideal intravenous agent should have a predictable onset of action, preferably in one arm-brain circulation time. The offset of action should be fast and predictable, leaving no or minimal hangover effect, with metabolism only to inactive metabolites. This drug should not accumulate in tissues and should have a context-insensitive half time when used by infusion.

Pharmacodynamically, the drug should have a high potency and efficacy and have minimal effects on other organ systems, such as cardiovascular and respiratory. Additional desirable qualities would be painless administration, non-teratogenic, and with a low incidence of toxicity and allergic reactions. This drug should be non-irritant to vasculature and should not cause harm in the case of accidental arterial injection or extravasation.

Logistical features include that the ideal intravenous agent should be inexpensive, easy to produce, and readily available. It should require minimal preparation or reconstitution at the clinical stage. It should have a long shelf-life and should not require complicated transport or storage requirements.

4.3 Which central receptors do the intravenous induction agents act on?

Propofol, thiopental, and etomidate mainly act by potentiation of the central gamma amino butyric acid (GABA) A receptor. GABA is an inhibitory neurotransmitter. In addition, propofol and thiopental potentiate the glycine receptor, which usually binds the inhibitory neurotransmitter glycine, while also inhibiting the central nicotinic acetylcholine receptor, which usually binds the excitatory neurotransmitter acetylcholine. Etomidate does not demonstrate these effects. In contrast, ketamine acts by inhibiting the NMDA receptor, which is usually bound by the excitatory neurotransmitter glutamate.

4.4 Which intravenous induction agent do you use most often?

Here you choose which of the intravenous induction agents to speak about. We will use propofol as an example.

In my day-to-day practice, I use propofol as my preferred intravenous induction agent.

4.5 Why is propofol your preferred option?

Propofol exhibits many features of the ideal intravenous induction agent. It is readily available in my hospital, and it does not require refrigeration for transport and storage. It is compatible with anaesthetic drugs in common use and does not require reconstitution prior to administration. This is a useful feature in time-critical situations. Also, its offset of action is relatively fast and predictable after a single dose, it is metabolized to inactive metabolites, and has little hangover effect. This makes it useful for short anaesthetic procedures and day-case surgery, and it can also be used as part of a total intravenous anaesthetic (TIVA) protocol. It has not been reported to cause severe adverse events if injected intra-arterially or in the case of accidental extravasation. Cough or laryngospasm are uncommon, and this makes propofol ideal for the placement of laryngeal mask airways.

4.6 What are the disadvantages of using propofol as an induction agent?

Propofol is presented as a lipid emulsion, and therefore should not be prepared long before its intended use as it offers a good medium for bacterial growth. It can also have an unpredictable onset time, which is not solely dependent on patient weight but also on other subjective factors such as the patient's level of anxiety preoperatively. This makes it an unreliable induction agent when the recommended dose of 1.0–2.5 mg/kg is administered in a time-critical setting, for example during rapid sequence intubation. In addition, it often causes pain on administration and may cause significant hypotension when a standard induction dose is given, particularly in haemodynamically compromised patients. Respiratory depression is commonly observed.

4.7 Can you compare and contrast propofol and thiopental as induction agents?

Propofol and thiopental have different strengths and weaknesses when used as induction agents. Propofol is ready for use as presented in the vial, while thiopental requires reconstitution from a yellow powder into a water-based solution prior to use. The time required for this, and the risk of dilution error, need to be considered. However, since thiopental is a water-based solution, it can be prepared some hours in advance and stored in a safe manner for emergency use as required. This is not recommended for propofol, which is a lipid emulsion.

In terms of onset of action, thiopental has a rapid and reliable onset of action in a dose of between 3 and 7 mg/kg, in one arm-brain circulation time. This is very useful during a rapid sequence induction. Propofol does not behave in the same manner, as described earlier, and so this would be a disadvantage in an emergency situation. On the other hand, if there is any doubt as to the patency or siting of the intravenous access available, thiopental should not be used as extravasation may cause severe skin injury, including necrosis. Propofol is safer than thiopental in cases of accidental arterial, subcutaneous, or intramuscular injection. Unlike propofol, thiopental is not suitable for total intravenous anaesthesia due to saturation of hepatic enzymes and active metabolites.

Specific contraindications exist for both propofol and thiopental. For example, thiopental cannot be used in patients with porphyria and propofol should be avoided in patients with severe egg allergies.

4.8 What are the advantages and disadvantages of etomidate as an induction agent?

Etomidate is an imidazole hypnotic used for induction of anaesthesia, often in haemodynamically compromised patients. This is because it is cardio-stable when compared with the other intravenous induction agents. In a dose of 0.2–0.3 mg/kg, it has a fast and reliable onset of action and therefore can be used for rapid sequence induction. It is presented as a clear, colourless solution in a glass vial, and does not require reconstitution prior to use.

The main concern with its use is related to transient suppression of adrenal steroid production, secondary to inhibition of the 11β-hydroxylase enzyme. This has been reported to last up to 72 hours after a single induction dose. Patients experience pain on injection and myoclonus is observed in about a third of patients. It may also cause an increased incidence of postoperative nausea and vomiting.

4.9 What are the advantages and disadvantages of ketamine as an induction agent?

Ketamine is quite different from the other intravenous induction agents as it causes dissociative anaesthesia. S-ketamine is preferred to its stereoisomer R-ketamine, due to a more favourable pharmacological profile. The drug is often presented as a racemic mixture.

Advantages of using ketamine include: it can be administered intravenously, intramuscularly, orally, nasally, and even rectally to induce anaesthesia; it is often used in hypotensive patients as it causes tachycardia, hypertension, and increased cardiac output; it preserves the protective airway reflexes, making it ideal for use in a pre-hospital setting. Specifically, in severe asthma, ketamine is the ideal choice of induction agent due to its bronchial smooth muscle relaxation effect.

Disadvantages of ketamine use include: a sometimes difficult to define onset of anaesthesia due to open-eyed staring associated with dissociative anaesthesia; increased salivation which may cause laryngospasm or make airway management more complex. Concerns regarding increased cerebral blood flow and increased intracranial pressure have resulted in caution being exercised when ketamine is used in head-injured patients. Ketamine can cause vivid and unpleasant dreams that can be lessened by the prior administration of benzodiazepines or opioids.

4.10 What other intravenous agents can be used to induce general anaesthesia?

Other intravenous agents include drugs of the barbiturate class, such as methohexital or phenobarbital. Although more commonly used as adjuvants, benzodiazepines such as midazolam or diazepam can be used to induce general anaesthesia.

Reference

Peck, T.E. and Hill, S. *Pharmacology for Anaesthesia and Intensive Care*, 4th edition. Cambridge University Press, 2014.

Answer to SOE 5

5.1 What do you understand by the term 'muscle relaxants'?

Muscle relaxants, or neuromuscular blockers, are drugs used in anaesthetic practice to cause blockade of the neuromuscular junction in skeletal muscle. These drugs do not affect cardiac or smooth muscle.

5.2 What types of muscle relaxants are you aware of?

Muscle relaxants are divided into depolarizing and non-depolarizing types.

5.3 Tell me about depolarizing muscle relaxants first.

Succinylcholine is the only depolarizing muscle relaxant in clinical use, causing Phase I neuromuscular blockade. It is presented as a clear, colourless solution in a concentration of 50 mg/ml, commonly in 2 ml vials. It does not require reconstitution prior to use but needs to be stored and transported at 4°C. It is also available in pre-filled syringes.

Its mode of action is through binding to post-synaptic nicotinic cholinergic receptors, blocking the action of acetylcholine. On binding, it causes depolarization of the muscle, visible to the naked eye as fasciculation. When used in a dose of 1–1.5 mg/kg, it has an onset time of 30–45 seconds making it ideal for use during a rapid sequence intubation. It is quickly metabolized by plasma cholinesterase usually within three to five minutes, and therefore, provides a short duration of muscle relaxation. There is no reversal agent for succinylcholine, and recovery is dependent on drug metabolism.

5.4 Describe the side effects of succinylcholine.

Succinylcholine apnoea may occur in patients with plasma cholinesterase abnormalities. Succinylcholine is also associated with malignant hyperthermia. It causes a rise in serum potassium and a transient rise in intracranial, intragastric, and intraocular pressure. It can also cause myalgia, commonest in young females mobilizing rapidly in the postoperative period. Another side effect of succinylcholine is bradycardia, often observed after a second dose and in children.

5.5 Classify the non-depolarizing muscle relaxants.

The non-depolarizing muscle relaxants can be classified based on their chemical structure. These can be grouped into the benzylisoquinoliniums and the aminosteroids. Drugs of the benzylisoquinolinium class include atracurium and mivacurium. The aminosteroid class includes vecuronium, rocuronium, and pancuronium.

5.6 Describe the pharmacology of your preferred muscle relaxant.

Here you may select the non-depolarizing muscle relaxant you use most frequently. We will use atracurium as an example.

My preferred muscle relaxant for elective use is atracurium. Atracurium besylate is a benzylisoquinolinium presented as a clear, colourless solution containing 10 mg/ml. It does not require reconstitution prior to use and should be transported and stored at approximately 4°C. The dose of atracurium for intubation is 0.3–0.6 mg/kg. The onset of action is between two to four minutes, and the duration is usually between 45 and 60 minutes. Top-up doses of 0.1–0.2 mg/kg can be used to maintain muscle relaxation. It can also be used as an infusion during long procedures or in the intensive care unit.

Pharmacokinetically, atracurium is given intravenously so bioavailability is 100%. It is moderately protein bound at about 82%. Atracurium is mainly metabolized through Hofmann degradation. This is a process of spontaneous breakdown to laudanosine and a quaternary monoacrylate at body pH and temperature. It means that the metabolism of atracurium is independent of renal or liver function. Additionally, atracurium is metabolized through ester hydrolysis via non-specific plasma esterases.

When administered as a fast bolus, atracurium may cause histamine release, which could precipitate bronchospasm, hypotension, or skin manifestations. Therefore, the use of atracurium in atopic individuals should be carefully monitored or avoided. Prolonged atracurium infusion in an intensive care setting is associated with critical illness myopathy.

5.7 Which drugs are used to reverse the action of muscle relaxants?

The action of non-depolarizing muscle relaxants can be reversed using neostigmine or sugammadex.

Neostigmine is a quaternary amine, used in anaesthetic practice as an intravenous preparation. The vial commonly contains 2.5 mg in one ml and does not require reconstitution prior to use. It forms a carbamylated enzyme complex with acetylcholinesterase, preventing it from hydrolysing acetylcholine. This increases the amount of acetylcholine available at the neuromuscular junction, to counter the effect of the muscle relaxant. The intravenous dose used to reverse the action of non-depolarizing muscle relaxants is 0.05 mg/kg. Neostigmine causes bradycardia and increased salivation via muscarinic receptors, and therefore should be given together with atropine or glycopyrrolate to mitigate these effects. It also causes increased intestinal motility.

Sugammadex is the first selective relaxant binding agent designed to reverse the action of the aminosteroid, non-depolarizing muscle relaxants rocuronium and vecuronium. It is a γ-cyclodextrin and dosing is dependent on the depth of neuromuscular blockade, varying from 2 to 16 mg/kg. It has a ring-like structure which envelops rocuronium and vecuronium in a lipophilic core, rendering them inactive. It is biologically inactive and has no chemical properties. Sugammadex, as well as the cyclodextrin-aminosteroid complex, are excreted via the kidneys unchanged.

5.8 How can the effect of muscle relaxants be monitored?

The effect of muscle relaxants can be monitored clinically using observation or using nerve stimulators. Observations such as the onset of spontaneous respirations and movement are easily performed. Nerve stimulators stimulate motor nerves using electrical current. This is usually done transcutaneously for monitoring muscle relaxant effects, aiming to produce an action potential which may result in muscle contraction. Often, the ulnar nerve is stimulated while observing the contraction of the adductor pollicis muscle. A supramaximal stimulus of 80 mA is applied, and various stimulation patterns are available. The commonest are the train-of-four (TOF) stimulation, tetanic stimulation and post-tetanic count, and double-burst stimulation. Acceleromyography is available on most modern nerve stimulators to quantify the TOF and TOF ratio.

Prior to the administration of a neuromuscular antagonist such as neostigmine, the measured TOF should be at least three out of four. Satisfactory recovery from neuromuscular blockade occurs when the TOF ratio is above 0.9.

5.9 What can potentiate or prolong the effect of muscle relaxants?

The effect of muscle relaxants can be potentiated by inhalational anaesthetic agents, and by antibiotics including aminoglycosides such as gentamicin, tetracyclines, and clindamycin. Additionally, lithium, local anaesthetics, and anti-epileptic medications have been reported to have this effect. Administration of magnesium can prolong the effect of muscle relaxants.

Drugs metabolized and excreted by the liver and the kidneys, such as rocuronium, may have a prolonged effect in patients with liver and/or renal impairment or failure. The effect of atracurium is prolonged in the presence of acidosis and hypothermia due to the slowing down of Hofmann degradation. Patients suffering from neuromuscular pathology may be more sensitive to the effect of muscle relaxants than the general population and include patients with amyotrophic lateral sclerosis, myasthenia gravis, or muscular dystrophies.

5.10 What are the indications for using muscle relaxants in anaesthetic practice?

Muscle relaxants are used to facilitate intubation and ventilation in the operating theatre and intensive care unit. They provide optimal surgical conditions as the patient does not move and their muscles are relaxed to facilitate access to body cavities, such as is required for abdominal or thoracic surgery.

5.11 What are the problems with using muscle relaxants in anaesthetic practice?

The dangers of using muscle relaxants include recognized generic side effects such as anaphylactic or anaphylactoid reactions, as well as specific effects of the particular agent. For example, succinylcholine is associated with hyperkalaemia and malignant hyperthermia, and atracurium is known to cause histamine release, which may precipitate bronchospasm and hypotension.

The use of muscle relaxants is associated with awareness during general anaesthesia and adequate depth of anaesthesia should be ensured when these drugs are used. Moreover, the administration of these drugs causes the patient to become apnoeic, and the anaesthetist must provide an open airway and appropriate oxygenation and ventilation during this time.

References

EMC medicine updates (n.d.). Available at: https://www.medicines.org.uk.

McCombe, K., Wijayasiri, L., and Patel, A. *MasterPass: The Primary FRCA Structured Oral Examination Study Guide 2*. Radcliffe Publishing Ltd., 2010.

Peck, T.E. and Hill, S. *Pharmacology for Anaesthesia and Intensive Care*, 4th edition. Cambridge University Press, 2014.

APPLIED ANATOMY

QUESTIONS

SOE 1 The larynx

1.1 Outline the anatomy of the larynx.
1.2 Name the laryngeal cartilages.
1.3 Describe the anatomy of the thyroid cartilage.
1.4 Outline the anatomy of the cricoid cartilage.
1.5 Outline the anatomy of the epiglottis.
1.6 What are the arytenoid cartilages?
1.7 Briefly describe the anatomy of the cuneiform and corniculate cartilages.
1.8 What is the nerve supply to the larynx?

SOE 2 The thoracic inlet

2.1 What different types of ribs are there?
2.2 Describe the anatomy of the first rib.
2.3 What is the clinical relevance of a first rib fracture?
2.4 What is the thoracic inlet?
2.5 What are the boundaries of the thoracic inlet?
2.6 What structures pass through the thoracic inlet?
2.7 Describe the course of the subclavian arteries.
2.8 Describe the anatomy of the subclavian veins.
2.9 What is the ideal location for the tip of a central venous catheter?

SOE 3 The diaphragm

3.1 Outline the anatomy of the diaphragm.
3.2 Describe the muscular attachments of the diaphragm.
3.3 What are the main openings in the diaphragm?
3.4 What is the innervation of the diaphragm?
3.5 What is a diaphragmatic hernia?
3.6 Briefly outline the different types of diaphragmatic herniae.

SOE 4 Abdominal wall

4.1 Describe the general structure of the abdominal wall.
4.2 What muscles are found in the anterolateral abdominal wall?

4.3 Name the muscles of the posterior abdominal wall.

4.4 Outline the nerve supply to the anterolateral abdominal wall.

4.5 What is the thoracolumbar fascia?

4.6 Name the structures labelled A–H, and V–Y in the accompanying image (Fig. 18.1) of a transverse section through the abdomen at the level of the third lumbar vertebra.

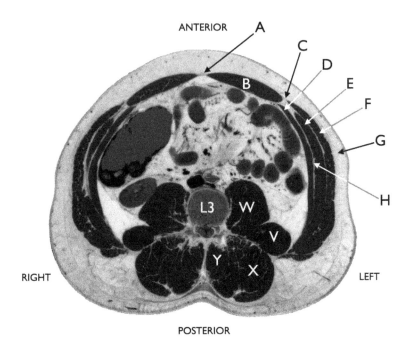

Fig 18.1 Transverse section through the abdomen at the level of the third lumbar vertebra (L3).

Image taken from the VH Dissector, Touch of Life Technologies (toltech.net). Used with permission.

SOE 5 Lumbar plexus

5.1 Tell me about the anatomy of the lumbar plexus.

5.2 Describe the anatomy of the femoral nerve.

5.3 What structures are innervated by the femoral nerve?

5.4 What are the borders and contents of the femoral triangle?

5.5 What is the femoral sheath?

5.6 What is the adductor canal?

5.7 Outline the course of the obturator nerve.

5.8 What is the lumbosacral trunk?

Answers to SOE 1

1.1 Outline the anatomy of the larynx.

The larynx is a complex hollow structure in the anterior neck at the level of the third to sixth cervical vertebrae. It is composed of a framework of nine articulating cartilages connected by ligaments and muscles. It connects the inferior part of the pharynx to the trachea and is lined by a ciliated mucous membrane. It functions as a sphincter protecting the air passages from aspiration, especially during swallowing. It is also the organ of phonation (voice production) and is required for coughing and straining.

1.2 Name the laryngeal cartilages.

The cartilaginous skeleton of the larynx is made up of three unpaired cartilages (epiglottis, thyroid, cricoid) and three paired cartilages (arytenoid, corniculate, cuneiform).

1.3 Describe the anatomy of the thyroid cartilage.

The thyroid cartilage is the largest of the laryngeal cartilages. It is a shield-shaped structure consisting of right and left laminae joined in the midline anteriorly to form the laryngeal prominence and widely separated posteriorly. The angle of fusion is more acute in the male (90°) compared with the female (120°). In the midline above the laryngeal prominence is the superior thyroid notch, and below it is the less distinct inferior thyroid notch. The superior and inferior cornua (horns) are projections from the respective borders of the thyroid cartilage. The superior cornu is attached to the hyoid bone (which is not regarded as part of the larynx) via the thyrohyoid membrane, and the inferior cornu forms an articulation with the cricoid cartilage.

1.4 Outline the anatomy of the cricoid cartilage.

The cricoid cartilage is the only cartilage in the respiratory tract that forms a complete ring. It is shaped like a signet ring with an anterior arch connected to a single posterior quadrilateral lamina. The anterior arch of the cricoid cartilage is connected to the thyroid cartilage above via the median cricoid ligament (usually referred to clinically as the cricothyroid membrane), and to the first tracheal ring below via the cricotracheal ligament. The cricothyroid membrane is relatively avascular and is a vital landmark for front of neck access (FONA) in emergency airway management.

1.5 Outline the anatomy of the epiglottis.

The epiglottis is a heart- or leaf-shaped elastic cartilage covered with mucous membrane. The inferior and narrowest end is connected to the thyroid cartilage via the thyroepiglottic ligament. The epiglottis projects posterosuperiorly to cover the laryngeal inlet. Its free posterior surface is concave from side to side and bears an elevation on its lower part termed the epiglottic tubercle. The mucous membrane covering the superior part of the epiglottis is reflected onto the pharyngeal part of the tongue to form the median glosso-epiglottic fold, flanked on either side by the lateral glosso-epiglottic folds. The recess formed on either side of the median gloss-epiglottic fold is termed the vallecula, which is an important landmark during endotracheal intubation.

1.6 What are the arytenoid cartilages?

The arytenoid cartilages are paired pyramidal-shaped cartilages that articulate with the superior border of the lamina of the cricoid cartilage. Each has an apex to which the corniculate cartilage is attached, an anterior vocal process to which the posterior part of the vocal ligament is attached, and a lateral muscular process to which the posterior and lateral cricoarytenoid muscles are attached.

1.7 Briefly describe the anatomy of the cuneiform and corniculate cartilages.

The cuneiform cartilages are small, paired elongated pieces of fibroelastic cartilage in the aryepiglottic fold which form small nodules visible at laryngoscopy.

The corniculate cartilages are paired conical nodules of fibroelastic cartilage, which form an articulation (or are sometimes fused with) the upper pole of the arytenoids. They are also visible at laryngoscopy in the posterior aryepiglottic fold posteromedial to the cuneiform cartilages (Fig 18.2).

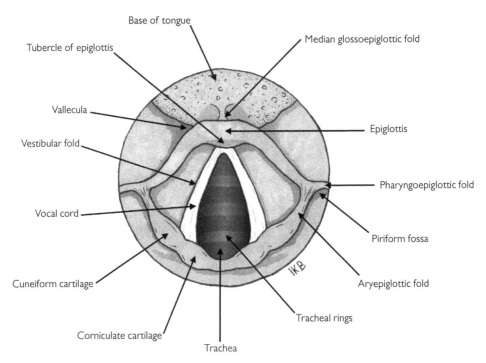

Fig 18.2 Typical laryngoscopic appearance of the larynx.

1.8 What is the nerve supply to the larynx?

The larynx is innervated entirely by branches of the vagus nerve (Fig 18.3). The vagus nerve exits the skull via the jugular foramen and descends into the neck in the carotid sheath. The superior laryngeal nerve arises from the inferior vagal (nodose) ganglion within the jugular foramen. Within the carotid sheath, it divides into the external and internal laryngeal nerves. The external laryngeal nerve supplies motor innervation to the cricothyroid muscle, and the larger internal laryngeal nerve provides sensory innervation to the larynx above the vocal cords (including the superior surface of the vocal cords).

The recurrent laryngeal nerve arises from the vagus nerve within the thorax. The right recurrent laryngeal nerve leaves the vagus nerve, crosses anterior to the subclavian artery, and then passes inferior and posterior to the artery to ascend in the neck in the tracheo-oesophageal groove. The left recurrent laryngeal nerve arises at the level of the aortic arch passing inferior then posterior to the arch to ascend in the tracheo-oesophageal groove (Fig 18.5). The recurrent laryngeal nerve provides sensory innervation to all the larynx below the vocal cords, and motor innervation to all the intrinsic muscles of the larynx except for the cricothyroid.

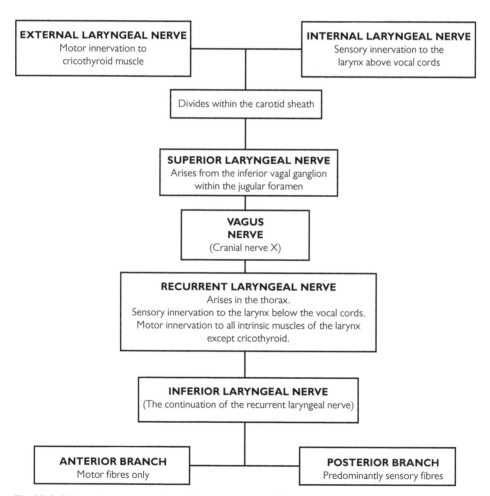

Fig 18.3 Schematic representation of the innervation of the larynx.

References

Burdett, E. and Mitchell, V. Anatomy of the larynx, trachea and bronchi. *Anaesthesia and Intensive Care Medicine*, 2011;12:335–339.

Ellis, H. and Lawson, A. *Anatomy for Anaesthetists*, 9th edition. Wiley Blackwell, 2013.

Saran, M., Georgakopoulos, B., and Bordoni, B. *Anatomy, Head and Neck, Larynx Vocal Cords*. [Updated 2021 Feb 7]. StatPearls [Internet]. StatPearls Publishing, Treasure Island (FL), 2022. Available at: https://www.ncbi.nlm.nih.gov/books/NBK535342/.

Standring, S. *Gray's Anatomy: The Anatomical Basis of Clinical Practice*, 41st edition. Elsevier, 2015.

Answers to SOE 2

2.1 What different types of ribs are there?

The ribs are either categorized according to their anterior attachment (into true, false, or floating ribs), or according to anatomical similarities between them, into atypical and typical ribs.

The first (upper) seven pairs of ribs are termed true (vertebrosternal) ribs because they attach directly to the sternum via their own costal cartilage. The eighth, ninth, and tenth ribs are termed false (vertebrochondral) ribs because they do not articulate directly with the sternum, but instead are joined by cartilage to the seventh costal cartilage. The eleventh and twelfth (lowest) pair of ribs are termed floating ribs because they have no anterior attachment; instead, their anterior end terminates in the musculature of the posterior abdominal wall.

Ribs one, eleven, and twelve are atypical ribs due to anatomical differences between them and the other ribs. Because ribs two and ten have some anomalous features some authors consider them also to be atypical. The remainder are classified as typical ribs.

2.2 Describe the anatomy of the first rib.

The first rib is the shortest, flattest, and most curved rib (Fig 18.4). It forms a 'C' shape, featuring a small round head, which forms an articulation with the body of the first thoracic vertebra, connected to the main shaft of the rib via a rounded neck. At the junction between the neck and the shaft, a prominent tubercle projects upwards and backwards and bears an oval facet that forms an articulation with the transverse process of the first thoracic vertebra. The first rib slopes forwards and downwards. Its anterior end forms a connection with the manubrium via its costal cartilage. The lower surface of the first rib is smooth and lies in apposition to the pleura, while the upper surface bears two grooves along which the subclavian vessels pass. These grooves are separated by the scalene tubercle, a bony projection near the centre of the inner border of the rib, which is the attachment for the anterior scalene muscle.

2.3 What is the clinical relevance of a first rib fracture?

First rib fractures are associated with high velocity impact, most commonly motor vehicle collision, and are strongly associated with life-threatening injuries, notably of the head, cervical spine, thorax, liver, and pelvis. There is a significant difference in the mechanism of injury in those sustaining first rib fractures compared with fractures of the other ribs.

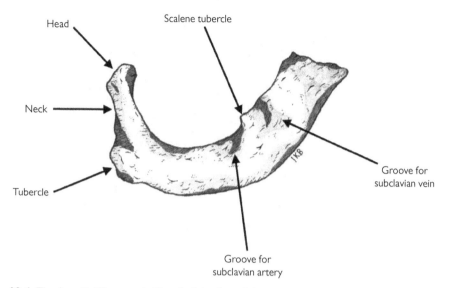

Fig 18.4 The first rib. The rounded head of the first rib bears a single articular facet. The neck is roughly cylindrical, and the tubercle at the junction between the neck and the shaft bears a single articular facet. While the other ribs contribute to the wall of the thoracic cavity, the first rib forms part of the roof of the thorax.

2.4 What is the thoracic inlet?

The thoracic inlet is the aperture at the top of the thorax (the superior thoracic aperture). It forms a junction between the root of the neck and the thoracic cavity. The anatomical thoracic outlet (inferior thoracic outlet) is the floor of the thoracic cavity. Almost completely closed by the diaphragm the thoracic outlet is the junction between the thoracic and abdominal cavities. Somewhat confusingly the term thoracic outlet is sometimes used clinically to refer to the anatomical thoracic inlet, because major vessels and nerves *exit* the thorax via this aperture.

2.5 What are the boundaries of the thoracic inlet?

The thoracic inlet is bounded by a kidney-shaped (reniform) bony ring orientated in an oblique transverse plane. The bony ring consists of: posteriorly the body of the first thoracic vertebra, laterally the first ribs and their costal cartilages, anteriorly the costal cartilages of the first ribs and the superior border of the manubrium (Fig 18.5).

2.6 What structures pass through the thoracic inlet?

The thoracic inlet transmits many vital structures. These can be organized into lists of nerves, muscles, vessels, and so on, but it is better (and easier) to present them using a diagram that can be reproduced in the examination (Fig 18.5).

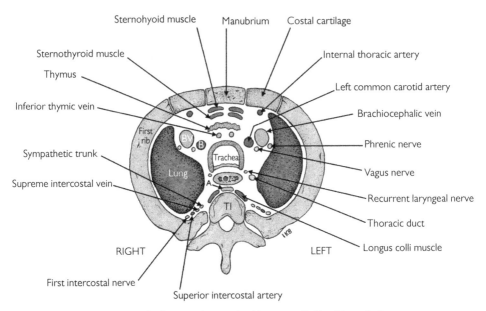

Fig 18.5 The thoracic inlet. A: Anterior longitudinal ligament, B: Brachiocephalic artery, BV: brachiocephalic vein, Oe: Oesophagus, T1: First thoracic vertebra.

2.7 Describe the course of the subclavian arteries.

The subclavian arteries are asymmetrically paired vessels. The right subclavian artery arises from the brachiocephalic trunk, also known as the brachiocephalic (or innominate) artery, whereas the left subclavian artery originates directly from the aortic arch. Each is divided into three parts for the purpose of description. The first (prescalene) part extends from the origin to the medial border of the anterior scalene muscle, the second (scalene) part is behind the anterior scalene muscle (and in front of the middle scalene muscle). The third (postscalene) part begins at the lateral border of the anterior scalene muscle and ends by becoming the axillary artery at the lateral border of the first rib. The second and third parts of the subclavian arteries are both intimately related to the pleura as they pass over its cervical part, which covers the apex of the lung.

2.8 Describe the anatomy of the subclavian veins.

The subclavian veins are paired, large central veins that pass through the inferior part of the cervical region. They return blood from the upper limbs to the central circulation. At the outer border of the first rib, each axillary vein becomes the subclavian vein. The subclavian vein crosses the groove on the upper surface of the first rib (Fig 18.4), initially arching cranially before curving caudally to join the internal jugular vein forming the brachiocephalic vein posterior to the sternoclavicular joint. The thoracic duct drains into the left subclavian vein close to its junction with the left internal jugular vein.

2.9 What is the ideal location for the tip of a central venous catheter?

Opinion is divided about the ideal target location for the tip of a central venous catheter. It is a widely held view that the mid superior vena cava (SVC) above the junction between the SVC and the right atrium is the ideal location. It is believed that keeping the catheter tip proximal to the pericardial reflection around the lower SVC reduces the risk of cardiac perforation and subsequent cardiac tamponade. The mid-SVC is at the level of the carina anatomically. Others are of the opinion that it is more important that the catheter tip is free-floating and not in contact with a vessel wall than it being above the pericardial reflection.

References

Agur, A.M.R. and Dalley1s, A.F. *Moore's Essential Clinical Anatomy*. Wolters Kluwer, 2019.

Craven, J. The thoracic inlet and first rib. *Anaesthesia & Intensive Care Medicine*, 2007;8:497–498.

Sammy, I.A. et al. Are first rib fractures a marker for other life-threatening injuries in patients with major trauma? A cohort study of patients on the UK Trauma Audit and Research Network database. *Emerg Med J*, 2017;34:205–211.

Standring, S. *Gray's Anatomy: The Anatomical Basis of Clinical Practice*, 41st edition. Elsevier, 2015.

Tempe, D.K. and Hasija, S. Quest to determine the ideal position of the central venous catheter tip. *Br J Anaesth*, 2017;118:148–150.

Answers to SOE 3

3.1 Outline the anatomy of the diaphragm.

The diaphragm is a musculotendinous septum that separates the thoracic cavity from the abdominal cavity. It consists of a peripheral muscular part with a complex origin, inserting into a central (trefoil shaped) tendon (Fig 18.6). The superior surface of the central tendon is fused with the fibrous pericardium and flanked on either side of the pericardium by a muscular dome. The right dome

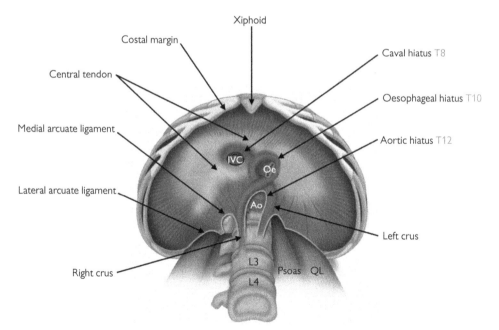

Fig 18.6 The diaphragm. The vertebral level of the major diaphragmatic apertures is indicated. Muscle fibres from the right crus (and in some individuals from the left crus) of the diaphragm form a sling around the oesophageal hiatus which may contribute to the integrity of the gastro-oesophageal junction. IVC: inferior vena cava, Oe: oesophagus, Ao: aorta, QL: quadratus lumborum.

Modified from Smith C.D. (2021) Diaphragm. In: Skandalakis LJ (Eds) *Surgical Anatomy and Technique*. Springer, Cham. https://doi.org/10.1007/978-3-030-51313-9_5 Used with permission from Springer.

of the diaphragm is higher than the left. This asymmetry is attributed to the presence of the liver on the right side. Key anatomical structures pass between the thorax and abdomen via several diaphragmatic apertures.

3.2 Describe the muscular attachments of the diaphragm.

The peripheral muscular part originates from multiple attachments (sternal, costal, and vertebral) around the circumference of the thoracic outlet:

1. The sternal part arises from the posterior surface of the xiphoid process.
2. The costal part arises from the inferior surface of the lower six costal cartilages and their associated ribs.
3. The vertebral (lumbar) part arises from the lumbar vertebrae (as the left and right crura) and the arcuate ligaments. The crura of the diaphragm are elongated tendinous structures arising from the bodies of the upper three (right) and first two (left) lumbar vertebrae, respectively. There is some variation in the precise level of the vertebral attachments, but the right crus is longer and larger than the left. The two crura are connected by the fibrous median arcuate ligament.

The medial and lateral arcuate ligaments are formed by a thickening of the fascia overlying the psoas and quadratus lumborum muscles, respectively (Fig 18.6).

3.3 What are the main openings in the diaphragm?

There are three major openings (apertures or foramina) in the diaphragm named according to the major structure transmitted through the opening.

1. The caval hiatus is an opening in the tendinous part of the right hemidiaphragm which transmits the inferior vena cava and the right phrenic nerve. It is at the level of the 8th thoracic vertebra.
2. The oesophageal hiatus is an opening in the right crus but to the left of the midline at the level of the 10th thoracic vertebra. The gastric vessels and gastric branches of the vagus nerve pass through, along with the oesophagus.
3. The aortic hiatus is found between the diaphragmatic crura anterior to the 12th thoracic vertebra. In addition to the aorta, the thoracic duct and azygous vein pass through this hiatus.

3.4 What is the innervation of the diaphragm?

Each half of the diaphragm is innervated by a phrenic nerve. The left and right phrenic nerves arise from spinal roots C3–C5 with the predominant contribution from C4. They are mixed motor and sensory nerves but are the sole motor supply to the diaphragm. In addition to pain and proprioception for most of the diaphragm, the phrenic nerves convey sensory information from the fibrous pericardium, mediastinal pleura, and the diaphragmatic peritoneum. These fibres are important in referred pain. The peripheral diaphragm receives sensory innervation from the intercostal (T6 or T7 to T11) and subcostal nerves (T12).

3.5 What is a diaphragmatic hernia?

Any defect in the integrity of the diaphragm may result in protrusion or herniation of abdominal contents into the thoracic cavity.

3.6 Briefly outline the different types of diaphragmatic herniae.

Diaphragmatic herniae may be either congenital or acquired.

Congenital herniae include posterolateral (Bochdalek) hernias, anterior (Morgagni) hernias, and central hernias. In rare cases, the diaphragm may be entirely absent. Bochdalek hernias are the commonest congenital hernias and are most frequently found on the left side.

The commonest acquired diaphragmatic hernia is a hiatus hernia, where there is herniation of abdominal contents into the thorax via the oesophageal opening of the diaphragm. Other causes include secondary trauma (blunt or penetrating), and iatrogenic diaphragmatic herniae.

References

Agur, A.M.R and Dalley, A.F. *Moore's Essential Clinical Anatomy*. Wolters Kluwer, 2019.

Chandrasekharan, P.K. et al. Congenital diaphragmatic hernia a review. *Maternal Health, Neonatology, and Perinatology*. 2017;3:6.

Ellis, H. and Lawson, A. *Anatomy for Anaesthetists*, 9th edition. Wiley Blackwell, 2013.

Standring, S. *Gray's Anatomy: The Anatomical Basis of Clinical Practice*, 41st edition. Elsevier, 2015.

Answers to SOE 4

4.1 Describe the general structure of the abdominal wall.

The abdomen is the part of the trunk between the thorax and pelvis. It is enclosed by the abdominal wall, a continuous cylindrical myofascial structure. For the purposes of description, the abdominal wall is divided into anterior and posterior walls linked by right and left lateral walls. The lateral abdominal wall extends forwards from the posterior axillary line. The junction between the anterior and lateral walls is indistinct, so the term anterolateral abdominal wall is used.

4.2 What muscles are found in the anterolateral abdominal wall?

Five bilaterally paired muscles are found in the anterolateral abdominal wall (Table 18.1). Laterally three flat muscle layers are found. From superficial to deep these are the external oblique, internal

Table 18.1 The origin and insertion of the muscles of the anterolateral abdominal wall. The muscle fibres of the external oblique descend in an inferomedial direction. The upper fibres of the internal oblique ascend in a superomedial orientation perpendicular to the fibres of the external oblique, while the lower fibres run parallel to those of the overlying external oblique. As the name suggests the fibres of the transversus abdominis run horizontally (except for the lowermost fibres)

Muscle	Origin	Insertion
External oblique	External surface of 5th to 12th rib	Anterior iliac crest Linea alba Pubic tubercle
Internal oblique	Anterior two-thirds of iliac crest anteriorly Thoracolumbar fascia posteriorly	Inferior border 10th to 12th ribs Linea alba Pubic crest and pubis as the conjoint tendon
Transversus abdominis	Internal surface 7th to 12th costal cartilages Thoracolumbar fascia Iliac crest Connective tissue deep to inguinal ligament	Rectus abdominis aponeurosis and ultimately the linea alba Forms the conjoint tendon with the lower part of the aponeurosis of the common aponeurosis of the internal oblique
Rectus abdominis	Pubic symphysis Pubic crest	Xiphoid 5th to 7th costal cartilages
Pyramidalis	Pubic crest	Linea alba

oblique, and transversus abdominis muscles. Anteriorly, on either side of the midline run two pairs of vertically orientated muscles: rectus abdominis and pyramidalis. An understanding of the anatomy of these muscles and their related fascia is essential for abdominal fascial plane blocks used in regional anaesthesia.

Rectus abdominis is a broad elongated muscle in the anterior abdominal wall extending from the pubic symphysis and pubic crest to the xiphoid process and fifth to seventh costal cartilages (Fig 18.7). It is mostly invested in a fascial sheath (the rectus sheath) formed in the midclavicular line from the aponeuroses of the external oblique, internal oblique, and transversus abdominis. The inferior termination of the rectus sheath is defined by the arcuate line which is found approximately at the midpoint between the umbilicus and the pubic crest. Each rectus abdominis has three or more tendinous intersections on its anterior aspect which reflect the segmental embryological origin of the muscle. They characteristically subdivide the rectus abdominis into several muscle bellies. Typically, these tendinous intersections occur at the level of the xiphoid, the umbilicus, and halfway between these two. In some individuals, a fourth intersection occurs inferior to the umbilicus. The absence of tendinous intersections posteriorly allows unimpeded spread of local anaesthetic injected into the posterior part of the rectus abdominis sheath. The left and right rectus abdominis muscles are separated by the linea alba, a tendinous raphe formed in the midline by fusion of the aponeuroses of the rectus sheath, extending from the xiphoid process above to the symphysis pubis below. The lateral border of each rectus abdominis is delineated by a further tendinous intersection, the linea semilunaris.

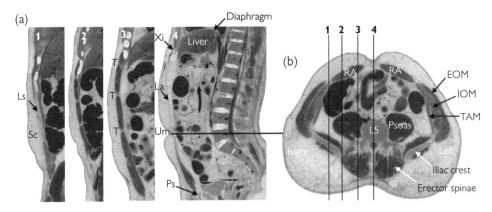

Fig 18.7 (a) Serial sagittal sections through the abdomen show the anterior abdominal wall. (b) Transverse section through the lower abdomen at the level of the fifth lumbar vertebra (L5). Planes 1-4 show the corresponding level of the sagittal sections. 1. Linea semilunaris (Ls), 2. Lateral rectus abdominis, 3. Medial rectus abdominis, 4. Median sagittal plane through linea alba (La), Rectus abdominis (RA) originates from the pubic symphysis (Ps) and pubic crest and inserts into the xiphoid (Xi). Tendinous intersections (T) are seen at the level of the xiphoid, umbilicus (Um) and approximately at the midpoint between these two levels. Sc, subcutaneous fat; EOM, external oblique muscle; IOM, internal oblique; TAM, transversus abdominis muscle. The diaphragm and its crura arising from the lumbar vertebrae are also shown in Fig 18.6. Pyramidalis is absent in this specimen.

Absent in approximately 20% of individuals, pyramidalis is a small triangular muscle that originates from the pubic crest and inserts into the linea alba. When present it is found in the rectus sheath anterior to the inferior portion of the rectus abdominis.

4.3 Name the muscles of the posterior abdominal wall.

The muscles of the posterior abdominal wall are iliacus, psoas (major and minor), quadratus lumborum, and the posterior part of the diaphragm.

4.4 Outline the nerve supply to the anterolateral abdominal wall.

The anterolateral abdominal wall receives innervation from the thoracoabdominal, subcostal, iliohypogastric, and ilioinguinal nerves (Table 18.2). The thoracoabdominal nerves arise from the anterior rami of spinal nerves T6–T12. They are the anterior continuation of the intercostal nerves. They enter the abdominal wall in the fascial plane between the internal oblique and transversus abdominis muscles (the transversus abdominis plane). The seventh and eighth thoracoabdominal nerves pass behind the rectus abdominis, then pass through it to provide cutaneous innervation to the upper abdominal skin. Nerves nine through eleven enter the rectus abdominis sheath at its lateral margin, again piercing the muscle to innervate the abdominal skin. Each thoracoabdominal nerve gives off a lateral cutaneous branch in the midaxillary line.

Table 18.2 Innervation of the anterolateral abdominal wall muscles. Except for the pyramidalis, all these muscles receive innervation from the thoracoabdominal nerves (the anterior rami of spinal nerves T7–T11) and the subcostal nerve (T12). The rectus abdominis receives a contribution from T6, while the transversus abdominis also receives a contribution from the first lumbar (ilioinguinal) nerve. When present pyramidalis is innervated from the subcostal nerve. EOM: external oblique muscle, IOM: internal oblique muscle, TAM: transversus abdominis muscle, RAM, rectus abdominis muscle.

Nerve and level of origin			Anterolateral abdominal muscles				
T6							
T7							
T8		Thoracoabdominal nerves					
T9							
T10			EOM	IOM		RAM	
T11					TAM		
T11							
T12	Subcostal nerve	Iliohypogastric					Pyramidalis
L1			Ilioinguinal				

The iliohypogastric and ilioinguinal nerves arise from the anterior rami of spinal nerve L1 with the iliohypogastric receiving a variable contribution from T12 (Fig 18.8). There is significant variability in the course of these nerves. Both ultimately enter the transversus abdominis plane passing through it for a variable distance before traversing the internal and external oblique muscles to provide cutaneous innervation of suprapubic skin (iliohypogastric) and the skin of the scrotum or labia majora and adjacent thigh (ilioinguinal).

4.5 What is the thoracolumbar fascia?

The thoracolumbar fascia is a complex arrangement of aponeuroses and fascial planes that separates the paraspinal muscles from the muscles of the posterior abdominal wall. It has an important functional role in contributing to the mechanical stability of the lumbosacral spine, and is an important landmark for fascial plane blocks.

4.6 Name the structures labelled A–H, and V–Y in the accompanying image of a transverse section through the abdomen at the level of the third lumbar vertebra:

A: Linea alba

B: Rectus abdominis muscle

C: Linea semilunaris

D: Transversus abdominis muscle

E: Internal oblique muscle

F: External oblique muscle

G: Subcutaneous fat

H: Transversus abdominis plane (TAP)

V: Quadratus lumborum muscle

W: Psoas major muscle

X: Erector spinae muscle (iliocostalis and longissimus)

Y: Multifidus muscle

References

Agur, A.M.R. and Dalley, A.F. *Moore's Essential Clinical Anatomy*. Wolters Kluwer, 2019.

Chin, K.J. et al. Essentials of our current understanding: abdominal wall blocks. *Reg Anesth Pain Med*, 2017;42:133–183.

Standring, S. *Gray's Anatomy: The Anatomical Basis of Clinical Practice*, 41st edition. Elsevier, 2015.

Willard, F.H. et al. The thoracolumbar fascia: anatomy, function and clinical considerations. *Journal of Anatomy*, 2012;221(6):507–536.

Answers to SOE 5

5.1 Tell me about the anatomy of the lumbar plexus.

The lumbar plexus is a bilateral neural network originating from the ventral rami of spinal nerves T12–L5. It forms within the psoas major muscle anterior to the transverse processes of the lumbar vertebrae. It supplies motor innervation to the lower limb and sensory innervation to the lower anterior abdominal wall, anteromedial thigh, and part of the external genitalia. The main branches of the lumbar plexus are shown in Fig 18.8.

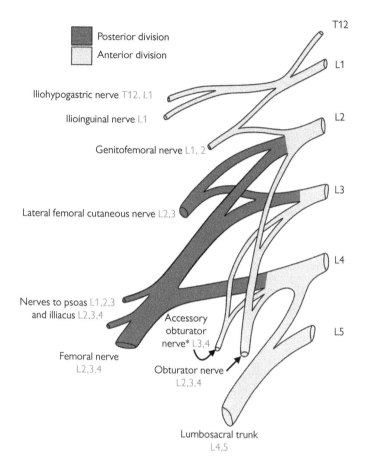

Posterior division
Anterior division

Iliohypogastric nerve T12, L1

Ilioinguinal nerve L1

Genitofemoral nerve L1, 2

Lateral femoral cutaneous nerve L2,3

Nerves to psoas L1,2,3
and illiacus L2,3,4

Accessory
obturator
nerve* L3,4

Femoral nerve
L2,3,4

Obturator nerve
L2,3,4

Lumbosacral trunk
L4,5

T12
L1
L2
L3
L4
L5

Fig 18.8 The lumbar plexus showing the typical arrangement of nerves. *The accessory obturator nerve is present in approximately 30% of individuals.

Adapted from Standring S (2020) 'Gray's Anatomy' 42 Ed, with permission from Elsevier.

5.2 Describe the anatomy of the femoral nerve.

The femoral nerve is the largest branch of the lumbar plexus. It is a mixed motor and sensory nerve. It arises from the posterior divisions of the anterior rami of spinal nerves L2, L3, and L4. It is the main nerve supplying the anterior compartment of the thigh. Once formed within the lumbar plexus the femoral nerve courses inferiorly through the psoas muscle, emerging from its lateral border deep (posterior) to the fascia iliaca. It descends in the groove between the psoas and iliacus. It then passes under the inguinal ligament to enter the femoral triangle where it divides into anterior and posterior divisions, which in turn give rise to the terminal muscular and cutaneous branches.

5.3 What structures are innervated by the femoral nerve?

Immediately proximal to the inguinal ligament the femoral nerve supplies a motor branch to pectineus. The anterior (superficial) division of the femoral nerve supplies motor innervation to sartorius and gives off two sensory nerves, the medial and intermediate cutaneous nerves of the thigh. The posterior division of the femoral nerve supplies motor innervation to the quadriceps (rectus femoris, vastus lateralis, vastus intermedius, and vastus medialis). The saphenous nerve is the only sensory branch of the posterior division of the femoral nerve. It conveys sensation from the medial side of the knee, leg (calf), and medial side of the ankle and foot as far as the first metatarsophalangeal joint.

5.4 What are the borders and contents of the femoral triangle?

The femoral triangle is a subfascial space in the anterosuperior thigh. It is bounded by the inguinal ligament superiorly, the medial border of sartorius laterally, and the medial border of adductor longus medially. Sartorius crosses adductor longus at the apex of the triangle. From lateral to medial, the floor of the femoral triangle consists of iliopsoas and pectineus. The roof of the femoral triangle consists of the fascia lata, the cribriform fascia, subcutaneous fat, and skin.

The contents of the femoral triangle from lateral to medial are the femoral nerve, the femoral artery, the femoral vein, the deep inguinal lymph nodes and associated lymphatic vessels.

5.5 What is the femoral sheath?

The femoral sheath is a conical shaped fascial tube, which invests the proximal part of the femoral vessels thereby creating the femoral canal, a further small fascial compartment between the medial wall of the femoral sheath and the femoral vein (Fig 18.9). The femoral sheath is continuous superiorly with the abdominal fascia, and generally terminates 3–4 cm distal to the inguinal ligament by merging with loose connective tissue. The femoral nerve does not lie within the femoral sheath.

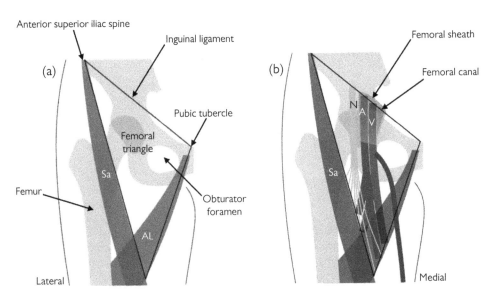

Fig 18.9 (a) The boundaries of the femoral triangle. (b) Diagrammatic representation of the femoral nerve N), femoral artery (A) and femoral vein (V) within the femoral triangle. The femoral sheath invests the proximal part of the femoral vessels. The femoral canal lies medial to the femoral vein within the femoral sheath, its superior opening is the femoral ring. AL: adductor longus, Sa: Sartorius.

Modified from original courtesy of Assoc Prof Craig Hacking, Radiopaedia.org, rID: 70536.

It lies deep to the fascia iliaca, whereas the femoral sheath is located superficial to the fascia iliaca (but deep to the fascia lata).

5.6 What is the adductor canal?

The adductor canal is an aponeurotic tunnel in the middle-third of the thigh extending from the apex of the femoral triangle to the adductor hiatus (an opening in the adductor magnus muscle). It lies between the anterior and medial compartments of the thigh, providing a conduit for the passage of the femoral artery, femoral vein, and two important branches of the femoral nerve: the nerve to vastus medialis and the saphenous nerve (which is the terminal branch of the femoral nerve).

5.7 Outline the course of the obturator nerve.

The obturator nerve arises from the lumbar plexus receiving fibres from the anterior divisions of the anterior rami of spinal nerves L2, L3, and L4. It descends through the psoas muscle to emerge from its medial border. The nerve runs posterior to the common iliac artery then lateral to the internal iliac artery and distal ureter to exit the pelvis through the obturator foramen via the obturator canal. After entering the thigh, it divides into anterior and posterior branches. It conveys motor fibres to obturator externus (but not obturator internus), adductor longus, adductor brevis, adductor magnus, and gracilis. The anterior obturator nerve carries sensory fibres from the medial thigh. The precise area of cutaneous sensation served by the obturator nerve in the thigh is not well understood.

5.8 What is the lumbosacral trunk?

The lumbosacral trunk is the most inferior component of the lumbar plexus. It carries some fibres from the ventral ramus of spinal nerve L4 and all the fibres from the ventral ramus of L5. Emerging from the medial border of psoas it descends in the pelvis to unite with the first sacral nerve to form the lumbosacral plexus.

References

Agur, A.M.R. and Dalley, A.F. *Moore's Essential Clinical Anatomy*. Wolters Kluwer, 2019.

Lumley, J.S.P., et al. (eds.). *Bailey & Love's Essential Clinical Anatomy*. CRC Press, 2019.

Standring, S. *Gray's Anatomy: The Anatomical Basis of Clinical Practice*, 41st edition. Elsevier, 2015.

Acknowledgements

Thank you to Isla K. Bresland for the original artwork in Figs. 18.2, 18.4 and 18.5 and Laura J. Weinkle MS, for providing VH dissector images used in the preparation of Figures 18.1 and 18.7.

CLINICAL MEASUREMENT

QUESTIONS

SOE 1 Pulse oximetry

1.1 How does the pulse oximeter work?

1.2 Which two particular wavelengths are used and why?

1.3 What do you understand by 'isobestic point' and why is it useful?

1.4 Draw a graph representing the different light absorption for deoxygenated and oxygenated haemoglobins.

1.5 What is the Beer–Lambert law and what is the importance of it for pulse oximetry?

1.6 What are potential sources of error, limitations of the technique, and problems in interpreting the results?

1.7 Can you put carboxyhaemoblobin (COHb) and methaemoglobin (MetHb) light absorption on a graph to demonstrate their absorption characteristics?

SOE 2 Arterial blood pressure measurement

2.1 What are the methods available for measuring arterial blood pressure?

2.2 Tell me about the different non-invasive methods first.

2.3 What are the key components of non-automatic intermittent non-invasive methods (NIMs)?

2.4 What methods are used to determine flow at systolic and diastolic pressures using NIMs?

2.5 What is the automatic, intermittent non-invasive blood pressure measurement method?

2.6 Tell me about currently available continuous non-invasive blood pressure measurement methods.

2.7 What are the components of an invasive arterial blood pressure measurement system?

2.8 What is the function of a transducer, and how does it work in the system?

2.9 What are the sources of error associated with arterial blood pressure measurement?

2.10 How is resonance important for causing errors in blood pressure measurement?

2.11 Tell me how damping affects the accuracy of blood pressure measurement.

SOE 3 Gas concentration measurement

3.1 What methods are available to measure gas concentration in a mixture of gases?

3.2 Explain to me the principle behind the paramagnetic analyser

3.3 What is the theoretical principle of infrared capnometry?

3.4 How does the infrared analyser measure the concentration of carbon dioxide?

3.5 What do you understand by the Beer–Lambert law?

3.6 Please draw and label a typical capnography trace seen in a spontaneously breathing patient.

3.7 Could you draw a capnography trace representing low cardiac output, oesophageal intubation, and malignant hyperpyrexia?

3.8 What types of capnograph do you know about and what are their advantages and disadvantages?

SOE 4 Computed tomography and magnetic resonance imaging

4.1 What is the principle behind computed tomography (CT)?

4.2 What are the components of the CT scanner?

4.3 What do you understand by the term computed axial tomography (CAT)?

4.4 How is it different from helical scanning?

4.5 How can CT imaging be enhanced?

4.6 What is the mechanism through which enhancement of the CT image occurs?

4.7 Explain how the magnetic resonance imaging (MRI) scanner generates a signal

4.8 What are the components of an MRI scanner?

4.9 What are the problems associated with providing anaesthesia for MRI investigations?

SOE 5 Neuromuscular blockade monitoring

5.1 What methods are available for monitoring muscle relaxation perioperatively?

5.2 What are the main patterns of nerve stimulation used clinically?

5.3 What are the indications for using the single twitch method?

5.4 Describe the characteristics of a train-of-four stimulation.

5.5 What do you understand by the train-of-four ratio?

5.6 What is the main clinical application of the train-of-four ratio?

5.7 How is double burst stimulation different from train-of-four stimulation?

5.8 What is tetanic stimulation?

5.9 What do you understand by post-tetanic count?

Answer to SOE 1

1.1 How does the pulse oximeter work?

A typical pulse oximeter consists of two parts: a peripheral probe and a processer/display unit. The probe contains two light-emitting diodes (LED) that trans-illuminate chosen tissues with monochromatic light at red (660 nm) and infrared (940 nm) wavelengths every 5–10 milliseconds from one side of the probe. A photodiode (PD) detects the transmitted light and converts it to an electrical signal. The functional haemoglobin saturation (SpO_2) is then calculated from the signal by the processing unit and displayed. One LED emits red and the other infrared light, but the PD is unable to differentiate between wavelengths. To overcome this problem only one LED trans-illuminates at a time, the LEDs switching on and off alternately. The pulses in the PD signal are then identified in time to give separate values for red and infrared absorbances.

1.2 Which two particular wavelengths are chosen and why?

Oxygenated haemoglobin or oxyhaemoglobin (HbO_2) and deoxygenated haemoglobin or deoxyhaemoglobin (Hb) have differential absorption spectra. Deoxyhaemoglobin absorbs light maximally in the red band of the spectrum (600–750 nm), while oxyhaemoglobin absorbs maximally in the infrared band (850–1000 nm). Absorbance at these two wavelengths is used to estimate arterial saturation (SaO_2), which is derived from the ratio of oxyhaemoglobin to the sum of oxyhaemoglobin plus deoxyhaemoglobin: $SaO_2 = OxyHb/(OxyHb + DeoxyHb)$. An accurate SaO_2 is measured directly by another device (co-oximeter) whereas the pulse oximeter is less accurate as it does not take into account the presence of other types of Hb (e.g., MetHb and COHb). In normal circumstances, SaO_2 correlates well with the value provided by the pulse oximeter which we refer to as SpO_2.

1.3 What do you understand by 'isobestic point' and why is it useful?

The isobestic point is the point (at 800 nm) where the absorption coefficients of oxygenated and deoxygenated haemoglobins are identical. The isobestic point may be used as a reference point where light absorption is independent of the degree of saturation.

1.4 Draw a graph representing the different light absorption for deoxyhemoglobin and oxyhemoglobin.

The candidate should draw two lines that cross at a wavelength of around 800 nm and label the axes as shown on the graph (see Fig 19.1).

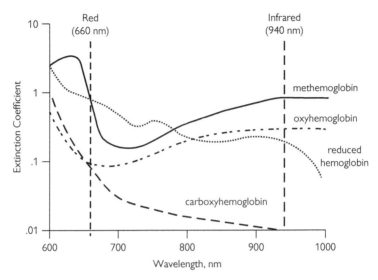

Fig 19.1 Light absorption curves of haemoglobin derivatives.

Reproduced from Jubran A (2015) 'Pulse Oximetry' Critical Care 19: 272, under the CC BY 4.0 license.

1.5 What is the Beer-Lambert law and what is the importance of it for pulse oximetry?

This is a combination of two laws describing the absorption of monochromatic light by a transparent substance through which it passes. **Beer's law:** the intensity of transmitted light decreases exponentially as the concentration of the substance increases. **Lambert's law:** the intensity of transmitted light decreases exponentially as the distance travelled through the substance increases.

As we are interested in whether oxygen is attached to haemoglobin or not, the relevant solutes are oxyhaemoglobin and deoxyhaemoglobin. The pulse oximeter performs mathematical calculations based on the Beer–Lambert law to determine the percentage of blood that is saturated with oxygen.

1.6 What are potential sources of error, limitations of the technique, and problems in interpreting the results?

1. The pulse oximeter is calibrated using volunteers, so calibration does not cover dangerously low hypoxic values. Hence the readings are less accurate at SpO_2 values below 70%.
2. Interference from ambient light. This can occur if the light is bright and direct, but the pulsed nature of the emissions is intended to allow detection of and compensation for any ambient light.
3. Loss of the pulsatile component. This occurs in conditions of hypoperfusion, hypothermia, peripheral vasoconstriction when there is a narrow pulse pressure, dysrhythmias that distort the points of maximum and minimum absorption, and venous congestion. These are all common reasons for a poor signal.

4. Movement artefact or electrical interference (neither are major problems).
5. Infrared absorption by other substances: such as dark nail varnish or nicotine staining.
6. More significant errors are associated with absorption by abnormal Hb and other substances:
    a. Carboxyhaemoglobin (COHb): This is seen in heavy smokers or in carbon monoxide poisoning. COHb has a similar absorption coefficient to HbO_2 and will give an abnormally high SpO_2 reading of about 96%.
    b. Methaemoglobin (MetHb): MetHb has identical absorption at both wavelengths and gives a saturation reading of around 84%.
    c. Dyes such as methylene blue or indocyanine green give falsely low readings.

7. Problems in interpretation.
    a. Pulse oximetry does not detect respiratory failure. A high FiO_2 may mask ventilatory failure by ensuring high SpO_2 readings despite a rising carbon dioxide (CO_2).
    b. In very anaemic patients, SpO_2 readings may show high saturations although oxygen delivery to the tissues may be impaired.

1.7 Can you put COHb and MetHb light absorption on a graph to demonstrate their absorption characteristics?

The candidate should add the curve for COHb clearly demonstrating the same absorption as OxyHb at the red-light spectrum. Then they should draw the curve for MetHb demonstrating that it absorbs both red and infrared light to the same degree as demonstrated in Figure 19.1.

References

Ebrahim, H. and Ashton-Cleary, H. *Maths, Physics and Clinical Measurement for Anaesthesia and Intensive Care.* Cambridge University Press, 2019: pp. 97–104.

Moyle, H.T. 'Uses and abuses of pulse oximetry. *Arch Dis Child*, 1996;74(1):77–80.

Answer to SOE 2

2.1 What are the methods available to measure arterial blood pressure?

All methods can be divided into invasive (direct) and non-invasive (indirect) methods, and the latter can be also subdivided into continuous and intermittent.

2.2 Tell me about the different non-invasive methods first?

These methods can be subdivided into three categories:
1. Non-automatic intermittent non-invasive methods (NIM)
2. Automatic intermittent NIM
3. Continuous NIM

2.3 What are the key components of non-automatic intermittent non-invasive methods (NIMs)?

There are three key components:
1. A cuff placed around a limb to occlude arterial flow. The width of the cuff should be 40% of the circumference of the part of the limb being used (or cover two-thirds of its length).

2. A method for measuring pressure within the cuff, e.g., a liquid manometer, an aneroid gauge, or an electronic pressure gauge.

3. A method to determine blood flow at systolic and diastolic pressures.

2.4 What methods are used to determine flow at systolic and diastolic pressures using NIMs?

1. **Palpation.** This method is easy to perform but may underestimate systolic pressure by 25%, and cannot measure diastolic or mean pressures.

2. **Doppler** can demonstrate flow at specific cuff pressures, and due to its sensitivity can measure flow at low pressures.

3. **Auscultation** using a stethoscope over the brachial artery to assess the pressures at which Korotkoff sounds are heard. Five Korotkoff sounds have been described. The first represents systolic pressure and the fifth tone when sounds disappear represents diastolic pressure.

4. **Oscillotonometry.** The Von Recklinghausen Oscillotonometer uses two overlapping cuffs, an occlusion and a sensing cuff. Systolic pressure is measured by deflating the occlusive cuff and measuring the pressure at the first vigorous needle oscillations. The mean pressure is measured from the pressure in the sensing cuff, while the occlusive cuff is deflated again, at maximum needle oscillation. Diastolic pressure is measured at the point where oscillations reduce. With this method, it is the systolic and the mean arterial pressure (MAP) that are most accurately estimated.

2.5 What is the automatic, intermittent non-invasive blood pressure measurement method?

DINAMAP (Device for Indirect Non-invasive Automatic MAP). This device is essentially an automated oscillotonometer. The modern DINAMAP uses one cuff for both sensing and occlusion functions. An electronic transducer detects the pulse pressure wave and cuff pressure simultaneously and is accurate to ± 2%. The microprocessor controls the inflation and deflation of the cuff. The cuff is automatically inflated 20–30 mmHg above the previous systolic pressure reading.

2.6 Tell me about currently available continuous non-invasive blood pressure measurement methods.

The two available methods are the Finapres and Radial Artery Compression method.

The Finapres utilizes the Penaz principle (volume-clamp method) which is very similar to how a pulse oximeter works. It measures finger arterial pressure and consists of a finger cuff with an inflatable bladder and an infrared photoplethysmograph that measures the absorption of infrared light to determine the volume of blood under the finger cuff. The cuff inflates and deflates periodically to keep the volume of blood in the finger the same irrespectively of the cardiac cycle phase. The blood pressure is then determined by the amount of pressure that the machine needs to apply in order to keep the plethysmograph as a flat trace. The accuracy of this method is not very good hence its use is not widespread.

The Radial Artery Compression method involves the application of a band that contains a cuff and a pressure sensor over the radial artery at the wrist level. The cuff is inflated to achieve maximal oscillations and then an algorithm derives systolic, diastolic, and MAP. Accuracy is very dependent on the correct position of the sensor over the artery.

2.7 What are the components of an invasive arterial blood pressure measurement system?

1. **Intra-arterial cannula**. 20–22-gauge cannula with parallel walls made of a special material (TeflonTM). This material reduces the risk of thrombus formation. The parallel sides ensure accurate pressure-wave transmission.
2. **Connection tubing**. The connection tubing between the transducer and the cannula in the patient is specifically designed to be relatively non-compliant to minimize damping and is different from conventional intravenous fluid tubing. Three-way taps can be added to allow for blood sampling and zeroing.
3. **Flush solution**. Normally 500 ml of 0.9% saline, pressurized to 300 mmHg.
4. **Transducer** that requires calibration and zeroing.
5. **Microprocessor, amplifier, and display**. The electrical signal from the transducer is amplified and analyzed. It is displayed on the monitor as a wave with accompanying numerical values of the blood pressure.

2.8 What is the function of a transducer, and how does it work in the system?

A transducer converts one form of energy into another. The arterial transducer converts mechanical energy into an electrical signal using a strain gauge. The strain gauge connects a diaphragm, which is in contact with the column of fluid, to a resistance wire. As the diaphragm moves in response to pressure changes, the length of the wire, and therefore its diameter and resistance changes proportionally, resulting in an electrical signal change.

2.9 What are the sources of error associated with invasive arterial blood pressure measurement?

There are several sources of error:

1. **Wave form morphology.** The more distal the artery where the blood pressure is measured the higher the systolic blood pressure and the lower the diastolic pressure readings. The MAP is not affected significantly.
2. **Zeroing.** The transducer should be exposed to atmospheric pressure and the pressure reading calibrated to zero several times a day to exclude errors due to calibration drift within the system.
3. **Levelling.** The transducer should be placed at the level of the heart for accuracy of measurements. If the transducer is placed 10 cm below the level of the heart, the blood pressure reading will be 7.5 mmHg higher than the true pressure and a similar amount lower if the transducer is placed above the level of the heart.
4. **Resonance.**
5. **Damping.**

2.10 How is resonance important in causing errors in blood pressure measurement?

Resonance is a phenomenon in which a system (e.g., the arterial blood measurement system) is subjected to an external oscillating force that causes it to oscillate at a greater amplitude. The frequency that causes the highest oscillation is termed the 'resonant frequency'. The natural frequency is the frequency at which a system oscillates freely once set in motion.

In clinical practice, resonance occurs when the frequency of the arterial waveform approaches the natural/resonant frequency of the invasive blood pressure monitoring system. If this happens, an increase in the amplitude of the waveform oscillation occurs, causing over-reading of systolic and under-reading of the diastolic blood pressure.

To maximize the natural frequency of the arterial blood pressure system, short, wide and stiff (non-compliant) cannula and tubing are used.

2.11 Tell me how damping affects the accuracy of blood pressure measurement

Damping is a decrease in the amplitude of an oscillation due to different factors within the system. Some damping is desirable for accurate measurement but too much damping is a problem. In any system, the damping coefficient (DC) could be between 0 (no damping) and 1 (critical damping). Zero damping is a theoretical situation when the system oscillates in response to an external stimulus (a step change seen with a system flush), and the amplitude of oscillations never changes. An under-damped system (DC 0-0.3) is unable to prevent oscillations in response to step change. In an over-damped system (DC > 1) the response is overly blunted and leads to inaccuracy. The causes of damping in the invasive blood pressure system include three-way taps, air bubbles, clots, excessively long tubing, and kinking of tubing/cannula. Overdamping causes underestimation of systolic and overestimation of the diastolic blood pressure. An optimally damped system has a DC of 0.64 with a rapid response time to a step change and minimal overshoot. See Figure 19.2.

References

Cross, M. and Plunket, E. *Physics, Pharmacology and Physiology for Anaesthetists*. Cambridge University Press, 2008: pp. 50–53.

Ebrahim, H. and Ashton-Cleary, H. *Maths, Physics and Clinical Measurement for Anaesthesia and Intensive Care*. Cambridge University Press, 2019: pp.159–173.

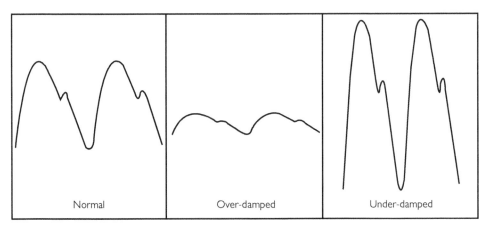

Fig 19.2 The effects of damping on the arterial waveform.

Answer to SOE 3

3.1 What methods are available for measuring gas concentration in a mixture of gases?

In routine anaesthetic practice, oxygen can be measured using a fuel cell or paramagnetic analyser, while carbon dioxide and anaesthetic agents require the use of an infrared analyser. Other methods used in industry or research include Raman gas analyzers, mass spectrometry, refractometry, ultraviolet absorption, piezoelectric absorption, and gas chromatography.

3.2 Tell me about the principle behind the paramagnetic analyser.

Gases that are attracted to a magnetic field are called paramagnetic as opposed to diamagnetic ones that are repulsed. Oxygen contains two unpaired electrons on separate atomic orbits that make it paramagnetic. The traditional paramagnetic analyser consists of a chamber with two spheres, filled with nitrogen, attached to each other in the form of a dumbbell. They are suspended on a filament allowing them to rotate. When gases enter the chamber, oxygen is attracted to the magnetic field making the dumbbells rotate. The degree of rotation corresponds to the concentration of oxygen in the sample.

3.3 What is the theoretical principle of infrared capnometry?

Any gas that contains two dissimilar atoms in its molecule can absorb infrared light at a specific wavelength. This is known as the Luft principle. Hence, an infrared gas analyser can measure the concentration of carbon dioxide, nitrous oxide, and all known anaesthetic agents.

3.4 How does the infrared analyser measure the concentration of carbon dioxide?

The infrared analyser contains several elements: *a hot wire* that emits infrared radiation, which is passed through a *filter* to obtain different frequencies for the measurement of different gases. After this, the infrared light enters the *sample chamber* via a special *sapphire window* that itself does not absorb the light. Expired gas enters the sample chamber via a different channel and CO_2 will absorb the infrared light. The higher the concentration of CO_2 the more absorption will occur. The degree of absorption is detected at the exit from the chamber by a *photodetector* and after processing, carbon dioxide concentration will be displayed on the monitor.

3.5 What do you understand by the Beer–Lambert law?

The Beer–Lambert law relates the degree of absorption with the concentration of gas (Beer) and the path length (Lambert) travelled by the infrared beam. Absorption (μ) = Path length × Concentration.

3.6 Please draw and label a typical capnography trace seen in a spontaneously breathing patient.

See Figure 19.3.

Phase I represents the inspiratory baseline, Phase II–IV are different stages of expiration: expiratory upstroke, expiratory plateau, end expiration, and expiratory downstroke. End expiration is the point where end-tidal concentration of CO_2 is measured and displayed on the monitor.

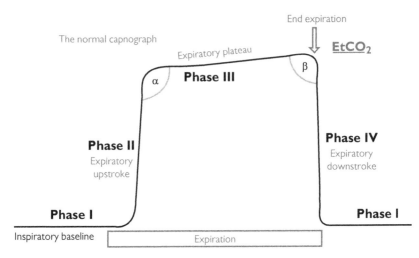

Fig 19.3 Normal capnography trace.

Reprinted from Manifold C et al (2013) 'Capnography for the nonintubated patient in the emergency setting' J Emerg Med 45(4):626–632, with permission from Elsevier.

3.7 Could you draw a capnography trace representing low cardiac output, oesophageal intubation, and malignant hyperpyrexia?

See Figure 19.4.

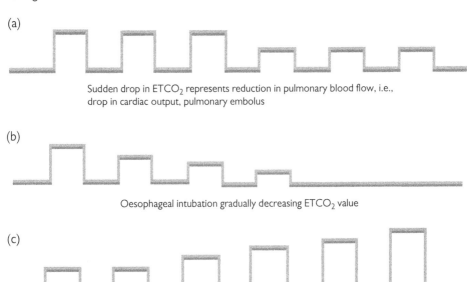

(a) Sudden drop in ETCO$_2$ represents reduction in pulmonary blood flow, i.e., drop in cardiac output, pulmonary embolus

(b) Oesophageal intubation gradually decreasing ETCO$_2$ value

(c) Typical ETCO$_2$ trace in hypoventilation or rarely malignant hyperpyrexia

Fig 19.4 Different capnography traces: (a) sudden drop in end-tidal CO$_2$; (b) oesophageal intubation; (c) steady rise in end-tidal CO$_2$.

Reprinted from Kerslake I and Kelly F (2017) 'Uses of capnography in the critical care unit' *BJA Education* 17(5):178–183 with permission from Oxford University Press.

3.8 What types of capnograph do you know about and what are their advantages and disadvantages?

Capnographs can be divided according to the method of gas sampling into *mainstream* and *sidestream* analyzers. Side stream analyzers take a sample from the main respiratory tubing closer to the patient end and require a flow of 50–100 ml/min. They are less bulky and can be used in non-intubated patients. Disadvantages include the need for a suction pump to draw the gas sample, possible blockage of the sampling line, the need for a water trap due to condensation as well as inaccuracies in neonates. Mainstream analyzers send the infrared signal from the measurement head that is mounted directly on the ventilation circuit and therefore does not require gas sampling avoiding all the problems listed above. Disadvantages include the facts that they are relatively expensive, bulky, and could be inaccurate if the sensor window is not kept clean.

References

Ebrahim, H. and Ashton-Cleary, H. *Maths, Physics and Clinical Measurement for Anaesthesia and Intensive Care*. Cambridge University Press, 2019: Chapter 6, pp. 86–96.

Kerslake, I. and Kelly, F. Uses of capnography in the critical care unit. *BJA Education*, 2017;17(5):178–183.

Answer to SOE 4

4.1 What is the principle behind computed tomography (CT)?

CT uses X-ray energy directed through the patient to an ionization chamber, acting as the detector on the opposite side of the apparatus. However, unlike in conventional X-rays that use a fixed X-ray tube, the whole CT emitter-detector unit rotates around the circular opening of a donut-shaped structure called a gantry, making multiple exposures of the patient's body to generate cross-sectional images (slices).

4.2 What are the components of the CT scanner?

The components of the CT scanner include an X-ray source which produces a fan of beams radiating out towards an array of detectors. Rather than ionization chambers, modern scanners use solid-state photodetectors that fluoresce visible light when exposed to X-ray energy. A photodetector then captures this visible light and converts it into an electric current that is conveyed to the computer producing a 2D image (slice), representing one full rotation around the body. The thickness of each slice can vary between 1 and 10 mm. The computer can analyze each slice individually or stack them together to create 3D images.

4.3 What do you understand by the term computed axial tomography (CAT)?

Traditionally, CT was known as computed axial tomography. In axial imaging, when a slice was acquired, the patient was then advanced through the scanner by a predetermined increment, a further slice was acquired and so on. The disadvantage of this method was that any reconstruction of images into other planes or thicknesses had to be planned before acquiring the required imaging data.

4.4 How is it different from helical scanning?

With helical scanning, the emitter-detector array spins continuously and the patient moves through the scanner continuously. This allows for multiplanar (any direction) reconstruction of the images. It is even possible to follow curving blood vessels and reconstruct them into a linear representation.

This allows accurate measurements to be made to plan endovascular procedures or assess for coronary vessel patency, for example.

4.5 How can CT imaging be enhanced?

CT imaging can be enhanced by the administration of contrast agents such as intravenous agents containing iodine or oral agents containing barium, for gastrointestinal imaging.

4.6 What is the mechanism through which enhancement of the CT image occurs?

There are two principal mechanisms: the photoelectric effect and Compton scattering. The photoelectric effect involves the absorption of a photon by an electron. This electron is then ejected from the atom having absorbed extra energy from the photon. This effect dominates at lower energy levels. In Compton scattering, the X-ray photon is not fully absorbed by interacting with the electron. Instead, it changes the frequency of the electron as a result of transferring part of its energy to it. The electron is then ejected from the atom. Compton scattering dominates at higher energy levels. High-density substances increase Compton scattering. A substance with a high atomic number (irrespective of density) increases photoelectric absorption. These two phenomena result in the radiopaque properties of iodine and barium.

4.7 Explain how the magnetic resonance imaging (MRI) scanner generates a signal.

Unlike CT, MRI does not involve X-rays but relies on the fact that all the protons of every nucleus of every atom have an inherent property of quantum spin state in addition to their positive charge and mass. This spin of the protons generates a magnetic field. The MRI scanner interferes with this magnetic field by first applying an electromagnetic current to align all the protons in the same direction and then by applying a short burst of radio waves knocking them off alignment. When the radio waves are turned off, the protons realign. This sends out radio signals, which are picked up by receivers. As hydrogen atoms are naturally abundant in the body, particularly in water and fat, most MRI scans essentially map the location of water and fat in the body.

4.8 What are the components of the MRI scanner and what is their function?

There are four main components of the MRI scanner: the main electromagnet, coils, an array of gradient magnets and a receiving coil. The main magnet applies a very strong magnetic field of 2–3 Tesla (Earth's magnetic field being 30–60 microTesla) to align the field and spin axes of the protons. Coils apply a radio frequency (RF) pulse in the region of the megahertz band, and this causes protons to resonate (hence the name of the scan). Proton resonance puts all the protons into an anti-parallel alignment and makes them rotate in phase. When the RF pulse is switched off the protons relax, losing their anti-parallel alignment (T1 relaxation) or phase alignment (T2 relaxation). Different tissues have different T1 and T2 relaxation which enables the scanner to determine their characteristics very precisely. The array of the gradient magnets superimposes a graded magnetic field in the x-, y-, and z-planes throughout the whole scanner, on top of the primary field. This makes the field strength slightly different in every single part of the body. This helps the scanner to distinguish the signals from the different tissues of the body. These gradient magnets are responsible for the characteristic loud noises in the scanning suite.

4.9 What are the problems associated with providing anaesthesia for MRI investigations?

The MRI scanner is a noisy machine and patients need isolating earphones to reduce noise even when conscious or under sedation. Long breathing circuits that are required when general anaesthesia is administered increase dead space and reduce lung compliance. All equipment should be MRI-compatible meaning no ferromagnetic items in the room. Cardiac pacemakers may malfunction, and metal cerebral aneurysm clips move. Before entering the vicinity of the magnet, patients and staff need to complete a rigorous checklist to ensure that they have no ferro-metallic objects in their bodies. Equipment such as IV poles, gas cylinders, laryngoscopes, and pens become potentially lethal projectiles if brought too close. This particularly applies to molybdenum steel oxygen cylinders that should be substituted with modern aluminium Kevlar wrapped cylinders. Special electrocardiographic (ECG) electrodes (made of carbon) should be placed close together and toward the centre of the magnetic field and the leads insulated from the patient's skin to avoid causing thermal injury.

References

Barash, P. *Clinical Anesthesia*, 8th edition. Wolters Kluwer, 2017: Chapter 33, p. 2202.

Ebrahim, H. and Ashton-Cleary, H. *Maths, Physics and Clinical Measurement for Anaesthesia and Intensive Care*. Cambridge University Press, 2019: Chapter 15, pp. 232–239.

Answer to SOE 5

5.1 What methods are available for monitoring muscle relaxation perioperatively?

Methods can be classified as: clinical signs, qualitative, and quantitative methods. Clinical methods were used before the wider introduction of nerve stimulators and included sustained head lift for five seconds, sustained 'tongue depressor test' and a maximum inspiratory pressure of −40 to −50 cmH$_2$O or greater. Qualitative methods require the use of peripheral nerve stimulators delivering an electrical stimulus to a peripheral nerve and subjective assessment of the response by clinicians. Quantitative methods use peripheral nerve stimulators that not only produce nerve stimulation, but also quantify and display the evoked response to nerve stimulation. The only quantitative method that is widely used clinically is acceleromyography.

5.2 What are the main patterns of nerve stimulation used clinically?

There are five patterns that could be used clinically for different purposes: single twitch, train of four (TOF), tetanic, post-tetanic count (PTC), and double burst stimulation (DBS). The stimulus that is delivered should be supramaximal to ensure recruitment of all the muscle fibres and is usually transcutaneous.

5.3 What are the indications for using the single twitch method?

This is the oldest method introduced in clinical practice and involves the application of a single supramaximal (20–30% over the maximal current) current to a peripheral nerve with a frequency ranging between 0.1 and 1 Hz (1/sec). It can be used to assess the onset of neuromuscular block at the induction of anaesthesia but cannot distinguish between using depolarizing and non-depolarizing agents. A decrease in twitch height will be apparent only after 75% or more receptors are blocked. Twitch depression will need to be more than 90% to provide good conditions for abdominal surgery. The major limitation to this technique is the need to measure a control twitch before administering the neuromuscular blocking agent.

5.4 Describe the characteristics of train-of-four stimulation.

In this method four identical supramaximal stimuli are delivered every 0.5 seconds (2 Hz) and repeated every 10–20 seconds. The number of twitches observed corresponds approximately to the percentage receptor blockade (0 twitches—100% blockade; 1 twitch—90%; 2 twitches—80%; 3 twitches—75%; 4 twitches < 75%). Unlike the single twitch method, TOF does not require a comparison of evoked response to a control response obtained before administration of a neuromuscular blocking drug.

5.5 What do you understand by the train-of-four ratio?

Comparing T4 (fourth twitch of the TOF) to T1 is known as the train-of-four (TOF) ratio. The response obtained before the administration of a muscle relaxant shows all four twitches the same amplitude. Hence, the TOF ratio is 1.0. When a non-depolarizing muscle relaxant is administered, T4 disappears first followed by T3, T2, and finally T1. This phenomenon is known as *fade*. On the contrary, when a depolarizing muscle relaxant is given all four twitches reduce in height equally before disappearing completely. No fade is observed. However, if repeated doses of a depolarizing agent are introduced, then a so-called Phase II block may develop that resembles the features of a non-depolarizing block, i.e., fade, will be observed.

5.6 What is the main clinical application of the train-of-four ratio?

The TOF ratio is mainly used for monitoring recovery from neuromuscular block. The TOF ratio must be 90% before it can be assumed that protective airway reflexes are intact. Traditionally it is accepted that the TOF needs to be at least 0.7 before successful reversal can be achieved when administering an anticholinesterase inhibitor, like neostigmine.

5.7 How is double burst stimulation different from train-of-four stimulation?

In DBS, two short bursts of tetanus at 50 Hz at a supramaximal current are applied to a nerve. Typically, each burst will have three impulses lasting 0.2 ms. Each impulse is delivered every 20 ms and the two bursts are separated by 750 ms. This method enables an anaesthetist to detect small degrees of residual neuromuscular block clinically by observing the DBS ratio which is similar to the TOF ratio (showing fade) but with more precision. This makes it more useful at the end of surgery.

5.8 What is tetanic stimulation?

Tetanic stimulation is an application of high-frequency electric stimuli for 5 sec most commonly at 50 Hz. This method is extremely painful and cannot be used on an awake patient. Tetanic stimulation produces fade in situations when the twitch response after TOF or DBS has returned to normal. It is therefore a more sensitive means of detecting low levels of receptor blockade.

5.9 What do you understand by post-tetanic count?

After an application of tetanic stimulation, single stimuli are produced at 1 sec intervals. As tetanic stimulation results in supranormal ACh release (post-tetanic facilitation), this transiently overcomes neuromuscular blockade. The observer counts the number of twitches that follow—the PTC. A PTC of less than 5 indicates profound block. A PTC of greater than 15 approximates to two twitches following TOF stimulation, at which point pharmacological reversal should be possible.

The technique is used to monitor significant degrees of block during types of surgery (e.g., neurosurgery, retinal surgery) when any patient movement could lead to complications.

References

Barash, P. *Clinical Anesthesia*, 8th edition. Wolters Kluwer, 2017: Chapter 33, p. 2202.

McGrath, C.D. and Hunter, J.M. Monitoring of neuromuscular block. *Cont Educ Anaesth Crit Care Pain*, 2006;6(1):7–12.

Miller, R.D. et al. *Miller's Anesthesia*, 8th edition. Elsevier, 2015: Chapter 53.

GENERAL ANAESTHESIA

SOE 1 Clinical history

A 73-year-old man is referred for a robot-assisted laparoscopic prostatectomy. He is 176 cm tall and weighs 99 kg. He has been a smoker for more than 50 years and was diagnosed with chronic obstructive lung disease five years ago. You are seeing the patient in the preoperative anaesthetic clinic one week before the scheduled surgery.

He is on the following daily medication:

Ipratropium bromide nebulization 4–6 per day

Salbutamol nebulization 4–6 per day

Budesonide nebulization 2 per day

Metoprolol 100 mg once per day

Valsartan 10 mg/amlodipine 160 mg combination tablets once per day

Simvastatin 40 mg once per day

Acetyl salicylic acid 150 mg once per day

1.1 How can you assess this patient's pulmonary function? Which pulmonary function tests would you require before accepting this patient for elective surgery?

1.2 Based on the patient's medical history, are there any other diagnostic tests you would require before accepting the patient for anaesthesia?

1.3 How can you optimize the patient's pulmonary function before surgery?

1.4 How would you handle the patient's medication up to the date of surgery?

SOE 2 Anaesthesia and postoperative management

2.1 How do you plan to monitor this patient during anaesthesia?

2.2 How do you estimate the patient's need for volume replacement during anaesthesia and surgery?

2.3 During anaesthesia, how can you try to minimize the increasing V/Q-mismatch developing during surgery?

2.4 Robotic pelvic surgery requires that the patient is on the operating table in the head down position for several hours. What complications do you expect from this positioning?

2.5 How and where do you plan to care for the patient postoperatively?

2.6 What is your plan for his pain management postoperatively?

SOE 3 Clinical history

You are the attending anaesthesiologist at 3 o'clock in the morning when you get an urgent call for a caesarean section. The patient is a 32-year-old primigravida at 30 weeks and three days of gestation. The patient has been a hospital inpatient on bed rest for the last three days due to proteinuria and elevated blood pressure. She has been treated with labetalol tablets. The obstetrician states that the baby should be delivered within one hour.

    3.1 What blood tests are necessary to perform safe surgery and anaesthesia for this patient?

    3.2 What other information would you need to plan your anaesthesia?

    3.3 How would the urgency and the blood test results influence your choice of anaesthesia for this patient?

    3.4 How would you care for this patient before surgery can be performed?

    3.5 Please describe the special risk factors of obstetric patients in general, and this patient specifically, regarding general anaesthesia and airway management.

SOE 4 Performance of anaesthesia and postoperative treatment

    4.1 What is HELLP-syndrome?

    4.2 How would HELLP-syndrome influence your choice of anaesthesia for this patient?

    4.3 You decide to move the patient to your ICU for treatment until you have a free operating theatre. When the patient arrives, the attending nurse calls you and states that the patient has a blood pressure of 160/115. The patient is also complaining of a strong headache. How would you proceed?

    4.4 As you arrive in ICU, the patient starts having seizures. How do you proceed?

    4.5 A caesarean section under general anaesthesia is successfully performed and the baby is taken care of by the paediatricians. What is your plan for the postoperative care of this patient?

SOE 5 Clinical history

You are responsible for the emergency orthopaedic list for this afternoon. The surgeon calls you about a patient whom she wants to operate on as soon as possible. The patient is seven years old. He was balancing on a concrete wall when he fell down. The child is being taken care of in the emergency room (ER) at the moment. The child is of foreign origin and the accompanying mother does not speak your language. The child himself presents as confused and agitated; awake, but not cooperating. He has obviously hit his head and has a bleeding scalp wound occipitally. He has an obvious dislocation of his right elbow and there is a strong suspicion that there is compromised circulation of the right hand. Distal neurological status is impossible to evaluate, due to a lack of cooperation.

The child looks otherwise healthy with no obvious operation scars. You estimate him to be of normal size and weight for his age.

    5.1 How do you evaluate the need for further diagnostic tests?

    5.2 How do you manage the lack of former medical history of the boy?

    5.3 To be able to examine the patient properly, he must be sedated. How do you proceed?

    5.4 The orthopaedic surgeon is pushing for a fast reduction of the dislocated elbow. Do you comply?

5.5 Which drugs would you use for rapid sequence induction (RSI) and intubation of this patient (assuming that you succeed in inserting an iv cannula)?

SOE 6 Performance of anaesthesia and postoperative treatment

You succeed in establishing two good iv cannulae, perform the RSI with propofol and rocuronium and intubate him uneventfully.

6.1 The boy is seven years old, is 125 cm tall and weighs 23 kg. What would be adequate doses of a) fentanyl (during preoxygenation), b) propofol (induction dose), c) rocuronium for the RSI?

6.2 You continue anaesthesia with sevoflurane. Which opioid would you choose as co-anaesthetic and why?

6.3 The surgeons identify an injury of the brachial artery, and the vascular surgeon repairs it with a patch procedure. After the repair, the patient has good pulsation in the radial artery. The surgeon asks you for a plexus block for postoperative pain management. How do you respond?

6.4 What is your plan for postoperative pain management after extubation?

6.5 The surgeon wants to inject bupivacaine in and around the operating area to prevent pain after extubation. What would be the maximum dose for a 23 kg child? Is there an alternative?

Answer to SOE 1

1.1 How can you assess this patient's pulmonary function? Which pulmonary function tests would you require before accepting this patient for elective surgery?

First of all, the patient should be asked about his exercise tolerance. It may be useful to take the patient for a walk in the hospital corridors and stairs to assess him during physical activity. Pulse oximetry during this exercise may give valuable information. Because of his long history of smoking, a chest X-ray is recommended. It is also possible to do an arterial blood gas (ABG) test to assess his PaO_2 and $PaCO_2$ levels and the level of renal compensation if he has respiratory impairment. When in doubt about the patient's pulmonary function, he should be referred for full spirometry including diffusion tests.

1.2 Based on the patient's medical history, are there any other diagnostic tests you would require before accepting the patient for anaesthesia?

This patient is planned to undergo a major surgical procedure. If he has a reduced exercise tolerance or the slightest suspicion of cardiac impairment, the anaesthesiologist should know more about this. The pre-anaesthetic evaluation starts with a physical examination including vital parameters such as pulse, and measurement of blood pressure. An electrocardiogram (ECG) is compulsory. The physical examination should also include listening to the heart sounds and lungs. If the physical examination, including heart auscultation and ECG, raises any suspicion of cardiac dysfunction, the patient should be referred to a cardiologist for further evaluation, such as echocardiography or exercise ECG.

1.3 How can you optimize the patient's pulmonary function before surgery?

The patient should be encouraged to quit or reduce smoking as much as possible. He could be referred to a physiotherapist to learn strategies for mucus clearance and atelectasis prevention and treatment. His pulmonary medication could be optimized by increasing the dose of inhaled budesonide up to the date of surgery. It is also possible to add an inhaled long-acting beta-agonist, for example, salmeterol. He should continue using ipratropium bromide and salbutamol inhalation up to the morning of surgery.

1.4 How would you handle the patient's medication up to the date of surgery?

See above for pulmonary medication. Continuation of acetyl salicylic acid depends on the indication for treatment. Normally, this platelet aggregation inhibitor will increase the risk of surgical bleeding marginally, given as a monotherapy. If the indication for this medication is stroke, TIA, or coronary disease, the surgeon should have a very good reason to ask for discontinuation. If it is discontinued, it should be stopped for five days before surgery. Regarding metoprolol, beta-blockers should never be discontinued before surgery because of a great risk of rebound hypertension and tachycardia. The combination therapy, valsartan/amlodipine, could be continued, but the anaesthesiologist should then be prepared for hypotension and a need for vasoactive medication during anaesthesia. In general, valsartan/amlodipine should not be given on the day of anaesthesia and surgery. Simvastatin should be continued up to the day of surgery.

Answer to SOE 2

2.1 How do you plan to monitor this patient during anaesthesia?

All patients that undergo general anaesthesia for major surgery should, as a minimum, have continuous ECG monitoring, pulse oximetry, capnography, and blood pressure monitoring. If the patient undergoes anaesthesia with volatiles, anaesthetic agent monitoring is mandatory. The patient above will normally be anaesthetised with neuromuscular blockers and should have neuromuscular monitoring, for example TOF (train-of-four). Monitoring of anaesthesia depth is recommended, for example BIS (Bispectral Index) or entropy. The above patient has pulmonary disease and possibly also cardiac disease, so invasive arterial pressure monitoring is recommended. This will also allow frequent ABG analysis perioperatively.

2.2 How do you estimate the patient's need for volume replacement during anaesthesia and surgery?

The most important parameters are urine output and blood pressure. An hourly urine production of 0.5 ml/kg is regarded as sufficient. In addition, blood loss and perspiration should be estimated regularly during the procedure and basal requirements should be replaced.

2.3 During anaesthesia, how can you try to minimize the increasing V/Q-mismatch developing during surgery?

The most important measure is to add a higher positive end-expiratory pressure (PEEP) than normal. Because the hydrostatic pressure in the heart, head, and neck region is increased because of the positioning, this will influence venous return and cardiac filling less than if the patient were flat on his back. It is useful to take regular arterial blood samples for gas analysis during surgery to monitor the arterial CO_2 level. The patient may need to be hyperventilated during this procedure to maintain normal $PaCO_2$ levels—minute volumes above 10 litres may be needed. If the patient's SaO_2 starts to deteriorate during surgery, this is most likely due to the development of atelectasis. Instead of increasing FiO_2 (which may actually worsen the degree of atelectasis), one could perform recruitment manoeuvres of the lungs.

2.4 Robotic pelvic surgery requires that the patient is on the operating table in the head-down position for several hours. What complications do you expect from this positioning?

The head-down position is a very demanding position regarding pulmonary function both during and after surgery. The abdominal contents will slide towards the head end and will compress the basal parts of the lungs. This will lead to atelectasis and shunting and an increased need for oxygen. In addition, this is a laparoscopic procedure and the gas used to insufflate the abdomen is normally CO_2. This is absorbed and has to be ventilated out of the body. There is also a considerable risk of oedema formation in the upper part of the body. This includes the risk of tracheal oedema which may compromise the work of breathing after anaesthesia. It is therefore essential that a cuff deflation test is performed before the patient is extubated, to ensure free air passage through the trachea. Conjunctival oedema is also very common after this procedure and the patient's vision may be impaired for some hours postoperatively because of this.

2.5 How and where do you plan to care for the patient postoperatively?

This patient is undergoing major surgery and will need postoperative surveillance for 24 hours in a high-dependency unit.

2.6 What is your plan for his pain management postoperatively?

Postoperative pain medication should be started before waking the patient from general anaesthesia. A robot-assisted laparoscopic procedure will normally not require the insertion of an epidural catheter, but in this case, it might be considered because of the patient's pulmonary condition. If an epidural catheter is inserted, it should be via a low thoracic approach to cover the operating area of Th 9/10 down to L 3/4.

All postoperative pain medication should start with paracetamol and a patient of this size should receive a loading dose of 1000 mg, given 6 hourly for the first 24 hours. In addition, a short-acting iv opioid should be prescribed, for example oxycodone or morphine to be given in the post-anaesthesia care unit (PACU). Depending on the need for oxycodone and/or morphine in the first hours postoperatively, one could either administer the patient a longer-acting opioid or step down to a less potent opioid, like tramadol.

Answer to SOE 3

3.1 What blood tests are necessary to perform safe surgery and anaesthesia for this patient?

Blood typing and screening, with cross-matching if necessary. Haemoglobin, platelet count, liver enzymes (AST, ALT, GGT), bilirubin. Electrolytes, including sodium, potassium, chloride, magnesium, and calcium. Osmolality, creatinine and urea, albumin.

3.2 What other information would you need to plan your anaesthesia?

It is necessary to know the patient's medical history: height and weight, other medical conditions, previous surgery or anaesthesia including any complications, medications, allergies. It is very useful to know all blood pressures measured during the pregnancy, and specifically the development of the BPs measured during the last three days. The amount of proteinuria is important. Even if a pregnant patient will never be properly fasted, it will be useful to know when and what the patient last ate and drank.

3.3 How would the urgency and the blood test results influence your choice of anaesthesia for this patient?

In the case of emergency delivery that has to be performed immediately, one has no other options but to choose general anaesthesia. Also, if the patient starts developing signs of coagulopathy, one should consider general anaesthesia as the method of choice. Otherwise, regional anaesthesia (spinal or epidural anaesthesia) will normally be preferred, unless the pregnant woman has special wishes to avoid this. There are also some specific medical conditions (for example adult (or Grown

Up) congenital heart disease (GUCH), neurologic diseases or spine malformations) where general anaesthesia might be preferred.

3.4 How would you care for this patient until surgery can be performed?

A patient with pre-eclampsia can deteriorate extremely quickly and must be monitored at all times. In an ideal world, such a patient should be transferred to an intensive treatment unit for optimization and monitoring while waiting for surgery. During this time, enough intravenous lines and a urinary catheter should be inserted. If the symptoms of pre-eclampsia are increasing, one should consider treatment with a magnesium sulfate infusion and antihypertensive treatment, for example with labetalol or hydralazine.

3.5 Please describe the special risk factors of obstetric patients in general, and this patient specifically, regarding general anaesthesia and airway management.

The pregnant patient in the third trimester has a considerably higher risk of airway complications than other patients. Due to progestogens, the lower oesophageal sphincter will be less competent than normal and the foetus will push abdominal contents towards the diaphragm and increase the risk of regurgitation of gastric contents into the oesophagus. In addition, gastric emptying will be delayed during the second half of the pregnancy, so that a pregnant patient after weeks 17–18 can never be considered fasted. The pregnant patient in the third trimester has a considerably higher risk of difficult intubation than other patients, due to a high incidence of airway oedema and therefore difficult visualization of the glottis at laryngoscopy. This is especially the case among patients with pre-eclampsia or eclampsia. Breasts increase in size during pregnancy, and might represent a mechanical difficulty at laryngoscopy.

Answer to SOE 4

4.1 What is HELLP-syndrome?

HELLP-syndrome is a complication of pregnancy. It is usually considered to be a variety of pre-eclampsia. HELLP stand for **H**aemolysis, **E**levated **L**iver enzymes, and **L**ow **P**latelets. It is a potentially life-threatening situation that is resolved by delivering the baby. It usually starts during the last three months of pregnancy (but up to 15% may start in the second trimester) or shortly after childbirth. Symptoms include tiredness, fluid retention/oedema, headache, nausea, upper right abdominal pain, blurry vision, nosebleeds, and seizures.

Untreated, HELLP-syndrome may lead to disseminated intravascular coagulation, placental abruption, kidney failure, seizures, and brain haemorrhage.

4.2 How would HELLP-syndrome influence your choice of anaesthesia for this patient?

The most important factors in decision making will be urgency, platelet count, and clinical condition of the patient. Normally, the method of choice would be spinal anaesthesia. When the platelet count is below 20,000 platelets/µl, spinal anaesthesia is absolutely contraindicated. At levels between 20,000 and 100,000 platelets/µl, the anaesthesiologist will have to consider the risks against the benefits. Normally, patients with pre-eclampsia and HELLP-syndrome are also oedematous, so that they might have a difficult airway. If a patient has HELLP-syndrome, one must also consider liver enzymes when choosing between different anaesthesia methods. Regarding urgency, if the patient is regarded as critically ill and/or having critically high blood pressure or seizures, general anaesthesia must be chosen in order to control blood pressure and seizure activity.

4.3 You decide to move the patient to your ICU for treatment until you have a free operating theatre. When the patient arrives, the attending nurse calls you and states that the patient has a blood pressure of 160/115. The patient is also complaining of a strong headache. How would you proceed?

The patient should receive antihypertensive treatment, either labetalol or hydralazine. Depending on the severity of hypertension, one could choose oral or intravenous treatment, but in the case discussed, iv treatment should be preferred. A magnesium sulfate infusion should be given to avoid seizures.

4.4 As you arrive in ICU, the patient starts having seizures. How do you proceed?

The onset of seizures is a medical emergency and the patient should be taken immediately to theatre for an emergency C-section. Anaesthesia of choice would be general anaesthesia, since this also prevents seizures. After anaesthesia induction, one should also perform aggressive antihypertensive treatment and start a magnesium sulfate infusion.

4.5 A caesarean section under general anaesthesia is successfully performed and the baby is taken care of by the paediatricians. What is your plan for postoperative care of this patient?

Patients with HELLP-syndrome, serious pre-eclampsia, and eclampsia must be treated in a high-dependency unit until blood values and blood pressure are normal. This includes aggressive iv antihypertensive treatment until the patient can be converted to oral therapy or blood pressure has returned to normal. Normally, the magnesium sulfate infusion should continue for 24 hours, and the patient must be monitored during this time. If a bleeding diathesis occurs, it is recommended that a thromboelastogram is performed for goal-directed therapy. Possible treatment could be a transfusion of platelets or plasma, or treatment with cryoprecipitate or concentrated fibrinogen. In addition, one should also consider treatment with low molecular weight heparin (LMWH) to avoid thromboembolic complications. Non-steroidal anti-inflammatory drugs (NSAIDs) should not be used as pain medication because they influence platelet function adversely. If paracetamol is used, a dose reduction should be considered in the presence of elevated liver enzymes. One possible adjuvant therapy is clonidine, since this drug also lowers blood pressure and is mildly sedative. Postoperative pain treatment with opioids should be discontinued within a few days or replaced by less potent opioids, such as tramadol.

Answer to SOE 5

5.1 How do you evaluate the need for further diagnostic tests?

There is no information given about how high the wall was. There is a possibility that the child has other injuries that are not as visible as the dislocated elbow, and a minimum diagnostic approach would be to make a thorough physical examination of the child, including a chest X-ray and a focused assessment with sonography in trauma (FAST) ultrasound examination to look for abdominal injury. The child´s confusion and agitation may be due to anxiety, but could also be a symptom of a head injury. On the other hand, one should try to keep the diagnostic tests as minimally invasive as possible.

5.2 How do you manage the lack of former medical history of the boy?

In normal cases, it is necessary to know all about the patient´s medical history: height and weight, other medical conditions, previous surgery or anaesthesia, medication, and allergies. In this case, we have to evaluate carefully if the time taken to get all this information will lead to a delay in treatment that would damage the boy further or put him in danger of losing future function. It would be paramount to try to establish cooperation with the mother, even though she does not speak your language, and try to get her to try to calm the patient down. In an ideal case, a translator should be summoned as soon as possible, either physically or by telephone.

5.3 To be able to examine the patient properly, he must be sedated. How do you proceed?

In this case, we have no former medical history and also no information about when the patient last ate and drank. He is anxious and in pain, so we must assume he is not fasted. In addition, there is a high probability that he might also have a head injury, due to his behaviour and a bleeding scalp wound. He also has no iv access, which makes titrated sedation impossible. If we try to sedate him, there is a high risk of aspiration of gastric contents to the lungs. The treatment of choice, in this case, would normally be to get informed consent from the mother, insert an iv cannula and intubate him following a RSI.

5.4 The orthopaedic surgeon is pushing for a fast reduction of the dislocated elbow. Do you comply?

Although delaying such a procedure may endanger the patient´s hand function, you have to be absolutely sure that the patient has no other injuries that may be more threatening. After intubation, you should order a full set of blood tests including acid-base status. Since it is impossible to rule out a head injury as a reason for the boy´s clinical condition, it is important to have a CT scan of the brain before the patient is exposed to a long stay in the operating theatre. As you have very little information about the injury mechanism and the patient is on the CT table already, it would be advisable to do a full-body CT scan to be sure that no injuries are missed.

5.5 Which drugs would you use for RSI intubation of this patient, assuming that you succeed in inserting an iv cannula?

The focus here should be on securing the airway as fast as possible. It could be wise to use a small dose of an opioid first to reduce pain and anxiety and to enable preoxygenation. Nitrous oxide in a 50% mix with 50% oxygen may also calm the boy down and enable at least some preoxygenation. Induction could be either with sodium thiopental or propofol, as both are potent induction drugs. Most important here, is that the dose is adequate enough for a fast, proper endotracheal intubation. The RSI could either be done with a depolarizing muscle relaxant or with a non-depolarizing one. A depolarizing muscle relaxant could have the problem that the dislocated elbow may damage the brachial artery or the nerves in the region of the fracture. A better solution might be to use a high dose of rocuronium, a non-depolarizing muscle relaxant which works almost as fast given in an adequate dose.

Answer to SOE 6

6.1 The boy is 7 years old, is 125 cm tall and weighs 23 kg. What would be adequate doses of a) fentanyl (during preoxygenation), b) propofol (induction dose), c) rocuronium for the RSI?

a. To ensure that this patient does not lose the ability to maintain the protection of his airway, one should be very cautious before intubation. On the other hand, a small dose of opioid may calm him down and might enable some preoxygenation. An adequate dose of fentanyl would be 1 µg/kg, so 25 µg would be sufficient. This could be divided into two doses.

b. Propofol should be given at a minimum dose of 2.5 mg/kg and the child might need up to 4 mg/kg if he is very agitated.

c. Rocuronium for RSI should be given at a dose of 1 mg/kg to a 7-year-old child. In very young children, the dose must be higher.

6.2 You continue anaesthesia with sevoflurane. Which opioid would you choose as co-anaesthetic and why?

Both continuous infusion of remifentanil and intermittent fentanyl boluses may be used. If you estimate the anaesthesia time to be very long, it might be better to use remifentanil to avoid the increase in context-sensitive half time seen with repeated doses of fentanyl.

6.3 The surgeons identify an injury of the brachial artery, and the vascular surgeon repairs it with a patch procedure. After the procedure, the patient has good pulsation in the radial artery. He asks you for a plexus block for postoperative pain management. How do you respond?

In general, you should be very careful when performing plexus anaesthesia in anaesthetised patients. In addition, if the dislocated elbow has injured the brachial artery, it might also have led to injury of a single nerve in the elbow area. A plexus catheter might mask the symptoms of such an injury and make it impossible to perform an examination of the peripheral neurologic status of the injured arm. Furthermore, we do not know the preoperative neurological status of the patient.

6.4 What is your plan for postoperative pain management after extubation?

The basis of all pain medication should be paracetamol. The patient should receive his first dose iv or rectally during surgery. The normal dose would be 80 mg/kg/day divided into three or (preferably) four doses. The first dose may be up to 40 mg/kg. If the CT scan of the brain was without pathology, an adequate dose of NSAID (e.g., diclofenac) may be considered. An adequate dose for a child of this size would be 25 mg two or three times a day. Before extubating the patient, an opioid should be administered, for example fentanyl 1–2 µg/kg. Later, oral medication should be offered as soon as tolerated; opioids should be given for as short a time as possible.

6.5 The surgeon wants to inject bupivacaine in and around the operating area to prevent pain after extubation. What would be the maximum dose for a 23 kg child? Is there an alternative?

The maximum recommended dose of bupivacaine is 2–2.5 mg/kg, so this child could safely have 50 mg of bupivacaine. This could either be injected as 10 ml of a 0.5% solution (5 mg/ml) or 20 ml of a 0.25% solution (2.5 mg/ml).

An alternative is for catheter placement locally with a lidocaine bolus of 1 mg/kg as a loading dose followed by an infusion of 15–50 µg/kg/min titrated to maximal pain relief.

chapter 71

CRITICAL INCIDENTS

QUESTIONS

The following chapter deals with critical incidents. These always feature in at least one of the afternoon clinical structured oral examination (SOE) questions. The questions are designed to allow the candidates to demonstrate to the examiners that they can be relied upon to stabilize a potentially catastrophic situation promptly and efficiently, at least until further help arrives. The examiners would be most interested in how YOU yourself would manage the scenario, rather than a discussion of possible options available. With this in mind, the model answers in this chapter have been written in the first person to give you, the candidate, a clear idea of the strategy you may use to excel in these questions.

Critical incident 1

You administer a general anaesthetic to a healthy, 35-year-old female for an elective right inguinal hernia repair. At induction, you also administer a dose of antibiotic. Ten minutes post-induction you cannot get a waveform or a reading from the pulse oximetry probe.

1.1 How would you proceed?

1.2 If you confirm that the pulse oximeter is working and that the airway is patent, what is your next step?

1.3 On assessment you notice that the lungs feel stiff, you auscultate expiratory wheeze and the capnograph is showing an upsloping trace. What are you thinking?

1.4 How would you manage intraoperative bronchospasm?

1.5 Your further assessment confirms tachycardia, hypotension, facial oedema, and a rash. What would be your specific management in this case?

1.6 What are the commonest causes of anaphylaxis in anaesthetic practice?

1.7 How could a drug error have caused anaphylaxis in this patient?

1.8 The patient stabilizes with your management. How would you proceed?

Critical incident 2

You are covering the delivery suite. One hour ago, you inserted an epidural for labour analgesia. The insertion was uneventful, and you started a continuous epidural infusion of 0.1% bupivacaine and 2 µg/ml fentanyl at 10 ml/hour. You are suddenly called by the midwife to assess the patient who has become very drowsy.

2.1 As you are going to attend to the patient, what do you think might be the cause for her drowsiness?

2.2 How would you approach the initial management of this patient?

2.3 The airway is patent, and the patient responds to voice. She is breathing at eight breaths per minute and oxygen saturation on air is 94%. How would you proceed?

2.4 Saturation improves to 100% on oxygen. The heart rate is forty-five (45) beats per minute and the blood pressure is 75/30 mmHg. There is no external blood loss. What is your plan now?

2.5 Your plans are in motion. How would you assess 'D' and 'E'?

2.6 What is the most likely diagnosis from your assessment?

2.7 How do you manage severe local anaesthetic toxicity?

2.8 How could this presentation progress from a cardiovascular and central nervous system point of view?

2.9 How would you manage these further complications?

Critical incident 3

You are covering the emergency department. You have just been called as a 35-year-old female patient is being brought in by ambulance after being involved in a motor vehicle accident. She was driving a car and was thrown through the windscreen and onto the tarmac by the collision. She was not wearing a seat belt.

3.1 As the anaesthetist, how would you prepare for her arrival in the emergency department as part of the trauma team?

3.2 On arrival, you notice that the patient is unresponsive, though she has a pulse. She has significant blood coming out of her ears, nose, and mouth. What is your plan?

3.3 How would you proceed to secure the airway?

3.4 The ENT surgeon has been called. However, the patient is now desaturating. What would you do?

3.5 You insert an endotracheal tube. On ventilation, there is no misting, no chest movement, and no end-tidal CO_2 trace. What would you do?

3.6 Your second attempt at intubation also fails. What would you do now?

3.7 Now you cannot ventilate. The oxygen saturation is dropping. What is your plan?

3.8 How would you perform a front-of-neck access?

3.9 How common is a Can't Intubate, Can't Oxygenate scenario?

Critical incident 4

A 65-year-old male patient after coronary artery bypass graft surgery is in the cardiac intensive care unit. On the second postoperative day, he tells the nursing staff that he remembers his operation. He complains of nightmares when sleeping and of flashbacks when he is awake. He finds these very disturbing and distressing. You are asked to review this patient as the colleague who anaesthetised this patient is away.

4.1 What anaesthetic complication is the patient describing?

4.2 What is the difference between 'explicit' and 'implicit' awareness?

4.3 How common is awareness as an anaesthetic complication?

4.4 What are the consequences of awareness?

4.5 What are the risk factors that predispose a patient to awareness?

4.6 What can the anaesthetist do to manage these risk factors?

4.7 What monitoring equipment can be used to reduce the risk of awareness?

4.8 As an anaesthetist, how would you manage this patient?

4.9 Which other specialists do you think this patient should be referred to?

Critical incident 5

A 55-year-old patient is admitted to the intensive care unit with status asthmaticus from the emergency department. Within 30 minutes of admission, the patient requires intubation and mechanical ventilation for worsening hypoxia and increasing hypercapnia. One hour after intubation, you are urgently called to the bedside as the patient has arrested. The intensive care nurse has started chest compressions.

5.1 What would you do first on arrival at the bedside?

5.2 As team leader, what are your priorities in managing this cardiopulmonary arrest?

5.3 What are the international recommendations in relation to chest compressions in adults?

5.4 The defibrillator has arrived, and the rhythm is ventricular fibrillation. What will you do now?

5.5 What would you do during the two-minute period post-defibrillation?

5.6 Once the two-minute period is up, what would you do?

5.7 The monitor again shows ventricular fibrillation. How would you proceed?

5.8 Considering the patient's history, what are the most likely causes for this cardiac arrest?

5.9 If at the third rhythm check the patient is still in ventricular fibrillation, what would you do?

Answer to Critical incident 1

1.1 How would you proceed?

Since this is a potentially emergency scenario, I would proceed using the ABCDE approach. A is for airway. Firstly, I would assess the patient clinically to gauge their condition, for example by looking at their colour and the temperature of their hands. I would ensure that the airway I have inserted, a laryngeal mask airway (LMA) or an endotracheal tube (ETT), is patent. I would check to see that it is not kinked; that the cuff is inflated adequately; and that it is still connected to the ventilator. I would also assess the oxygen supply to the ventilator and the fraction of inspired oxygen being delivered to the patient according to the gas analyser. Finally, I would assess the pulse oximetry probe to confirm that it is working well, for example, by double-checking it on myself; and I would make sure that it is properly positioned on the patient's finger or ear. It would make sense to increase the delivered oxygen to 100% until the emergency is resolved.

1.2 If you confirm that the pulse oximeter is working and that the airway is patent, what is your next step?

The next step would be to assess B, Breathing. Clinically, I would observe and palpate the patient's chest to assess for bilateral, equal chest expansion on ventilation. I would also auscultate the chest using a stethoscope for air entry and added sounds, such as crackles or wheezing. Switching to a manual mode of ventilation would allow me to get a 'feel' for lung compliance. In terms of monitoring, I would look at the capnography waveform to look for evidence of obstruction or bronchospasm, and to note the end-tidal carbon dioxide level to assess ventilation and perfusion. I would also review the ventilator settings to ensure that they are appropriate.

1.3 On assessment you notice that the lungs feel stiff, you auscultate expiratory wheeze and the capnograph is showing an upsloping trace. What are you thinking?

All the signs are pointing to bronchospasm. This could be due to underlying disease, such as asthma or COPD (chronic obstructive pulmonary disease); or to an acute event such as aspiration of gastric contents or anaphylaxis.

1.4 How would you manage intraoperative bronchospasm?

I would simultaneously need to treat the bronchospasm while looking for its underlying cause. Supportive treatment would include delivering 100% oxygen to the patient; consider changing a LMA to an ETT since higher ventilatory pressures and PEEP (positive end expiratory pressure) may be needed; increasing ventilatory pressures and PEEP while watching carefully for barotrauma complications such as pneumothorax; and using bronchodilators. Bronchodilators can be administered via the inhalational route such as isoflurane or sevoflurane; or intravenously such as salbutamol, magnesium, or ketamine.

Looking for the underlying cause of the bronchospasm would include a complete assessment of the patient including heart rate and blood pressure monitoring; clinical assessment such as looking for skin rashes or oedema; a review of the patient's past medical history and allergies; and a detailed consideration of all patient interventions and drug administration since induction and immediately before.

1.5 Your further assessment confirms tachycardia, hypotension, facial oedema, and a rash. What would be your specific management in this case?

Taking all the mentioned features together indicates a diagnosis of severe anaphylactic or anaphylactoid reaction. In addition to the supportive measures above, I would urgently administer adrenaline (epinephrine). This can be given intramuscularly as 0.5 milligrams of a 1:1000 dilution or intravenously using a 1:10,000 dilution. The intravenous dose can be titrated to effect in 50 µg aliquots. I would also give a crystalloid fluid bolus of between 500 and 1000 millilitres. Additional medications would include an antihistamine, such as chlorphenamine 10 mg intramuscularly or slowly intravenously, followed by 200 mg of hydrocortisone intramuscularly or slowly intravenously.

In relation to the cause of this reaction, I would stop any colloid infusions as these may trigger anaphylaxis. I would also review which medications had been administered to the patient and correlate this with any patient history of allergy. I would also take blood immediately and after two hours for serum tryptase levels.

1.6 What are the commonest causes of anaphylaxis in anaesthetic practice?

In anaesthetic practice, the commonest cause of anaphylaxis is muscle relaxants, followed by natural rubber latex and antibiotics. It has also been reported with the use of colloid infusions, barbiturates, benzodiazepines, local anaesthetic agents, povidone-iodine, chlorhexidine, and NSAIDs.

1.7 How could a drug error have caused anaphylaxis in this patient?

Drug errors can happen for a number of reasons, and some may cause anaphylaxis. For example, the patient could have received an antibiotic preoperatively that she had a history of allergy to. This history of allergy may have been missed or may have been noted and subsequently forgotten. This could also have happened due to communication errors between the team members during ordering, preparation, labelling, or administration of the antibiotic.

1.8 The patient stabilizes with your management. How would you proceed?

I would discuss with the surgeon the possibility of postponing surgery, in view of this critical incident. I would then need to decide whether it would be safe for me to wake the patient up, taking into consideration her haemodynamic stability and any airway compromise. I could check for airway swelling by performing a leak test by deflating the cuff of the endotracheal tube. I would then plan for the patient to have an overnight stay in a high dependency or intensive care unit, depending on her condition, due to the possibility of a delayed-onset recurrence of the anaphylactic reaction. I would arrange for a serum tryptase level to be repeated at approximately 24 hours from the initial event as a baseline level. Later, I would counsel the patient regarding this incident and refer her for allergy testing.

Reference

Lott, C. et al. European resuscitation council guidelines 2021: Cardiac arrest in special circumstances. *Resuscitation*, 2021;*161*:152-219.

Answer to Critical incident 2

2.1 As you are going to attend to the patient, what do you think might be the cause for her drowsiness?

Her drowsiness can be due to epidural-related causes, obstetric-related causes, or unrelated to the epidural analgesia or obstetric condition. Epidural-related drowsiness can be caused by a high epidural block; a subdural block; an inadvertent spinal (subarachnoid) block; local anaesthetic toxicity; or anaphylaxis to the bupivacaine or fentanyl used. Obstetric causes for drowsiness include ante-partum haemorrhage; amniotic fluid embolism; intracerebral events such as haemorrhage or thrombosis; or even post-ictal, for example after an eclamptic seizure. Unrelated causes could be hypotension, for example, secondary to a vasovagal syncopal episode; dehydration or sepsis; hypoglycaemia; pulmonary embolism; or as a result of cardiac pathology. The patient may also have self-administered non-prescribed medication.

2.2 How would you approach the initial management of this patient?

As in any emergency situation, I would initially manage this patient using an ABCDE approach. Firstly, I would stop the epidural infusion and ensure that this was correctly connected to the epidural catheter. Then I would move on to assessing the airway, by checking if the patient can speak to me and by assessing for any added airway sounds such as snoring, gurgling, stridor, or wheeze. After this, I would assess her breathing by checking the respiratory rate, assessing the patient's use of accessory muscles, examining the chest, and by attaching a pulse oximeter. I would start the patient on oxygen, targeting a saturation above 96%.

2.3 The airway is patent, and the patient responds to voice. She is breathing at eight breaths per minute and oxygen saturation on air is 94%. How would you proceed?

I would administer oxygen via facemask or non-rebreathing mask, targeting saturations above 96%. I would then move on to assessing and managing the circulation. I would position the patient in the full left lateral position, to reduce aorto-caval compression and protect the airway. I would check baseline parameters of heart rate, blood pressure, and capillary refill time. I would consider urinary catheterization for fluid charting if this was not already done. I would check the patency of intravenous cannulae and decide on the need for intravenous fluids depending on the patient's haemodynamic status. Finally, I would also look for any visible blood loss, particularly in the perineum.

2.4 Saturation improves to 100% on oxygen. The heart rate is forty-five (45) beats per minute and the blood pressure is 75/30 mmHg. There is no external blood loss. What is your plan now?

I am pleased to note the improvement in oxygen saturation, but I am very worried about the patient's cardiovascular status. I would ask for a three-lead electrocardiogram (ECG) monitor immediately and would arrange to obtain a formal 12-lead ECG for assessment of the heart rate, rhythm, and ECG morphology. In the meantime, I would like to treat this symptomatic bradycardia and hypotension using either 600 μg of intravenous atropine or a titrated dose of ephedrine intravenously, starting with a 6 mg bolus. I would also give a fluid bolus of 500 ml of Ringer's lactate. I would constantly monitor the heart rate and blood pressure response to my treatment and would escalate to using intravenous adrenaline, in 50 μg boluses, if the response to atropine and ephedrine is insufficient. Finally, I would take routine blood tests, including a crossmatch and toxicology screen, to send to the laboratory, as well as an arterial blood gas for analysis. I would ask a member of staff to bring the local anaesthetic toxicity protocol and the 20% lipid emulsion in case this is a situation of local anaesthetic toxicity.

2.5 Your plans are in motion. How would you assess 'D' and 'E'?

I would assess Disability by performing a formal AVPU (Alert, Verbal, Pain, Unresponsive) or Glasgow Coma Scale score. I would examine the pupils for size, symmetry, and for their reaction to light. I would examine the patient for any focal neurological deficits. I would ask a member of the team to measure a bedside glucose test to exclude hypoglycaemia or hyperglycaemic states such as diabetic ketoacidosis or hyperosmolar non-ketotic coma. For exposure, I would measure her temperature and expose her respectfully to look for any signs of rash, oedema, trauma, track marks, or injury. I would check the epidural pump for signs of any malfunction or human error in programming, by checking the settings and information available on the pump such as the volume infused. I would also ask the midwife to set up continuous foetal monitoring and liaise with the obstetricians regarding the progress of labour. I would finally take an AMPLE history from the person accompanying the patient in labour and the attending midwife. This would involve asking about allergies and medications, including any self-administered drugs, past medical history, last meal, and the events leading up to the state of drowsiness.

2.6 The patient's partner and midwife report that the patient complained of dizziness associated with tinnitus and a metallic taste in the mouth prior to her reduced level of consciousness. What is the most likely diagnosis?

From my assessment and the associated history, this lady is probably drowsy due to local anaesthetic toxicity.

2.7 How do you manage severe local anaesthetic toxicity?

I would ensure that the local anaesthetic infusion is stopped and disconnected from the patient. I would call for additional help since this patient can deteriorate further, even into cardiac arrest. I would ensure that the airway is maintained, and that oxygen is administered. If I think that the airway is at risk, then I would plan for endotracheal intubation. I would also keep an eye on her breathing pattern, to ensure that this is adequate. If not, then I would need to plan for assisted ventilation. Continuous monitoring of the cardiovascular system is also important, to treat any complications that arise. I would liaise with the obstetricians regarding the progression of labour and delivery options.

Lipid emulsion can be given in severe local anaesthetic toxicity. This is given as an initial bolus of 1.5 ml/kg over one minute of a 20% lipid emulsion. A maximum of two repeat boluses, five minutes apart, can be given if the patient is still unstable. Therefore, a maximum of three bolus doses can be given. A 20% lipid emulsion infusion should also be started at a rate of 15 ml/kg/

hour. The rate can be doubled to 30 ml/kg/hour after five minutes if the patient is still unstable. The maximum dose of lipid emulsion is 12 ml/kg and should not be exceeded.

2.8 How could this presentation progress from a cardiovascular and central nervous system point of view?

From a cardiovascular point of view, this presentation could progress to further arrhythmias including heart block, ventricular tachycardia, ventricular fibrillation, or even cardiac arrest. From a central nervous system aspect, the situation could deteriorate with worsening levels of consciousness or seizures.

2.9 How would you manage these further complications?

Heart block and bradyarrhythmias can be treated with atropine, adrenaline, or pacing. Tachyarrhythmias can be treated with amiodarone or DC cardioversion. Lidocaine should not be considered an alternative to amiodarone in this scenario. CPR would require starting advanced life support (ALS) algorithm management. Seizures can be treated with benzodiazepines, or even small boluses of thiopental or propofol under anaesthetic monitoring.

In all these situations, it must be kept in mind that complications of local anaesthetic toxicity may be refractory to treatment, so prolonged support may be necessary. Lipid emulsion infusion should be continued throughout CPR, and it should be noted that recovery from a local anaesthetic-induced cardiopulmonary arrest can take longer than one hour, so CPR may need to be continued for longer than in other pathologies. Finally, the patient should be transferred to an intensive care unit for monitoring once the acute event is managed. If she has received lipid emulsion, the patient should be observed for development of acute pancreatitis.

References

Association of Anaesthetists. Management of severe local anaesthetic toxicity. London: The Association of Anaesthetists of Great Britain & Ireland. 2010. Available at: http://dx.doi.org/10.21466/g.MOSLAT2.2010.

Lott, C. et al. European resuscitation council guidelines 2021: Cardiac arrest in special circumstances. *Resuscitation*, 2021;*161*:152-219.

Answer to Critical incident 3

3.1 As the anaesthetist, how would you prepare for her arrival in the emergency department as part of the trauma team?

This is an emergency situation and as the anaesthetist of the trauma team, I will be in charge of taking care of the airway. In view of the mechanism of injury, there is a good chance that this woman will have airway, face, or neck injuries with an increased possibility of a difficult airway. Keeping this in mind, I would wear personal protective equipment such as a suitable mask, face shield, a gown or apron, and gloves. I would then check my equipment and prepare for difficult ventilation and intubation. I would prepare facemasks, laryngeal mask airways, endotracheal tubes, direct and videolaryngoscopes, bougies, stylets; and I would ask for the fibreoptic scope and front-of-neck access kit to be directly available. I would also prepare suction apparatus, a bag-valve-mask, a Mapleson C circuit, and a ventilator. I would check that I have full oxygen cylinders or piped oxygen available. Also, I would prepare anaesthetic drugs like propofol or ketamine; muscle relaxants for a rapid sequence induction such as succinylcholine or rocuronium; opiates like fentanyl or morphine; and inotropes such as noradrenaline (norepinephrine) and adrenaline. Finally, I would ask for assistance—for example, a skilled emergency nurse or second anaesthetist to help me.

3.2 On arrival, you notice that the patient is unresponsive, though she has a pulse. She has significant blood coming out of her ears, nose, and mouth. What is your plan?

This information confirms that the patient requires securing of the airway and that this airway may be difficult to manage. In view of the history and the presenting findings, she may have facial fractures distorting anatomy and her neck will also need to be protected until cervical spine injuries can be excluded. My first priority will be to oxygenate the patient, using a non-rebreathing oxygen mask at 15 l/min initially if she is breathing well, or ventilating her using a bag-valve-mask or anaesthetic circuit with 100% oxygen if she is not. Manual inline stabilization of the neck will need to be in place at all times. To secure the airway, there is a number of options. An awake fibreoptic intubation is not suitable as the woman is unresponsive. In view of airway soiling with blood, an inhalational induction is also not ideal. Therefore, the options remaining are a rapid sequence induction and intubation using an oral endotracheal tube or a tracheostomy. I would not insert a nasal endotracheal tube because of the possibility of a base of skull fracture. I would also plan to clear the airway of blood using suction. I would start monitoring the patient with pulse oximetry, capnography, ECG, and non-invasive blood pressure, until an arterial line is inserted by a member of the trauma team. Prior to giving any anaesthetic drugs, I would formally assess the woman's Glasgow Coma Scale score and pupils. Finally, I would ask for further anaesthetic or ENT backup in case the intubation and ventilation attempts are unsuccessful.

3.3 How would you proceed to secure the airway?

Please note that there is more than one option for this question. Below is an example.

My first choice would be for an intravenous induction and oral endotracheal intubation using videolaryngoscope, suction, and a gum elastic bougie. If she is haemodynamically stable, my preferred hypnotic would be thiopental and if there are no contraindications, my preferred muscle relaxant would be succinylcholine. I would like to have a skilled assistant helping me, and I would want the difficult airway trolley to be available in the emergency room. I would ask for ENT assistance in case intubation or ventilation becomes difficult. Prior to induction, I would confirm that the emergency trolley can tilt head-down, and that suction is working. If available, I would use a pre-induction checklist.

3.4 The ENT surgeon has been called and you are about to start your induction. However, the patient is now desaturating. What would you do?

At this point, I think that if oxygenation is failing by using a facemask, a bag-valve-mask, or an anaesthetic circuit, then the patient needs intubation urgently. I would follow my Plan A, which is a rapid sequence induction with thiopental and succinylcholine, cricoid pressure, and oro-tracheal intubation.

3.5 You insert the endotracheal tube. On ventilation, there is no misting, no chest movement, and no end-tidal CO₂ trace. What would you do?

I would confirm that the patient still has a pulse and that the tube is not blocked or obstructed. If a pulse is present and the tube is patent, then I would consider that the endotracheal tube is misplaced, probably in the oesophagus, and I would remove it. I would focus on oxygenation of the patient, using a facemask or a laryngeal mask airway, until I can prepare for a second intubation attempt. For this second attempt, I would further optimize the patient's position if possible; I would consider removing cricoid pressure to improve the laryngeal view; and/or change the videolaryngoscope blade to a different size or shape.

3.6 Your second attempt at intubation also fails. What would you do now?

If the second attempt at intubation is unsuccessful, I would inform the team of a 'cannot intubate' scenario and I would shift my focus to oxygenation of the patient. My preferred approach would be a second-generation LMA such as an i-gel®, ProSeal™, or Supreme™. I would suction blood through the LMA's suction port. I would ensure that further senior anaesthetic and ENT help is on the way and that they understand the emergency of the situation. I would ask my assistant to open the difficult airway trolley and to prepare the fibreoptic bronchoscope as well as the front-of-neck access kit. If oxygenation of the patient is successful using an LMA, then I would consider *one* further attempt at intubation through the LMA, using a fibreoptic scope.

3.7 Now you cannot ventilate. The oxygen saturation is dropping. What is your plan?

I would now inform the trauma team that this is a 'cannot intubate, cannot oxygenate' scenario. Oxygenation is now the ultimate priority and I would prepare for front-of-neck access. I would ensure that the patient has adequate muscle relaxation, giving a second dose of succinylcholine, with atropine if necessary. Again, I would ensure that expert help is on the way.

3.8 How would you perform a front-of-neck access (FONA)?

Please note that there are options for this question. Below is one example.

I have been trained to do the scalpel-bougie-tube technique for FONA. If I can palpate the cricothyroid membrane, then I would use the scalpel to make a horizontal incision through the skin at this level. I would then make a vertical incision through the cricothyroid membrane itself, and turn the scalpel 90 degrees, to allow the bougie to be introduced into the airway. Once the bougie is in the trachea, an endotracheal tube can then be railroaded into the airway. If I cannot palpate the cartilages of the neck, then I would start with a long midline incision in the skin, to allow me to identify the cartilages and cricothyroid membrane directly. I would then proceed as described already. Once the endotracheal tube is in place, I would remove the bougie and inflate the cuff. Then, I would attach a capnograph and ventilate using 100% oxygen. To further confirm tube placement, I would look for bilateral chest expansion and misting, and would auscultate for bilateral air entry on ventilation. I would also hope that the pulse oximetry would show improving oxygenation values.

3.9 How common is a 'can't intubate, can't oxygenate' scenario?

The Fourth National Audit Project in the United Kingdom states that a 'Can't Intubate, Can't Oxygenate' (CICO) scenario happens about once every 10,000–50,000 general anaesthetics in surgical practice. This rises to once every 100-500 inductions of general anaesthesia performed in the emergency department. This scenario is more common in the obese population, and less so in the paediatric population. Rates in obstetric patients are quoted as 1:250 for a difficult obstetric intubation and 1:500 for a failed obstetric intubation.

References

Cook, T. et al. Major complications of airway management in the UK: results of the Fourth National Audit Project of the Royal College of Anaesthetists and the Difficult Airway Society. Part 2: intensive care and emergency departments. *Br J Anaesth*, 2011;*106*(5):632–642.

OpenAirway. *Algorithms*. 2020. Available at: https://openairway.org/algorithms/.

Answer to Critical incident 4

4.1 What anaesthetic complication is the patient describing?

The patient is describing awareness during anaesthesia. This is defined as recalling or remembering events or perceptions while a general anaesthetic is administered and is the result of memory formation.

4.2 What is the difference between 'explicit' and 'implicit' awareness?

Explicit awareness is conscious awareness, so patients may spontaneously remember intraoperative events when they should have been anaesthetised. This type of awareness may also be apparent in response to patient questioning or may be triggered by some event or speech.

Contrary to this, implicit awareness is not consciously remembered, but can affect the patient's actions at some time in the future. One example may be a great fear of future anaesthetics without being able to explain why. Therefore, in implicit awareness, memories are formed without the patient being consciously aware of them, but these manifest as changes in patient behaviour postoperatively.

4.3 How common is awareness as an anaesthetic complication?

Awareness during general anaesthesia has been reported in about 0.1–0.2% of cases. The incidence of awareness is higher than this in the paediatric population, secondary to underdosing of anaesthetic agents. Obstetric patients similarly have a higher incidence of awareness than the general population due to lack of opioid use at induction in view of neonatal concerns, higher likelihood of difficult airway and concerns regarding the effects of high doses of inhalational agents on uterine tone. Patients undergoing cardiac surgery are also at higher risk of awareness, reported at around 1.1–1.5% mainly associated with the use of cardiopulmonary bypass. Additionally, patients undergoing general anaesthesia for major trauma surgery are at increased risk of awareness due to the issues associated with general anaesthesia in haemodynamically unstable patients.

4.4 What are the consequences of awareness?

Consequences of awareness for the patient can be intraoperative or postoperative. There may also be consequences for the staff involved.

Intraoperative concerns include pain, experiencing paralysis, and associated features of anxiety, panic, helplessness, and feelings of impending doom. Postoperative sequelae include disturbed sleep, nightmares, flashbacks, and onset of psychological or psychiatric disorders. These could include depression, anxiety, and post-traumatic stress disorder.

Consequences for staff include litigation and feelings of guilt, or doubt in relation to professional competence. This is one example of the second victim effect of an adverse event.

4.5 What are the risk factors that predispose a patient to awareness?

Risk factors for patient awareness during general anaesthesia include patient characteristics, features of the anaesthetic technique, and the surgical procedure being undertaken.

Patient characteristics include a past history of awareness, a history of difficult intubation and a history of substance abuse or chronic use of high dose opioids. Paediatric and obstetric patients are at higher risk of awareness than the general adult population. Genetic variation in the response to anaesthetic agents, including resistance, may make some patients more susceptible than others to experiencing awareness.

Anaesthetic techniques involving use of muscle relaxants increase the risk of awareness during general anaesthesia. Vigilance for proper equipment function is very important for example ensuring that inhalational anaesthetic vaporizers are not empty, and that intravenous anaesthesia pumps and tubing are not disconnected from the intravenous access point. Underdosing of anaesthetic drugs, for example in a haemodynamically compromised patient, may also predispose to awareness.

In relation to surgical procedures, patients undergoing cardiac, trauma, and emergency surgery—including caesarean delivery—are at higher risk of awareness.

4.6 What can the anaesthetist do to manage these risk factors?

Anaesthetists need to be aware of this important complication of general anaesthesia and during preoperative assessment, consider whether the patient is at a higher risk as mentioned previously. In terms of the anaesthetic technique, premedication with benzodiazepines, avoiding underdosing with hypnotic agents, and using muscle relaxants only when necessary, can reduce the risk of awareness. When using inhalational anaesthetics, a minimum alveolar concentration (MAC) of at least 0.8-1 should be maintained. During total intravenous anaesthesia (TIVA), the anaesthetist should be vigilant for any disconnection or pump malfunction. All equipment must be checked prior to use. Intraoperative patient monitoring is very important, as is the maintenance of a detailed and accurate anaesthetic record.

4.7 What monitoring equipment can be used to reduce the risk of awareness?

Monitoring of patient parameters is essential as intraoperative awareness can present with tachycardia and hypertension. Clinical monitoring of the patient could uncover signs such as sweating, lacrimation, or dilated pupils. Where the patient has not received a muscle relaxant, the respiratory rate may also be an important indicator of awareness.

Basic monitoring, such as capnography and end-tidal inhalational agent concentration when using inhalational anaesthetics, is essential. In addition, a nerve stimulator could help to maintain a sufficient level of muscle relaxation for optimal surgical conditions without inducing complete paralysis. Cerebral electrical activity monitoring can also be helpful in this regard, using for example Bispectral index (Aspect Medical Systems) or Narcotrend (Monitor Technik) for spontaneous activity. Evoked activity monitors, using auditory evoked potentials for example, can also be used.

4.8 As an anaesthetist, how would you manage this patient?

This patient is reporting explicit awareness. I would take his complaints seriously and be empathic in my approach.

I would initially take a detailed account of the patient's experience and his current complaints and concerns. Then, I would look at his anaesthetic record to determine the details of the case, what drugs were administered and their timings, as well as his intraoperative haemodynamic status. Following that, I would try to provide the patient with an explanation for his symptoms and advise that the hospital will be providing the necessary assistance. I would reassure him in terms of future anaesthetics.

I would then write detailed documentation of my interaction with the patient in his records and would refer him to the appropriate specialists for follow up care. A management plan may include regular in person, telephone, or online reviews. It would be important to inform the Head of the Anaesthesia Department of this incident, who will coordinate with the hospital authorities, including possibly the hospital lawyers. The anaesthetist who was involved in the case should also be informed and offered any necessary support. Additionally, the responsible surgeon caring for the patient and the nursing staff on the cardiac intensive care unit need to be aware of the diagnosis and management plan.

4.9 Which other specialists do you think this patient should be referred to?

The patient may benefit from professional counselling, as well as possible review by a psychologist or psychiatrist. A named medical or nursing practitioner would be needed to coordinate outpatient care.

References

Brice, D.D., Hetherington, R.R., and Utting, J.E. A simple study of awareness and dreaming during anaesthesia. *Br J Anaesth*, 1970;42(6):535–542.

Ghoneim, M.M. and Weiskopf, R.B. Awareness during anesthesia. *Anesthesiology* 2000; 92:597.

Hardman, J.G. and Aitkenhead, A.R. Awareness during anaesthesia. *Continuing Education in Anaesthesia Critical Care & Pain*, 2005;5(6):183–186.

Nunes, R.R. et al. Risk factor for intraoperative awareness. *Revista Brasileira de Anestesiologia*. 2012;62(3):369–374.

Sandhu, K. and Dash, H. Awareness during anaesthesia. *Indian J Anaesth*, 2009;53(2):148–157.

Answer to Critical incident 5

5.1 What would you do first on arrival at the bedside?

On arrival at the bedside, I would ensure that it is safe to approach and that there are no hazards to the staff and the patient. I would wear personal protective equipment and encourage colleagues to do the same. Then, I would confirm cardiac arrest by briefly pausing chest compressions (not more than 10 seconds) —I would look for any signs of life including cardiac output by checking for a pulse and observing patient monitoring such as the arterial line, pulse oximeter, and capnography waveforms. Once this has been confirmed, I would ask the nurse to restart chest compressions and I would call for additional help and equipment, most importantly for the defibrillator.

5.2 As team leader, what are your priorities in managing this cardiopulmonary arrest?

The role of the team leader is to ensure the delivery of effective and efficient cardiopulmonary resuscitation (CPR) following the ALS algorithm using a coordinated team approach. My priorities would be the delivery of high-quality chest compressions with minimal interruptions, early rhythm analysis, and defibrillation if indicated, oxygenation through asynchronous ventilation since the patient is intubated, and consideration of the likely and possible causes of this cardiac arrest. The ALS algorithm proposes the use of the 4Hs and 4Ts for thinking about the reversible causes of cardiac arrest, namely: Hypoxia, Hypovolaemia, Hypo-/hyperthermia, Hypo-/hyperkalaemia/metabolic; Thrombosis—coronary or pulmonary, Tension pneumothorax, Tamponade—cardiac, and Toxins.

5.3 What are the international recommendations in relation to chest compressions in adults?

In adults, chest compressions should be delivered to the lower half of the sternum at a rate of 100–120 compressions per minute using a two-handed technique. Interruptions should be minimal, not longer than five seconds and ideally for planned interventions, such as rhythm recognition, defibrillation, or intubation. Chest compressions should be at a depth of between five and six centimetres and time should be allowed for the chest to recoil completely after each compression. Ideally, they should be performed on a firm surface. To ensure high-quality chest compressions at all times, the rescuer performing compressions should be changed as often as required. The recommended ratio of chest compressions to ventilations in adults is 30:2, unless the airway has been secured. In this case, chest compressions can be uninterrupted while ventilations should be given at a rate of ten per minute. Use of mechanical devices for chest compressions is only recommended if delivery of high-quality manual chest compressions is not possible or if staff safety is compromised. These mechanical devices are only recommended for use by trained teams familiar with the devices.

5.4 The defibrillator has arrived, and the rhythm is ventricular fibrillation. What will you do now?

Ventricular fibrillation is a shockable rhythm. I would advise restarting chest compressions to minimize interruptions and plan to deliver a safe shock. In my hospital, I would give the first shock at 200 J as we have biphasic defibrillators available. If I had additional help, I would delegate safe defibrillation to a member of the team so that I could focus on leading the CPR. Once the shock is delivered, I would ensure that chest compressions are restarted for a two-minute period.

5.5 What would you do during the two-minute period post-defibrillation?

During this two-minute period, I would consider the reversible causes of cardiac arrest. I would ensure that the endotracheal tube is in the correct position and that the ventilator is on a mandatory ventilation mode delivering 100% oxygen to address hypoxia. I would confirm that a capnography monitor is attached to the ventilator circuit and check for an accumulation of PEEP which may need to be released by disconnecting the circuit. To address hypovolaemia, I would deliver a crystalloid bolus of 500 ml through the intravenous access available. To assess for metabolic problems, I would request a sample from the arterial line for blood gas analysis and would confirm the patient's temperature using a temperature probe. To exclude tension pneumothorax, I would confirm the position of the trachea and auscultate the lungs during ventilation. I would examine the lower limbs for signs of thrombosis. Ultrasound may be helpful in the diagnosis of pneumothorax, cardiac tamponade, or lower limb thrombosis if a skilled operator is available. To consider a toxic cause for the arrest, I would check the patient's drug chart and infusion pumps for any malfunctions.

5.6 Once the two-minute period is up, what would you do?

My next step would be to pause chest compressions for rhythm analysis.

5.7 The monitor again shows ventricular fibrillation. How would you proceed?

I would ask for chest compressions to resume to minimize interruptions. I would then plan to deliver a second shock at 360 J, since we use a biphasic defibrillator in my hospital. I would recommend charging the defibrillator during chest compressions, following international guidelines to reduce the time with no chest compressions. Once the second shock has been safely delivered, I would ensure that chest compressions are restarted for a two-minute period.

5.8 Considering the patient's history, what are the most likely causes for this cardiac arrest?

The patient was admitted with status asthmaticus and required early intubation on admission to the intensive care unit. The arrest happened within 30 minutes of intubation. Therefore, the most likely causes related to this pathology would be hypoxia, hypovolaemia, tension pneumothorax, or metabolic derangement such as hypokalaemia. If an expiratory wheeze is auscultated on chest examination during ventilation, I would consider administering medication to help resolve the bronchospasm such as ketamine, magnesium, and/or intravenous salbutamol. I would also want to exclude anaphylaxis or anaphylactoid reactions by looking for skin rashes, as well as facial and tongue oedema.

5.9 If at the third rhythm check the patient is still in ventricular fibrillation, what would you do?

As before, I would restart chest compressions to minimize interruptions. I would then plan for the delivery of a safe shock at 360 J. Once this has been safely administered, I would advise the team to restart chest compressions. I would also advise the administration of 1 mg adrenaline and 300 mg amiodarone via the intravenous route.

References

BLS

Olasveengen, TM. et al. European resuscitation council guidelines 2021: basic life support. *Resuscitation*, 2021;*161*:98–114.

ALS

Soar, J. et al. European resuscitation council guidelines 2021: Adult advanced life support. *Resuscitation*, 2021;*161*:115–151.

Special Circumstances

Lott, C. et al. European resuscitation council guidelines 2021: Cardiac arrest in special circumstances. *Resuscitation*, 2021;*161*:152–219.

European Resuscitation Council Guidelines. 2021. Available at: https://cprguidelines.eu/

SOE question 1 ARDS

A 50-year-old patient is admitted to the intensive therapy unit (ITU) with Type 2 respiratory failure, after a week of feeling short of breath at home. He is febrile, tachycardic, and hypotensive. His chest X-ray shows the involvement of all four quadrants. He has been intubated and is now ventilated.

The ventilator settings are as follows:

FiO_2: 0.5, synchronized intermittent mandatory ventilation (SIMV), tidal volume: 450 ml, frequency 25 breaths per minute, positive end-expiratory pressure (PEEP): 7 cmH$_2$0.

His saturation is currently 97%, with a PaO_2 of 95 mmHg (12.7 kPa). $PaCO_2$ is 40 mmHg (5.3 kPa) with a pH of 7.38.

1.1 Discuss the clinical condition, and early management of such a patient.

SOE question 2 Discussion of ventilation strategies

2.1 What ventilator settings are used for patients with ARDS? How is this different from other lung pathologies, such as a lobar pneumonia?

2.2 What is the role of proning in ARDS?

2.3 When would higher PEEP be contraindicated in ventilated patients?

SOE question 3 Pancreatitis – acute presentation

A 60-year-old patient is referred to ITU with suspected pancreatitis. He requires high-flow oxygen with a non-rebreathing mask, to maintain an oxygen saturation of 95%. He requires boluses of fluid to maintain adequate blood pressure, and to maintain good urine output.

3.1 How would you manage such a case in intensive care, and how would you monitor the progress of such a patient?

SOE question 4 Pancreatitis – management of complications

4.1 What are the complications of pancreatitis?

4.2 The patient develops a fever, with a further rise of inflammatory markers. What complications would you suspect? How would you distinguish between these?

4.3 When would one consider surgery for complicated pancreatitis?

SOE question 5 Acute kidney injury

5.1 A patient develops acute kidney injury (AKI). What are the possible causes for this?

5.2 What investigations are necessary?

5.3 What forms of renal replacement therapy may be used? What are the advantages of each form?

Answer to SOE question 1 ARDS

1.1 Discuss the clinical condition, and early management of such a patient.

The patient is likely to have moderate ARDS, as defined by a P/F ratio of 190 (PaO_2 in mmHg/FiO_2), and chest X-ray findings. The latest criteria for ARDS, the Berlin Criteria (2012), are:

1. acute onset within 1 week or less
2. bilateral opacities consistent with pulmonary oedema must be present and may be detected on CT or chest radiograph
3. a P/F ratio < 300 mmHg with a minimum of 5 cmH_2O PEEP (or CPAP)
4. 'must not be fully explained by cardiac failure or fluid overload', in the physician's best estimation using available information — an 'objective assessment' (e.g. echocardiogram) should be performed in most cases if there is no clear cause such as trauma or sepsis.

In the past, a pulmonary capillary pressure of less than 18 cmH_2O was necessary, but this requires the use of a pulmonary artery catheter. Furthermore, the previous definition meant that if there were a cardiac cause, then ARDS was excluded. The new criteria allow a degree of cardiac impairment, but respiratory failure should not be attributable only to cardiac causes.

ARDS may be graded into mild (P/F ratio 200–300), moderate (P/F ratio 100–200) and severe (P/F ratio < 100).

Early management of ARDS is supportive, with a view to providing a protective ventilation strategy. This means a low-tidal volume, of around 6–8 ml/kg of **ideal** body weight and keeping plateau pressures less than 30 cmH_2O.

Answer to SOE question 2 Discussion of ventilation strategies

2.1 What ventilator settings are used for patients with ARDS?

The only strategy that is evidence-based is a low-tidal volume protocol. This is based on the ARDSNet trial (2000). This strategy allows for high levels of arterial CO_2, titrated to a pH of around 7.2–7.35.

ARDS is also a PEEP-responsive disorder, so patients require a higher level of PEEP. The exact setting for PEEP is debatable; so far, no specific strategy has been proven to be superior.

Oxygen supplementation should be as limited as possible, titrated to an arterial oxygen pressure (PaO_2) of 60–80 mmHg (8–10 kPa), and oxygen saturation levels of 88-92%.

ARDS is a diffuse alveolar disease, meaning that all areas of the lung will be affected. In non-diffuse disorders such as lobar pneumonia, there is also a shunt, which may be as significant or even more than in a patient with ARDS. However, there is also normal lung tissue. The application of PEEP may overdistended this lung tissue and cause harm. Also, tidal volumes may be set higher than for ARDS patients, although it would still be better to limit tidal volumes to 8 ml/kg.

2.2 What is the role of proning in ARDS?

Proning is reserved for patients who are still hypoxic, with a P/F ratio of less than 150, despite maximal treatment.

Proning helps by redistributing ventilation/perfusion matching. It reduces transpulmonary pressures, and hence reduces ventilator induced lung injury (VILI).

2.3 When would higher PEEP be contraindicated in ventilated patients?

PEEP may cause haemodynamic instability, by decreasing venous return to the heart. Hypovolaemic patients need appropriate fluid resuscitation before applying high levels of PEEP.

With regards to respiratory disorders, PEEP is contraindicated in the presence of:

- Pneumothorax
- Asthma
- Bronchopleural fistula

Reference

The ARDS Definition Task Force. Acute respiratory distress syndrome: the Berlin definition. *JAMA*, 2012;307(23):2526–2533.

Answer to SOE question 3 Pancreatitis – acute presentation

3.1 How would you manage such a case in intensive care unit, and how would you monitor the progress of such a patient?

Treatment of acute pancreatitis is mainly supportive. A systematic approach would help to ensure best management.

The airway is rarely of concern, but respiratory support might be needed; this may be through non-invasive or invasive ventilation. It is common for patients with pancreatitis to have moderate or large pleural effusions. Unless there is severe compromise, there is no benefit from draining such effusions, as they would recur.

Cardiovascular support with fluids and inotropes such as noradrenaline (norepinephrine) is common.

Metabolically, the patients will have deranged glucose control and low levels of calcium.

Antibiotics should not be started prophylactically, but in severe cases, broad-spectrum cover, including antifungals, would be needed.

Nutrition is also a contentious issue. It is advisable to start with nasojejunal feeding, but if this is not tolerated, then parenteral nutrition would be an option.

Patients who require large amounts of fluid for resuscitation are at risk of developing abdominal compartment syndrome and might benefit from monitoring of abdominal pressures.

If gallstone pancreatitis is suspected, and the patient is in shock, an urgent endoscopic retrograde cholangiopancreatography (ERCP) might be indicated.

Monitoring is, first of all, done clinically. If the patient is very tachypnoeic, or if oxygen requirements are high, then this might alert the physician to the need for further ventilatory support.

A CT scan is helpful to assess and grade the pancreatitis and observe for necrosis. If this is done too early, then the full picture might not be evident, so a CT scan 48 hours after admission might be indicated. This may be repeated every 7–10 days to assess disease progression.

Inflammatory markers do not prove very useful, as sustained inflammation means that white blood cell count, CRP, ESR will remain high. However, the trend in these values will be more useful. Furthermore, a case may be made for measuring procalcitonin, as this might rise when there is an infective process.

Answer to SOE question 4 Pancreatitis – management of complications

4.1 What are the later complications of pancreatitis?

Complications of pancreatitis may be non-specific or specific.

Complications that are non-specific include multiorgan failure especially cardiovascular, respiratory, and renal. Pancreatitis is also a risk factor for intra-abdominal compartment syndrome.

With destruction of the pancreas, diabetes mellitus ensues, and the patient would require long term insulin. Malabsorption of food and nutrients results from the loss of pancreatic enzymes, and patients would need supplementation (e.g. Pancrelipase).

The main local complication specific to pancreatitis is pancreatic pseudocyst, which might become infected.

4.2 The patient develops a fever, with a further rise of inflammatory markers. What complications would you suspect? How would you distinguish between these?

There is a number of infections that may occur in any patient in ITU, including patients with pancreatitis, such as hospital-acquired pneumonia and sepsis. However, the main two infective complications specifically associated with pancreatitis are infected pancreatic pseudocyst or infected pancreatic necrosis.

Infected pancreatitis usually occurs within one to two weeks and carries a high mortality. This is usually due to a number of micro-organisms. It is difficult to monitor, as it might be mimicked by a worsening of the pancreatitis. A CT scan would help in diagnosis.

A pseudocyst that has become infected usually occurs later, in three to four weeks. It is less severe, and carries a lower mortality.

4.3 When would one consider surgery for complicated pancreatitis?

Surgery is not indicated for most cases of pancreatitis, as there is a high risk of complications postoperatively, with a mortality of up to 60%.

However, there are particular situations that may require intervention. For instance, pancreatitis due to gallstones, with shock, may benefit from ERCP. Other indications may be for endoscopic drainage of pseudocysts, or even endoscopic or percutaneous necrosectomy. Open laparotomy during pancreatitis is ill advised.

Answer to SOE question 5 Acute kidney injury

5.1 A patient develops acute kidney injury (AKI). What are the possible causes for this?

AKI may be classified using the RIFLE criteria: based on serum creatinine and urine output. Acute renal failure (ARF) is defined as a creatinine greater than three times baseline, and anuria for more than 12 hours.

Causes for AKI may be broadly classified as: prerenal, renal, and postrenal.

Hypovolaemia and low cardiac output are prerenal causes of renal failure. However, if prolonged, there will be sustained damage to the kidneys.

Renal causes of AKI are varied. In intensive care, the commonest causes are urological infections, sepsis, and drugs (such as aminoglycosides, vancomycin, contrast medium, chemotherapeutic agents).

Postrenal causes of AKI would need to affect both kidneys, such as urinary catheter obstruction. However, if there is only one functioning kidney, then any form of obstruction may lead to renal failure.

5.2 What investigations are necessary?

Investigations will be required to identify possible reversible causes and grade the severity of the AKI.

Radiological investigations include an ultrasound of the kidney, to check for obstructive uropathy. A CT scan might be useful to check for masses, cysts, or ischaemia of the kidneys.

If nephrotoxic drugs have been given, such as aminoglycosides or vancomycin, it is useful to check plasma levels.

Serum creatinine is useful to diagnose AKI, but is not particularly helpful in assessing severity, especially in patients with loss of muscle mass. Serum urea is more useful, as this has a direct impact on the clinical status of the patient. Serum potassium needs to be checked. Arterial (or venous) blood gases will show if the kidneys still retain some function; in overt renal failure there will be metabolic acidosis, and a decrease in bicarbonate.

The decision to dialyse such a patient is not based on creatinine level, but on serum potassium, urea, and presence of metabolic acidosis.

5.3 What forms of renal replacement therapy may be used? What are the advantages of each form?

There are two forms of dialysis modalities in ICU: intermittent haemodialysis (IHD) and continuous renal replacement therapy (CRRT).

Intermittent haemodialysis, also known as conventional dialysis, usually lasts for three to four hours per session, although this may be prolonged even to eight hours (slow low-efficiency dialysis, SLED). It is cheaper than CRRT and offers a faster resolution of electrolyte disturbances. Furthermore, there are some toxins and drugs that are eliminated with IHD but not CRRT, for instance metformin.

CRRT is performed continuously, only stopping to change the filters and solutions. It is more effective than IHD and allows for better management of fluid balance. It also causes hypotension, but this is less marked than with IHD.

The choice between IHD and CRRT depends on a number of factors. Availability, the experience of staff, and clinical status of the patient are all important variables that one must consider.

References

Chacko, J. Renal replacement therapy in the intensive care unit. *Indian J Crit Care Med*, 2008;12(4):174–180.

London Health Sciences Centre. Principles of CRRT. Available at: https://www.lhsc.on.ca/critical-care-trauma-centre/principles-of-crrt.

SOE question 1 Chest X-ray interpretation 1

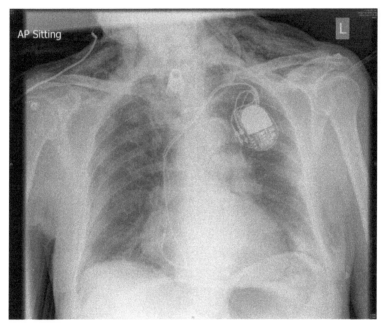

Fig 23.1 A chest X-ray taken after a tracheostomy insertion in theatre.

1.1 Comment on this chest X-ray.
1.2 What is the cause of the main acute abnormality?
1.3 What advice would you give?

SOE question 2 Chest X-ray interpretation 2

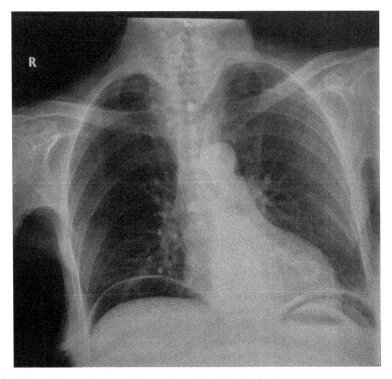

Fig 23.3 A chest X-ray taken erect in a patient with abdominal pain.

    2.1 Comment on this chest X-ray.
    2.2 What are the likely causes of the main acute abnormality?
    2.3 What treatment will the patient need?

SOE question 3 CT scan interpretation

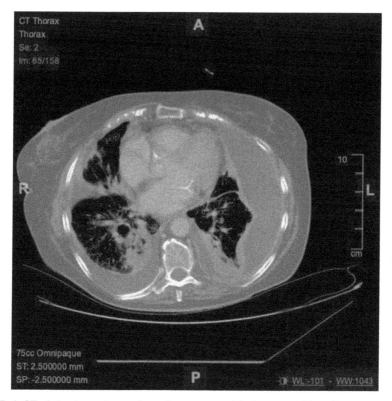

Fig 23.5 A CT of the thorax in a patient who presents with shortness of breath.

3.1 Comment on this CT scan.
3.2 What are the possible causes for the abnormalities seen?
3.3 What treatment might be considered?

SOE question 4 MRI scan interpretation

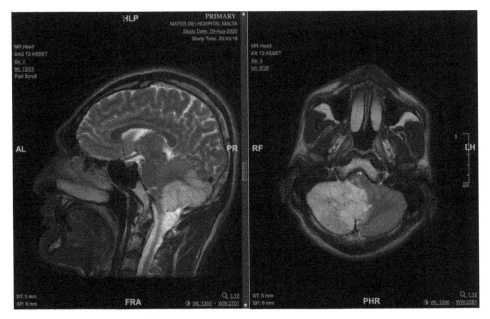

Fig 23.7 An MRI of the brain of a patient who is found unconscious.

4.1 Comment on this MRI. What type of MRI is this?

4.2 What deficit will the patient have? What other areas of the brain might also be affected?

4.3 What complication needs to be checked for?

SOE question 5 Echocardiogram interpretation

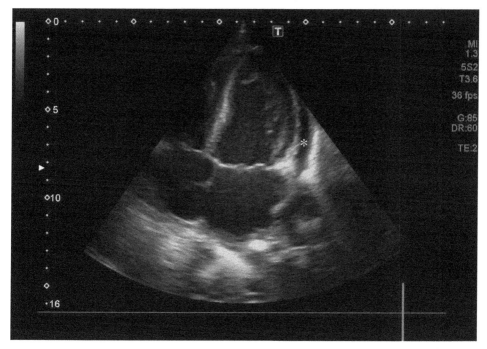

Fig 23.9 An echocardiogram of a patient with SLE (lupus).

5.1 Comment on this echocardiogram. What view is this?

5.2 What is the area marked with an asterisk?

5.3 What ECG findings would you expect in this patient?

Answer to SOE question 1 Chest X-ray interpretation 1

1.1 Comment on this chest X-ray. See Figure 23.2

It is important to use a systematic and logical approach to read and interpret a chest X-ray. A number of such approaches exist, such as starting centrally from the mediastinum, and moving out to the lung fields, or the RIPE/ABCDE approach.

The image is a chest X-ray, taken in an AP direction with the patient sitting, as given on the image. The main abnormality is the presence of subcutaneous emphysema [1], which is localized to the neck.

The trachea appears central [2], and there is no mediastinal shift [3]. There is the presence of a calcified aorta [4], which would indicate an elderly patient. On very close inspection, there seems to be a small pneumomediastinum as evidenced by a sliver of air around the heart shadow [5].

The lung fields appear congested [6].

There do not seem to be any masses in the lung fields, nor are there any obvious rib fractures.

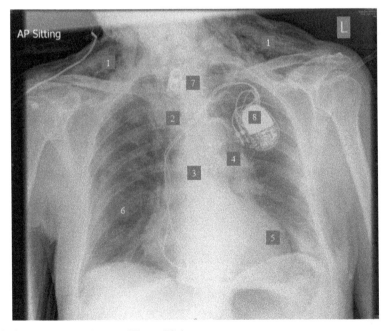

Fig 23.2 Annotated chest X-ray of Figure 23.1.

There is no endotracheal tube, but there is a tracheostomy tube inserted [7]. There is also a pacemaker [8], which is a dual chamber pacemaker. There is no central line in place.

1.2 What is the cause of the main acute abnormality (subcutaneous emphysema)?

The main abnormality appears to be subcutaneous emphysema, localized to the neck.

There may be several causes for this. The main obvious cause from this image seems to be the tracheostomy tube insertion.

Other causes not pertinent to this case would be trauma, but there are no obvious rib fractures in this image. Also, there are no central lines in place, but this does not exclude any attempts. There is a pacemaker, and from the image it is not possible to judge when this was inserted.

1.3 This is a patient who has just had a tracheostomy inserted. What advice would you give?

The clinical picture needs to be considered. If the patient is not distressed, then careful observation may be all that needs to be done.

Positive pressure ventilation with intermittent positive-pressure ventilation (IPPV) or manual bagging should be limited, although this is not absolutely contraindicated.

Drainage of the emphysema is not usually possible.

Answer to SOE question 2 Chest X-ray interpretation 2

2.1 Comment on this chest X-ray.

See Figure 23.4

The image is a chest X-ray, taken most probably in a posteroanterior (PA) view, with the patient erect. There is obvious air under the diaphragm, a tell-tale sign of an intestinal perforation [1], present on both sides.

The trachea appears central [2], and there is no mediastinal shift [3]. The cardiac shadow appears normal and not enlarged [4].

The lung fields look normal [5].

2.2 What is the cause of the main acute abnormality (air under the diaphragm)?

Air under the diaphragm (pneumoperitoneum) is usually due to intestinal perforation. This is typically at the duodenum (peptic ulcer, e.g. with NSAID use), but may be elsewhere. Pneumoperitoneum may also be due to gas-forming organisms. Of course, it may also be found after a laparotomy, or after perforation during an endoscopic procedure, so the clinical picture is very important.

2.3 What treatment will the patient need?

Unless this is a postoperative patient, surgery is usually required. The most likely site of intestinal perforation would be a duodenal ulcer but could also be from other causes of intestinal perforation, such as diverticular disease.

References

Lee, C.H. Images in clinical medicine. Radiologic signs of pneumoperitoneum. *N Engl J Med*, 2010;362(25):2410.

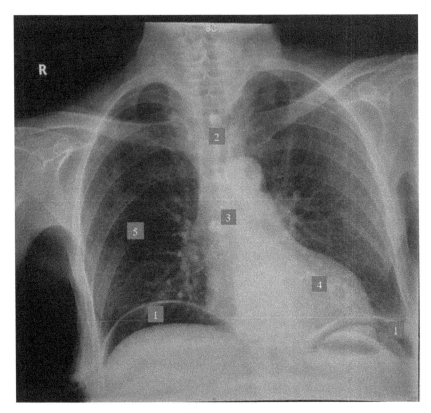

Fig 23.4 Annotated chest X-ray of Figure 23.3.

Ramachar S.M. and Melanta, K. R gas under diaphragm. *Int J Surg Case Rep*, 2016;28:314–316.

Sureka, B., Bansal, K., and Arora, A. Pneumoperitoneum: what to look for in a radiograph? *J Family Med Prim Care*, 2015;4(3):477–478.

Answer to SOE 3 CT scan interpretation

3.1 Comment on this CT scan.

See Figure 23.6

CT images are rarely labelled, but the convention is to have the right side of the body on the left side of the screen, and vice versa: this is similar to a chest X-ray. Whenever possible, compare the two sides of the image, and check for asymmetry, as in the case of a thoracic CT scan.

It is also useful to check if intravenous contrast has been given (vessels appear bright), or if there are any artefacts (such as metal surgical clips).

This CT scan is a non-contrast image of the mid-thoracic cavity, at the level of the left atrium [1].

There are two main abnormalities. On the right side, there are consolidated areas of the middle lobe [2], and a moderate pleural collection [3]. On the left side, there is a large pleural collection [4], with a split-pleural sign [5]. This is highly indicative of an empyema, with thickened pleural membranes.

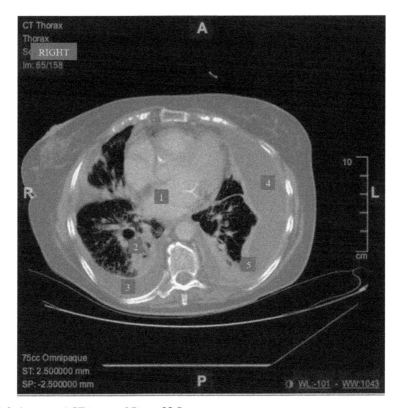

Fig 23.6 Annotated CT image of Figure 23.5.

3.2 What are the possible causes for the abnormalities seen?

There is a number of causes for the CT image shown. Highly probable is a widespread infective process, such as would occur in an immunocompromised patient. Another possibility would be an infiltrative process, such as metastatic disease.

This patient had cavitating lesions, with a 9th rib fracture, likely pathological. This would point to a carcinoma, most likely a squamous cell type.

3.3 What treatment might be considered?

Antibiotics are definitely needed. One could start with a broad-spectrum antibiotic, until microbiology results with sensitivities are available.

Such a large empyema would need drainage. However, this should be done under radiological guidance, to ensure drainage of a possibly separated empyema.

References

Kraus, G.J. The split pleura sign. *Radiology*, 2007 243(1):297–298.

Tobler, M. Empyema imaging. *Emedicine Medscape*. Available at: https://emedicine.medscape.com/article/355892-overview

Answer to SOE 4 MRI scan interpretation

4.1 Comment on this MRI. What type of MRI is this?

See Figure 23.8

There exists a variety of different MRI modalities, especially for investigating the brain, such as T1- and T2-weighted imaging, diffusion weighted imaging (DWI), perfusion weighted imaging (PWI), FLAIR.

At the very least, you should understand the difference between T1- and T2-weighted imaging. Cerebrospinal fluid (CSF) will appear dark on a T1-weighted image, and bright on a T2-weighted image. Similarly, if in view, the eyeballs will appear dark on a T1-weighted image, and bright on a T2-weighted image.

This is very important, as it would determine where the abnormality is. On a T2-weighted image, oedema will appear as bright white.

Also, MRI images are rarely labelled, but the convention is to have the right side of the brain on the left side of the screen, and vice versa: this is similar to a chest X-ray.

This MRI is composed of a parasagittal view [1], and an axial view of the posterior fossa [2]. Both are a T2-weighted images as evidenced by CSF in the sulci being bright [3].

There is a hyperdense lesion in the right cerebellum [4], which would indicate oedema. In this context, the most likely cause is a cerebrovascular event like a stroke. This is an example of a posterior inferior cerebellar artery occlusion, also known as a lateral medullary syndrome or Wallenburg syndrome.

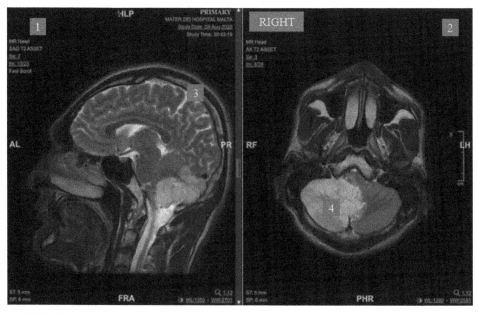

Fig 23.8 Annotated MRI image of Figure 23.7.

4.2 What deficit will the patient have? What other areas of the brain might also be affected?

Cerebellar symptoms: ataxia, nystagmus, vertigo, nausea, vomiting.

Other areas that might be involved are supplied by the vertebral artery, such as: midbrain, giving rise to dysphagia and/or Horner's syndrome; trigeminal areas; spinothalamic tract.

4.3 What complication needs to be checked for?

Compression of the IV ventricle, which is already evident in this case. This would cause hydrocephalus and might necessitate insertion of a ventricular drain.

References

Learning Neuroradiology. The basics. Available at: https://sites.google.com/a/wisc.edu/neuroradiology/image-acquisition/the-basics

Saleem, F. and M Das, J. *Lateral Medullary Syndrome*. StatPearls [Internet]. StatPearls Publishing, Treasure Island (FL), 2020. Available at: https://www.ncbi.nlm.nih.gov/books/NBK551670/.

Answer to SOE 5 Echocardiogram interpretation

5.1 Comment on this echocardiogram. What view is this?

See Figure 23.10.

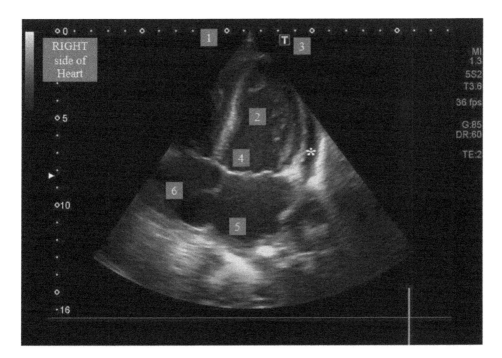

Fig 23.10 Annotated echocardiogram image of Figure 23.9.

The echocardiogram shown is a 4-chamber apical view, with the ultrasound probe being placed at the apex beat (5th intercostal space, laterally) [1]. With the index of the ultrasound probe pointing posteriorly [3], the left ventricle [2] will appear on the right-hand side of the screen.

The mitral valve [4] is closed, and the left ventricle [2] still has not contracted. This indicates that this image has been taken at the start of systole.

The left and right atria [5, 6] also appear slightly enlarged when compared to the left and right ventricle. At end-systole, the left atrium should be 30-40 mm: in this patient, this was 37 mm.

5.2 What is the area marked with an asterisk?

This is fluid (black) in the pericardial space: a pericardial effusion. This is small. There is no compression on the ventricle, at least in this view, so it is not a tamponade.

With the present clinical information, it is likely that this is an effusion related to pericarditis.

5.3 What ECG findings would you expect in this patient?

The ECG features of pericarditis include:

- widespread concave ST elevation in most of the leads, with PR depression
- sinus tachycardia

References

Pericarditis. Life in the fast lane. 2021. Available at: https://litfl.com/pericarditis-ecg-library/.

Xanthopoulos, A. and Skoularigis, J. Diagnosis of acute pericarditis. e-*Journal of Cardiology Practice*, 2017. Available at: https://www.escardio.org/Journals/E-Journal-of-Cardiology-Practice/Volume-15/Diagnosis-of-acute-pericarditis.

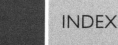

INDEX

For the benefit of digital users, indexed terms that span two pages (e.g., 52–53) may, on occasion, appear on only one of those pages.

Page prefix Q related to questions, A to answers.